BRITISH MEDICAL BULLETIN

British Medical Bulletin is published four times each year, in January, April, July and October.

Subscriptions and single-copy orders should be sent to: Longman Group Ltd, PO Box 77, Harlow, Essex CM19 5BQ. Tel: 0279 623760 Subscription rates for 1994 are: £126 (UK, £6 postage), £126 (Europe, £8 postage), $207 (USA, $15 postage) or £126 (RoW, £11 postage) Single copies will be available at £49.95 (UK)

NEXT ISSUE

BRITISH
MEDICAL BULLETIN

VOLUME FIFTY
1994

CHURCHILL LIVINGSTONE
EDINBURGH, LONDON, MADRID, MELBOURNE,
NEW YORK AND TOKYO

CHURCHILL LIVINGSTONE
Medical Division of Longman Group Limited

Distributed in the United States of America by Churchill
Livingstone Inc., 650 Avenue of the Americas, New York,
NY10011, and by associated companies, branches and
representatives throughout the world.

ISSN 0007-1420
ISBN 0-443-05153-4

Published by Longman Group Ltd.
Printed in Great Britain by Bell and Bain Ltd., Glasgow

This journal is indexed, abstracted and/or published online in the following media:
Adonis, Biosis, BRS Colleague (full text), Chemical Abstracts, Colleague (Online),
Current Awareness in Biological Science, Current Contents/Clinical Medicine,
Current Contents/Life Science, Excerpta Medica/Embase, Index Medicus/Medline,
Medical Documentation Service, Reference Update, Research Alert, Science
Citation Index, Scisearch, SIIC-Database Argentina), UMI (Microfilms), USSR
Academy of Sciences

Notes to users in the USA: Authorisation to photocopy items for internal or personal use
is granted by Longman Group UK Ltd provided that the appropriate fees are paid directly
to Copyright Clearance Center, 27 Congress Street, Salem, MA 01970, USA. For more
information, please contact CCC. For territories outside North America, permission should
be sought direct from the copyright holder. This consent does not extend to other kinds of
copying, such as copying for general distribution, for advertising and promotional purposes,
for creating new collective works, or for resale.

British Medical Bulletin is published quarterly in January, April, July and October by
Churchill Livingstone c/o Mercury Airfreight International Ltd Inc, 2323 Randolph
Avenue, Avenel, New Jersey 07001. Subscription price is $222.00 per annum. Second Class
Postage paid at Rahway NJ (USPS No. 011-369). Postmaster: Send address corrections to
British Medical Bulletin c/o Mercury Airfreight International Ltd Inc, 2323 Randolph Avenue,
Avenel, New Jersey 07001.

Genetics of Malignant Disease

Scientific Editor: *B A J Ponder*

1994 Vol. 50 No. 3

Professor B Ponder chaired the committee which included Mr J Northover, Dr N Hastie, Dr D T Bishop and Dr J Birch which planned this number of the British Medical Bulletin. We are grateful to them for their help and particularly to Professor B Ponder for his work as Scientific Editor.

British Medical Bulletin is published by Churchill Livingstone for The British Council, 10 Spring Gardens, London SW1A 2BN

British Medical Bulletin (1994) Vol. 50, No. 3, pp. 517–526
© The British Council 1994

Cancer genetics

W F Bodmer

Imperial Cancer Research Fund, London, UK

The fundamental ideas on the causes of cancer have been known for some time. They can now be interpreted in terms of the notion that cancer is essentially a genetic disease at the cellular level. The aim of this introductory article is to provide a brief overview of these ideas and the evidence for them, as well as some of the implications for future approaches to the prevention, early detection and treatment of cancer.

Percival Pott, the distinguished British surgeon, identified about 200 years ago the first environmental, and perhaps first occupational, cause of cancer, namely cancer of the scrotum amongst chimney sweeps, due to their exposure to soot. The other major ideas on causes, which originated around the turn of this century, include abnormalities of differentiation, viruses, effects of the immune system, chromosome abnormalities and, finally and most importantly, somatic mutations. These ideas can all now be combined into the one main notion that cancer arises from a series of changes in the expression of genes, mostly genetic mutations, that lead progressively from the normal to the malignant cell.

Most cancers, especially of the solid tissues, increase markedly in incidence with age. This is consistent with the idea that cancer is due to the successive accumulation of a series of genetic changes. The slope of the line relating the logarithm of cancer incidence to the logarithm of age, provides a crude estimate of the number of independent steps. Such data suggest that at least 4–6 critical steps are involved in the development of a malignant cancer.

There are now many lines of evidence for specific genetic changes in cancer cells. Firstly, the cellular genetic basis for a cancer implies a clonal origin. This was first clearly shown by studying the expression of X-linked genes in cancers from females, and showing that only the genes from one X-chromosome were in general expressed in a tumour. Subsequently, many observations of specific mutations in cancers have confirmed this fundamental principle. The facts that many carcinogens are also mutagens, and that inherited deficiencies in the ability to repair

DNA damage greatly increase susceptibility to cancer, also strongly support its genetic origins.

Each cancer, therefore, is the result of an independent evolutionary process at the somatic cell level, involving the usual mechanisms of mutation and selection but without the intervention of a sexual process. The accumulation of the successive mutations that result in a cancer must take place step-wise, with each mutation having a selective advantage and so leading to an expanded cellular population, within which the next mutation giving rise to a further selective advantage and further cellular expansion, takes place. The clue to understanding cancer is to define the set of individual genetic steps that constitute this somatic evolutionary process and, through understanding their functions, to define effectively the nature of the selective advantages associated with each step. (For further background, see[1,2] and other chapters in this issue.)

THE PHILADELPHIA CHROMOSOME, TRANSLOCATIONS AND DOMINANT ONCOGENES

The first clear cut evidence for a specific change in a cancer was the discovery in the early 1960s by Noel and Hungerford of the Philadelphia Chromosome in chronic myelogenous leukaemia (CML). This was interpreted by Janet Rowley some 10 years later, after the development of chromosome banding techniques, as a specific translocation between chromosomes 9 and 22, posing the question as to what the nature of the specific changes at the break points was, and how this influenced the development of CML. The fact that this translocation is seen in all the cells of a CML and is virtually diagnostic of CML, but has never been seen in normal cells supports convincingly the clonal origin of at least this form of leukaemia and the key role of the translocation in its progression.

The interpretation of the Philadelphia Chromosome depended on the discovery of the dominant oncogenes carried by the oncogenic retroviruses, as first identified by Peyton Rous in 1910. The work of Varmus and Bishop and others showed that their transforming ability was determined by genes they carried which were homologous to normal nuclear genes. These are the dominant oncogenes. They are dominant because they can carry out their function in the presence of the unaltered normal version of the corresponding gene. It was soon shown by a variety of approaches that the dominant oncogenes identified in the retroviruses could be mutated in cancers by conventional genetic mechanisms unconnected with any role for viruses. Thus, for example, the ras family of oncogenes is mutated in specific positions in a wide variety of human solid tumours, such as of the colon and rectum. The work of Waterfield and others showed that some of these dominant oncogenes coded for variant growth factors or their receptors. Subsequent work has shown that other oncogenes include genes involved either in the signalling process (for example, transmission of the signal to the nucleus) following attachment of a growth factor to its receptor, or transcription factors involved in receiving these signals, and so initiating changes in cellular behaviour.

It was natural to ask the question as to whether any of the identified oncogenes might be involved in mediating the effects of specific translocations, such as the Philadelphia Chromosome. Thus, somatic cell genetic techniques were used to map the oncogenes. One of the first fruits of this genetic mapping was the assignment of the c-abl oncogene to chromosome 9, immediately suggesting, admittedly as a very long shot, that this might be involved in the 9/22 translocation of the Philadelphia Chromosome. That this indeed was the case, was shown by Heisterkamp, Groffen and others. This led to the identification of the partner gene, bcr, on Chromosome 22 and the identification of a totally novel fusion gene formed from the combination of abl and bcr, which explains the effect of the Philadelphia Chromosome on CML. Now, through the use of the polymerase chain reaction, identification of this fusion gene provides the most sensitive assay for residual leukaemic cells after treatment. Subsequently, a large number of other translocations have been explained in similar ways, mostly occurring in leukaemias and lymphomas, and identifying a range of new dominantly acting novel fusion genes as critical events in tumourigenesis.

FAMILIAL CANCER AND TUMOUR SUPPRESSOR GENES

There is a simple and fundamental idea suggested by Knudson[3] in 1971, which forms the basis for the search for a totally different class of genetic changes in cancers that are essentially recessive in their action. Knudson pointed out that if a cancer is due to a series of genetic changes at the somatic level, then sometimes one of those changes may be inherited in the germline and so be present in every cell in the body.[3] In that case such an individual will have cells that are already one step along the carcinogenic pathway, and it is that head start which can be the basis for a dominantly inherited cancer susceptibility. He suggested, in addition, that a further genetic step which occurs somatically could be another mutation in the same gene, knocking out fully its function. In other words, while the familial inherited susceptibility behaved as a dominant, the effect at the somatic cell level contributing to tumour progression, was recessive. This, therefore, predicted a class of genetic changes in tumourigenesis which were recessive at the somatic cell level, suggesting functions which normally prevented the development of a cancer. His ideas were consistent with the data of Harris, Klein,

Stanbridge and others, who had suggested from somatic cell hybridisation studies that the non-transformed cellular state is generally dominant in somatic cell hybrids. These ideas, therefore, defined a class of genetic changes which have been called tumour suppressor mutations.

Knudson chose as his model retinoblastoma,[8] of which about 40–50% of cases are clearly inherited as Mendelian dominants. A few percent are associated with a small visible deletion on Chromosome 13 which, using the polymorphic enzyme esterase D, led to the localisation of the retinoblastoma gene to this position on Chromosome 13. The observation by Sparkes and others that retinoblastomas from such familial cases sometimes lost expression of one of their esterase D alleles was the precursor to the introduction by Cavenee and colleagues in 1983[4] of the search, using restriction fragment length polymorphisms, for allele loss, or loss of heterozygosity as it is often referred to, in cancers. Cavenee et al[4] argued that if Knudson's ideas were correct, markers which were heterozygous on a chromosome carrying a tumour suppressor gene should often become homo- or hemizygous in a tumour. This is because a common mechanism for the second somatic change that Knudson[8] had predicted would be chromosome loss by non-disjunction, or homozygosity resulting from mitotic recombination. Both of these genetic events would be revealed by tumours carrying only one allele detected by a heterozygous DNA probe on Chromosome 13, while the surrounding normal tissue still showed the presence of two alleles. Using this approach, Cavenee and his colleagues demonstrated such changes in a high proportion of both sporadic and familial retinoblastomas and so ushered in the era of loss of heterozygosity studies in cancers as an approach to identifying the position of potential tumour suppressor genes. Knudson's ideas were thus dramatically confirmed. Soon after, Dryja and colleagues cloned the retinoblastoma gene itself, one of the first examples of the use of genomic analysis for positional cloning of a gene of unknown function. Now it could be confirmed that familial retinoblastomas were really due to an inactivating mutation in the Rb gene and, furthermore, that such mutations were also found in sporadic retinoblastomas. Intriguingly, Rb mutations are also commonly seen in, for example, breast carcinomas, although these tumours do not apparently arise in members of retinoblastoma families. Subsequent work has suggested that the Rb gene product is somehow involved in aspects of the control of the cell cycle.

Following this work a number of other tumour suppressor genes, identified through familial cancers, have been cloned, as described in other chapters in this issue. A notable example is the APC gene, whose mutation gives rise to familial adenomatous polyposis (FAP), one of the first described familial dominantly inherited cancer susceptibilities, in this case to colorectal cancer. Affected individuals develop from a few hundred to several thousand adenomatous polyps in their large bowel and rectum, usually starting in their early teens. The gene was localised using RFLP analysis following the identification of an individual with polyposis who had a deletion of chromosome band 5q21. The APC gene was then identified using positional cloning techniques by Nakamura, Vogelstein, White and others. It codes for a 2843 amino acid protein, whose function is somehow connected with cellular adherence and which is mutated in at least 70–80% of all colorectal carcinomas. Exactly as predicted by Knudson for a tumour suppressor gene, the vast majority of mutations are nonsense or frameshift mutations following small deletions, and a high proportion of tumours are homo- or hemizygous for mutations, or are heterozygous for two different mutations. So far more than 300 APC mutations have been sequenced and these are beginning to provide important clues to the mechanisms underlying colon tumour carcinogenesis (*see* for example [5–7]).

The evidence suggests, as might be expected for a gene associated with a familial cancer susceptibility, that APC mutation is one of the earliest steps in the development of a colorectal carcinoma. It seems possible that the polyps in an FAP individual develop spontaneously without further genetic changes, simply as a result of a gene dosage effect. The pattern of mutations observed in the germline and somatically is remarkably similar. A high proportion of changes are small deletions, probably due to replication slippage, and most of the point mutations are C to T transitions expected to occur with relatively high frequency at methylated C positions due to spontaneous deamination. A relatively small proportion of the mutations involve GC to TA transversions, suggesting that external mutagens do not play a major role in colorectal carcinogenesis. Some of the germline mutations occur extraordinarily frequently, such as the 5 base pair deletion at codon 1309, which accounts for 10–15% of all the observed mutations. Indeed, the data on APC mutations in families provide for the first time a basis for the proper estimation of human germline mutation rates using classical mutation – selection balance theory. This suggests that, for example, the mutation rate for simple single base pair transversions is of the order of 5×10^{-9} per generation, while the mutation rate to the commonest deletion is a thousand times more frequent than this and that to the commonest C to T transition is 40–50 times more frequent.

Perhaps the most notable class of genetic mutations detected by allele loss studies is that of the p53 gene, discussed in detail in this issue by David Lane. This was first identified through the cytogenetic observation of loss of the chromosome arm 17p in colorectal carcinomas, and then through allele loss studies by Vogelstein and his colleagues, who provided the first evidence for specific mutations of p53 in colon carcinomas. Subsequently, p53 mutations have been found in approximately 50% of a very wide range of human cancers. As in the analysis of APC mutations, the pattern of sequenced p53 mutations, which now total well over 1000, provides interesting clues to environmental carcinogenesis. Thus, a particular GC to TA transversion is found with exceptionally high frequency in liver cancers, presumably associated with mutagens connected with the fungal toxin aflotoxin B1. Similarly, more than 40% of p53 mutations found in lung carcinomas, largely associated with cigarette smoking, are GC to TA transversions, whereas the frequency of such mutational events in colorectal carcinomas is exceedingly low. This strikingly confirms the role of carcinogens in cigarette smoke in initiating lung carcinomas and, in contrast, the lack of a role for mutagenic carcinogens in the etiology of colorectal carcinomas.[8] This approach to the analysis of environmental effects heralds in a new era of the genetic epidemiology of cancer.

Recently, two members of a new category of mutations have been described that explain certain non-polyposis hereditary colon carcinomas and that also arise in sporadic tumours of a variety of different types. These are genes controlling the first two steps of mismatch repair, originally identified in *Eschericheae coli*, and whose human homologues are hMSH2 and hMLH1 (for review *see*[7]; *see also*[9,10]). These genetic mutations raise intriguing questions as to the basis for their selection at the somatic level, and the role of increased mutation rates in carcinogenesis. While the increase in mutation rates may explain an inherited increase in cancer risk, it seems unlikely that an increase in mutation rate is a strong selective factor during the somatic evolution of a cancer. There is already evidence to suggest that the prognosis of tumours with a mutator phenotype is better than average, and that these events may to some extent be an early alternative to APC mutations. The data emphasise a further interesting aspect of the genetic epidemiology of cancer, namely the opportunity to study the pattern of genetic changes in tumours in relation, for example, to tumour grade, prognosis, location (for example right versus left-sided colon carcinomas), geography, diet and genotype.

The tumour suppressor genes and other genes identified through studies of familial cancers may, it appears, include a wide range of functions from control of the integrity of the genome, such as is the case for p53, hMSH2 and hMLH1, or control of surface interactions associated with cellular adhesion molecules, such as the DCC gene identified by Vogelstein, perhaps the APC gene and the wide range of observations suggesting changes in the expression of molecules controlling surface interactions, such as the integrins and E-cadherin.[11]

APPLICATIONS TO CANCER IMMUNOLOGY AND EARLY DETECTION

The development of understanding of the immune mechanism of T-cell recognition, especially by cytotoxic T-cells, clearly shows that potential targets can include intracellular changes and not only cell surface changes as was at one time assumed to be the case. Thus, a wide range of genetic mutations in dominant oncogenes and tumour suppressor genes may create targets for recognition by immune cytotoxic T-cells. Evidence for such immune responses comes from the observation of relatively frequent changes in surface expression of HLA Class I molecules in a variety of carcinomas. This is one of the mechanisms by which a tumour may evolve to escape from immune attack.[12] In this context, it is intriguing that early observations suggest that tumours with a mutator phenotype may often carry mutations of the β2 microglobulin gene which eliminate HLA Class I expression. This could be due to the fact that such mutating tumours give rise to many potential determinants for recognition by the immune system which are simply a by-product of a high mutation rate and not specifically selected for during tumour progression.[13] There is clearly now an opportunity for developing new approaches to tumour immunotherapy and even anti-tumour vaccination based on our understanding of the mechanisms of T cell immunity, the evidence from changes in HLA expression that immune responses are generated by human tumours, and the discovery of the genetic changes in tumours that provide the potential targets for immune recognition.

Early diagnosis is another interesting and potentially important application of the discovery of the genetic changes in tumours. Mutations, such as in the ras oncogene, present in tumour cells shed (for example) into the stool or into the urine, should be detectable by sensitive PCR based techniques and provide a means of early detection of tumours.[14] It has already been shown that DNA extracted from stool samples of colorectal carcinoma patients with known ras mutations can reveal the presence of these mutations.[15,16] However, undoubtedly much further work is needed to explore these possibilities and develop the sensitivity and specificity of the assays.

A NEW CANCER GENETIC EPIDEMIOLOGY

Another aspect of the new genetic epidemiology of cancers is simply to establish the relative frequency of different types of cancer susceptibility genes in the population. Inherited dominant familial cancers, such as retinoblastoma or FAP, or recessive cancer susceptibilities connected with repair deficiencies, are each individually comparatively rare. Nevertheless, for example, the population incidence of FAP appears to be about one in 7000 births, which is comparable to that for some of the commoner inherited congenital abnormalities. The frequency of FAP has been clearly established by population based registers, particularly in Denmark, and so the frequency of other familial cancers can, to some extent, be assessed in comparison with that of FAP. The data suggest that at most a few percent of the commoner cancers (such as colorectal and breast) are truly familial, though these, nevertheless, pose a significant problem for appropriate counselling and care as discussed elsewhere in this issue. There may, however, in addition, be a class of genetic polymorphisms which give rise to significantly increased susceptibility to cancer, but each with relatively low penetrance. Such genes will not give rise to obvious familial clustering, but may, nevertheless, contribute significantly to the overall population based genetic contribution to cancer susceptibility. One example of such a class of genes would be heterozygotes for clear cut mutations in DNA repair enzymes, which have long been suggested possibly to be at increased risk of cancers although they have no gross abnormality in DNA repair.

It may also be the case that mutations exist in genes, such as APC, which have relatively minimal effects, but nevertheless give rise to a significantly increased cancer susceptibility. It should be possible to detect such mutations by looking at the frequency of normal polymorphic variants in such genes in populations of cancer patients as compared to controls. Thus, the principle of linkage disequilibrium, by which two mutations in a gene which are very close to each other are held together for many generations in a population, would lead to a distortion in the frequency of a normal marker within such a gene in cancer patients, due to its association with the mutation involved in the cancer susceptibility. The discovery of such genetic variation would lead to an approach to cancer prevention targeted to genetically identified susceptible individuals. There is, of course, no doubt that the introduction of such a targeted prevention programme would have to be undertaken with great care to avoid raising unnecessary concern and to ensure cost effectiveness.

There is a completely different category of inherited cancer susceptibilities connected with systemic effects, such as differences in immune response, in repair proficiency as already discussed, and in the rate of metabolism of potential carcinogenic compounds. Thus, there have been many studies carried out on the association between HLA and certain cancers on the assumption that immune response, for example, to a virus such as EBV or HPV associated with a cancer, may influence cancer incidence. Amongst the most persistent of such associations is indeed the first HLA and disease association ever carried out, namely with Hodgkin's lymphoma. The association is not very strong, but is nevertheless significant and is consistent with the long standing idea that Hodgkin's disease may be associated with a virus, but one that has yet to be clearly identified.[17] There have been many suggestions that variations in, for example the P450 enzyme systems, might be associated with cancer incidence due to differential metabolism of potential carcinogens, including cigarette smoke. Now that so many of the genes for these enzymes have been cloned there is an increasing opportunity to look for inherited cancer susceptibilities associated with such systemic effects,[18] as discussed by Forman and Wolf in this issue.

The ideas developed by Boveri and Little in the early years of this century, that cancer is essentially a genetic disease at the cellular level, have been abundantly confirmed by modern molecular and cellular biology; and indeed they underlie the most exciting advances in the fundamental understanding of cancer. They also provide the basis for a wide variety of new approaches to the prevention, early detection and treatment of cancer.

REFERENCES

1 Bodmer W. Somatic cell genetics and cancer. Cancer Surv 1988; 7: 239–250.
2 Bodmer W. Cancer genetics and the human genome. Hospital Practice 1991; 26: 101–117.
3 Knudson AG. Mutation and cancer: statistical study of retinoblastoma. Proc Natl Acad Sci USA 1971; 68: 820–823.
4 Cavenee WK et al. Expression of recessive alleles by chromosomal mechanisms in retinoblastoma. Nature 1983; 305: 779–789.
5 Cottrell, S et al. Molecular analysis of APC mutations in familial adenomatous polyposis and sporadic colon carcinomas. Lancet 1992; 340: 626–630.
6 Mori T, Nagase H, Aoki T et al. The APC (adenomatous polyposis coli) gene a novel mutation in an fap patient and a ddei polymorphism in 5' noncoding region. Hum Mutat 1993; 2 (N3): 240–243.
7 Bodmer WF, Bishop T, Karran P. Genetic steps in colorectal cancer. Nature Genet 1994; 6: 217–219.
8 Harris RA. p53 – at the crossroads of molecular carcinogenesis and risk assessment. NY Acad Sci 1993; 262: 1980–1981.
9 Bronner CE et al. Mutation in the DNA mismatch repair gene homologue hMLH1 is associated with hereditary non polyposis colon cancer. Nature 1994; 368: 258–261.
10 Papadopoulos N, Nicolaides NC, Wei YF et al. Mutations of a mult homolog in hereditary colon-cancer. Science 1994; 263: 1625–1629.
11 Pignatelli M. Models of colorectal tumor differentiation. Cancer Surv 1993; 16: 3–13.
12 Bodmer W et al. Tumour escape from immune response by variation in HLA expressions and other mechanisms. New York Academy of Sciences 1993; 690: 42–49.
13 Bicknell D, Rowan A, Bodmer W. Microglobulin gene mutations: A study of established colorectal cell lines and fresh tumours. Proc Natl Acad Sci USA 1994 (In press).
14 Bodmer W. Hereditary colorectal cancer: a commentary. Proceedings of the 4th International Symposium on Colorectal Cancer 1989, Kobe, Japan. Springer-Verlag 1989; 37–42.
15 Sidranksky D et al. Identification of ras oncogene mutations in the stool of patients with curable colorectal tumors. Science 1992; 256 (5053): 102–105.
16 Smith-Ravin J et al. Detection of C-Ki-ras mutations in faecal samples from sporadic colorectal cancer patients. Gut 1994 (In press).

17 Tonks S et al. An international study of the association between HLA-DP and Hodgkin's disease. Proceedings of the Eleventh Int. Histo. Workshop and Conference 1991. Oxford: Oxford University Press, 1992; 2: 539–543.

18 Zhong et al. Relationship between gstm 1 genetic-polymorphism and susceptibility to bladder, breast and colon cancer. Carcinogenesis 1993; 14: 1821–1824.

British Medical Bulletin (1994) Vol. 50, No. 3, pp. 527–535
© The British Council 1994

The inherited component of cancer

D F Easton

*Section of Epidemiology, Institute of Cancer Research, Surrey, UK**

All cancer types exhibit familial clustering, suggestive of a significant inherited component; however, to date only a few of the genes responsible have been identified and the inherited component, if any, underlying most common cancers has not been well defined. Amongst the important known susceptibility genes are those dominant genes conferring a high risk of breast and ovarian cancer (BRCA1), colon cancer (hMSH2 and hMLH1), and melanoma (MLM). All these genes confer a high lifetime risk of the disease concerned, but are rare and only account for a small minority (less than 5%) of cases. However, there are also commoner genes conferring lower risks but accounting for a more substantial fraction of cancer cases; those so far identified include the ataxia-telangiectasia gene and the HRAS1 minisatellite locus.

In their review of the causes of cancer in 1981, Doll and Peto[1] wrote 'At present, the relevance of genetic susceptibility to the common types of cancer remains obscure'. Whilst there is still a great deal of truth in this statement, much has been learnt over the intervening 13 years about inherited susceptibility to cancer. Before 1980, the only cancers known for certain to have an inherited basis were those occurring in rare familial syndromes clearly conforming to Mendelian inheritance, such as hereditary retinoblastoma and colon cancer in polyposis coli. An inherited component to common cancers was inferred firstly, from some anecdotal families with extraordinarily large numbers of cases and, secondly, from epidemiological studies indicating that most common cancers occur more frequently in close relatives of cancer patients

*Present address: Genetic Epidemiology, Dept of Medical Informatics, University of Utah, Salt Lake City, Utah 84108, USA.

with the same type of cancer. More recently, however, the inherited basis of certain families with a high risk of common cancers has been confirmed with the identification of predisposing mutations, or the localisation of susceptibility genes by linkage analysis. These include: BRCA1, causing susceptibility to early onset breast cancer and ovarian cancer;[2,3] p53, responsible for the majority of families with the Li-Fraumeni syndrome;[4] hMSH2 and hMLH1, causing non-polyposis colorectal cancer, endometrial cancer and a number of other cancers;[5–7] and MLM causing familial melanoma.[8]

In this chapter we review briefly the evidence for genetic susceptibility to common cancers, and consider in somewhat greater detail susceptibility to breast cancer.

FAMILIAL RELATIVE RISKS

One of the most important measures of the contribution of inherited factors to disease is the relative risk of the disease to close relatives of affected individuals, usually first degree relatives, compared to the risk in the general population. Table 1 summarises these 'familial relative risks' for some of the common cancers for which reasonably precise estimates are available, usually from case-control studies. For most cancers, the familial risks are of the order of 2–3-fold, though sometimes higher amongst early onset cases, as for breast and colon cancer. The major exceptions would appear to be testis cancer and thyroid cancer, and perhaps also chronic lymphocytic leukaemia, multiple myeloma and laryngeal cancer, which show higher relative risks. It is also possible that certain histological subtypes may show stronger familial risks, such as lobular breast cancer[9] but these have not been studied extensively.

The rather moderate familial risks are sometimes taken as evidence that there is little variation in cancer susceptibility, but this argument is falacious; such familial risks can disguise surprisingly large genetic effects. To take a simple example, suppose that the familial relative risk of 2 for, say, pancreatic cancer were due to a single gene (which is admittedly rather unlikely), then there are a variety of single gene models which could explain this familial risk.[10] It could, for example, be explained by a rare dominant gene with frequency 0.0002, which increased the disease risk 75-fold in carriers (if the lifetime population risk were 1%, this would translate into a risk of about 50% in carriers). Under this model, the gene would account for only about 3% of cases. At the other extreme, the familial risk could be due to a much more common dominant gene with a frequency of 15%, conferring a lifetime risk of 3% in carriers compared to 0.15% in non-carriers. In the latter case, the gene would account for about 85% of cases. What both these

Table 1 Relative risks to first degree relatives of selected common cancers*

Cancer	Estimate	References
Breast	2.1	Schildkraut et al[23]
aged <45	3.6	Claus et al[24]
Colon	3.4	Macklin[25]
		Lovett[26]
Ovary	3.6	Schildkraut and Thompson[27]
Endometrium	2.7	Schildkraut et al[23]
Lung	3	Tokuhata and Lilienfeld[28]
		Ooi et al[29]
Stomach	2.6	Macklin[25]
Melanoma	2.5	see Easton and Peto[10]
Prostate	1.9	Steinberg et al[30]
Testis	9	Forman et al[31]
Thyroid	8.2	Stoffer et al[32]

*Most of these estimates are based on the largest available studies, and not on comprehensive overviews of all available data.

models have in common is that the ratio of disease risks in carriers to non-carriers is much higher than the familial relative risk (being 75-fold in the first case and 20-fold in the second); in fact it can be shown that, for a familial relative risk of 2, this ratio must always be at least 9-fold.

Known cancer susceptibility genes include examples of both rare, high penetrance genes accounting for a small proportion of cases, such as p53, BRCA1 and the HNPCC genes; and of low risk genes accounting for the majority of cases, such as the HLA linked susceptibility genes causing nasopharyngeal carcinoma and perhaps also Hodgkin's disease. In practice, most of the familial risks are probably the result of mutation in several different genes each causing an increased risk (genetic heterogeneity), as has been clearly shown in the case of breast and colon cancer, or perhaps the result of several genes acting synergistically. This does not alter the argument that there are large variations in susceptibility, but it makes the genes themselves much harder to identify.

Reliable determination of the correct genetic model only becomes possible once the genes responsible become isolated by linkage analysis, and this stage has not been reached yet for most cancers. However, some indication of the genetics of some of the commoner cancers has been possible by more detailed analysis of the pattern of inheritance using segregation analysis. For example, a number of segregation analyses have indicated that familial breast cancer is best explained by a rare dominant gene conferring a high risk, but accounting only for a small minority of cases; in the largest such study by Claus et al[11] the high risk allele has a population frequency of 0.3%, confers a risk of about 67% by age 70 and would account for about 15% of cases below age 50 and 8% of cases below age 70. Similar evidence for a high risk dominant gene has been found for prostate cancer,[12] colon cancer (Bishop D T, personal communication), and lung cancer.[13] The lack of similar evidence for other cancers may simply reflect the fact that no sufficiently large systematic family studies have yet been performed.

The evidence for a rare dominant gene in these studies is derived chiefly from the observation that individuals with two or more affected relatives suffer a much higher cancer risk than individuals with just one affected relative, which is better explained by a rare gene conferring a high risk than a common gene conferring a moderate risk or a polygenic model. However, these analyses merely indicate that some of the familial clustering is likely to be due to a highly penetrant gene; they do not rule out the possibility of several genes being involved, perhaps conferring a range of risks.

COLON CANCER

One example of a cancer in which several genes affect susceptibility is provided by colon cancer, for which 3 genes predisposing to a high risk of colon cancer have now been identified. These are the APC gene in which colon cancer occurs as a consequence of polyposis coli,[14] and the 2 genes hMSH2 and hMLH1 which are responsible for families with the hereditary non-polyposis colon cancer syndrome (HNPCC),[5-7] in which there is also a high risk of endometrial cancer and a number of other cancers. APC mutations are rare and only account for a tiny proportion of colon cancer cases, particularly since many polyposis cases are successfully treated by surgery to prevent cancer developing. As yet there are no systematic studies to estimate the prevalence of hMSH2 and hMLH1 mutations amongst colon cancer patients, but it seems likely that the proportion will be low (perhaps 1 or 2%,[15] though higher amongst young cases). It has been suggested that these genes account for most familial colon cancer, but this is probably more a reflection of the families tested so far.[7] The HNPCC genes also confer a high risk of other cancers which is not seen in all colon cancer families, and some families appear to be unlinked to either locus.[16] It seems much more likely that the existing genes account for the majority of large high risk families but that other genes, conferring a lower risk and perhaps more restricted to colon cancer, explain smaller families.

BREAST CANCER

It is instructive to consider susceptibility to breast cancer in some detail, because it has been more thoroughly studied than any other common cancer, and many of the complexities which have arisen in respect of familial breast cancer probably also apply to other cancers.

To date 5 genes have been shown to be involved in breast cancer susceptibility. Moreover, these genes do not account for all high risk breast cancer families, so at least one and, more probably, several genes remain to be identified. The known genes are summarised in Table 2; they differ markedly in the risks of breast cancer they confer, the proportion of breast cancer cases which they explain, and the other cancers which they cause. Germline p53 mutations appear to cause the highest breast cancer risk, over 50% by age 50, as well as substantial risks of childhood sarcomas, brain tumours and a number of other cancers. However, p53 mutations are rare and cause less than 1% of breast cancer cases, even below age 50.[17,18] Germline mutations of the androgen receptor (AR) gene are an even rarer cause of breast cancer, having been shown only to cause male breast cancer in 2 families.[19]

The BRCA1 gene causes a somewhat lower risk of breast cancer than p53, but mutations in BRCA1 are probably much more common than p53 mutations, so BRCA1 accounts for a much higher proportion of breast cancer cases. BRCA1 mutations also confer a lifetime risk of ovarian cancer in excess of 50%, and may in fact account for most familial clustering of ovarian cancer. The BRCA1 gene has not yet been cloned, so direct estimates of the gene frequency of BRCA1 are not yet possible. However, Ford et al (personal communication) have used population data on the familial associations between breast and ovarian cancer to estimate that BRCA1 mutations will account for about 5% of all breast cancer cases, below age 50 and 1% over age 50; the corresponding estimates for ovarian cancer are 5% and 2%.

The other 2 genes are examples of more common susceptibility alleles causing more moderate risks. Individuals affected with the recessive disorder ataxia-telangiectasia (AT) have a grossly elevated risk of lymphomas and many other cancers at a young age, but heterozygous carriers of AT mutations also appear to suffer an excess cancer risk, particular of breast cancer where the relative risk is about 8-fold, equivalent to an absolute risk of about 11% by age 50.[20] This is much lower than the risk conferred by either p53 or BRCA1; however, given the high frequency of AT mutant alleles in the population (about 0.5%) could be responsible for a higher proportion of breast cancer cases (about 7%),

Table 2 Genes predisposing to breast cancer*

Gene	Chromosomal location	Breast Cancer risk by age:		Risk of any cancer by age:		Proportion of breast cancers due to gene		Associated cancers
		50	70	50	70	<50	50+	
P53	17p	40%	?	80%	?	<1%	–	Sarcomas, brain
BRCA1	17q	45%	59%	58%	85%	5%	1%	Ovary, colon?, prostate?
BRCA2	?	?	?	?	?			Male breast, prostate
AT	11q	11%	30%	15%	46%	7%	7%	ALL?
HRAS	11p	3%	10%	9%	9%			ALL?
AR	Xq	??	(Male BC only)			<<1%		

*Modified from Easton et al.[33]

particularly at older ages. An example of an even lower penetrance gene is provided by HRAS1 minisatellite locus. A certain class of rare alleles at this locus is associated with an approximately 2-fold increased risk of breast cancer and a number of other common cancers.[21] These alleles have a population frequency of about 6%, and are therefore responsible for about 1 in 11 of these cancers. Such low risk effects are of course, of more mechanistic than practical importance, unless they can be shown to interact with the effects of other genes or environmental exposures.

Of all the genes so far identified, only BRCA1 explains a substantial fraction of 'familial breast cancer', accounting for about half of all multiple case families.[22] Thus, only BRCA1 has any detectable influence on the familial risks or the segregation analysis. The other genes are either too rare (p53, AR) or confer too low a risk (AT and HRAS) to have a measurable familial effect. For the same reason, only BRCA1 of the currently identified genes has been mapped by linkage analysis; the other effects have been detected either by direct sequencing or in the case of AT because an associated phenotypic marker.

CONCLUSIONS

The exact contribution of the known cancer susceptibility genes to overall cancer incidence is still somewhat unclear, and large population based studies of mutation rates in different cancers at different ages will be required to provide more precise estimates (thus far only available for p53). However, it seems likely that the currently known high risk genes account for perhaps 0.5–1% of all cancer cases. This figure will of course rise as other susceptibility genes are identified; given the known familial risks and the results of segregation analysis, this seems likely that such genes will be found for breast cancer (in addition to BRCA1), prostate cancer, and lung cancer and perhaps also colorectal cancer not due to the HNPCC genes. (Given the size of the familial relative risks, it seems likely that genes for testis cancer and thyroid cancer should also be mappable, though these may not cause high lifetime risks.) Taken together, these 'high risk' genes could account for anything up to about 5% of incident cancers. The likelihood, however, is that many more susceptibility genes exist which cause lower risks; but these genes will only be detected by direct sequencing of candidate genes.

REFERENCES

1   Doll R, Peto R. The causes of cancer: quantitative estimates of avoidable risks of cancer in the United States today. Oxford: Oxford University Press, 1981.
2   Hall JM, Lee MK, Morrow J et al. Linkage analysis of early onset familial breast cancer to chromosome 17q21. Science 1990: 250; 1684–1689.
3   Narod SA, Feunteun J, Lynch HT et al. Familial breast-ovarian cancer locus on chromosome 17q12–23. Lancet 1991; 338: 82–83.

4   Malkin D, Li FP, Strong LC et al. Germline mutations in a familial syndrome of breast cancer, sarcomas and other neoplasms. Science 1990; 250; 1233–1238.

5   Leach FS, Nicolaides NC, Papadopoulos N et al. Mutations of a mutS homolog in hereditary nonpolyposis colorectal cancer. Cell 1993; 75; 1215–1225.

6   Bronner CE, Baker SM, Morrison PT et al. Mutation in the DNA mismatch repair gene homologue hMLH1 is associated with hereditary nonpolyposis colon cancer linked to chromosome 3p. Nature 1994; 368; 258–261.

7   Papadopoulos N, Nicolaides NC, Wei Y-F et al. Mutation of the mutL homolog associated with hereditary colon cancer. Science 1994; 263; 1625–1629.

8   Cannon-Albright LA, Goldgar DE, Meyer LJ et al. Assignment of a locus for familial melanoma, MLM, to chromosome 9p13–p22. Science 1992; 258; 1148–1152.

9   Cannon-Albright LA, Thomas A, Goldgar DE et al. Familiarity of cancer in Utah. Cancer Res 1994; 54; 2378–2385.

10   Easton DF, Peto J. The contribution of inherited predisposition to cancer incidence. Cancer Surv 1990; 9; 395–416.

11   Claus EB, Risch N, Thompson WD. Genetic analysis of breast cancer in the Cancer and Steroid Hormone Study. Am J Hum Genet 1991; 48; 232–242.

12   Carter BS, Beaty TH, Steinberg GD, Childs B, Walsh PC. Mendelian inheritance of familial prostate cancer. Proc Natl Acad Sci USA 1990; 87; 8751–8755.

13   Sellers TA, Baily-Wilson JE, Elston RC et al. Evidence for Mendelian inheritance in the pathogenesis of lung cancer. J Natl Cancer Inst 1990; 82; 1272–9.

14   Bodmer W, Bishop DT, Karran P. Genetic steps in colorectal cancer. Nature Genet 1994; 6: 217–219.

15   Nishisho I, Nakamura Y, Mishoshi Y et al. Mutation of chromosome 5q21 genes in FAP and colorectal cancer patients. Science 1991; 253; 665–669.

16   Lewis CM, Cannon-Albright LA, Burt RW, Disario J, Samowitz W, Skolnick MH. Linkage analysis of colorectal cancer to chromosome 2 in Utah kindreds. Am J Hum Genet 1993; 53; A23.

17   Borresen A-L, Anderson TI, Garber J et al. Screening for germline TP53 mutations in breast cancer patients. Cancer Res 1992; 52; 3234–3256.

18   Sidransky D, Tokino T, Helzlsouer K et al. Inherited p53 mutations in breast cancer. Cancer Res 1992; 52; 2984–2986.

19   Wooster R, Mangion J, Eeles R et al. A germline mutation in the androgen receptor in two brothers with breast cancer and Reifenstein Syndrome. Nature Genet 1992; 2; 132–134.

20   Swift M, Reitnauer PJ, Morrell D, Chase CL. Breast and other cancers in families with ataxia-telangiectasia. N Engl J Med 1987; 316; 1289–1294.

21   Krontiris TG, Devlin B, Karp DD, Robert NJ, Risch N. An association between the risk of cancer and mutations in the Hras1 minisatellite locus. N Engl J Med 1993; 329; 517–523.

22   Easton DF, Bishop DT, Ford D, Crockford GP, Breast Cancer Linkage Consortium. Genetic linkage analysis in familial breast and ovarian cancer: results from 214 families. Am J Hum Genet 1993; 52; 678–701.

23   Schildkraut JM, Risch N, Thompson WD. Evaluating genetic association between ovarian, breast and endometrial cancer: evidence for a breast-ovarian relationship. Am J Hum Genet 1989; 45: 521–529.

24   Claus EB, Risch N, Thompson WD. Using age at onset to distinguish between subforms of breast cancer. Ann Hum Genet 1990; 54: 169–177.

25   Macklin MT. Inheritance of cancer of the stomach and large intestine in man. J Natl Cancer Inst 1960; 24: 551–571.

26   Lovett E. Family studies in cancer of the colon and rectum. Br J Surg 1976; 63: 13–18.

27   Schildkraut JM, Thompson WD. Familial ovarian cancer: a population-based case-control. Am J Epidemiol 1988; 128; 456–466.

28   Tokuhata GK, Lilienfeld AM. Familial aggregation of lung cancer in humans. J Natl Cancer Inst 1963; 30; 289–312.

29 Ooi WH, Elston RC, Chen VW, Bailey-Wilson JE, Rothschild H. Increased familial risk for lung cancer. J Natl Cancer Inst 1986; 76; 217–222.
30 Steinberg GS, Carter BS, Beaty TH, Childs B, Walsh PC. Family history and the risk of prostate cancer. Prostate 1990; 17; 337–347.
31 Forman D, Oliver RTD, Brett AR et al. Familial testis cancer: a report of the UK family register, estimation of risk and an HLA class I sib-pair analysis. Br J Cancer 1992; 65; 255–262.
32 Stoffer S, Van Dyke DL, Vaden Bach V, Weiss L. Am J Med Genet 1986; 25; 775–782.
33 Easton DF, Ford D, Peto J. Inherited susceptibility to breast cancer. Cancer Surv 1994; (in press).

British Medical Bulletin (1994) Vol. 50, No. 3, pp. 536–559
© The British Council 1994

Identification and characterisation of cancer genes

C M Steel

School of Biological and Medical Sciences, University of St Andrews, Fife, UK

Cancer genes have been subdivided into oncogenes and tumour suppressors though the distinction is not entirely valid. In many cases their effects can be demonstrated by induction or reversal of a transformed phenotype following transfection into a suitable host cell but full characterisation requires isolation by positional cloning and analysis of function at the molecular level. Almost all have been ascribed some function within the complex pathways of signal generation, receipt and response that regulate cell growth and differentiation. However, few, if any, tumours result from just a single mutation and the key to a real understanding of the molecular basis of malignancy must be studies, currently in their infancy, of interactions between the various genes implicated in the initiation and progression of cancer.

Understanding the molecular basis of carcinogenesis requires more than a list of gene sequences consistently altered in a given type of tumour. Most importantly we need to know the normal cellular function of each implicated gene and how that function is changed by the particular mutations observed. Eventually we may build a comprehensive picture of the interactions between multiple mutant gene products and so explain the phenotype of disordered growth, impaired differentiation and resistance to therapy that characterises a typical advanced cancer. That goal has yet to be attained for any tumour and this chapter is, of necessity, concerned chiefly with techniques that can illuminate individual elements of what is clearly a very complex process.

DIRECT FUNCTIONAL ASSAYS FOR MOLECULAR CARCINOGENESIS

Transfection/transformation

The fact that the basic lesion in malignancy resides in the genetic material of the cell has been beyond dispute for decades but attribution of blame at the molecular level required 3 developments; first a simple assay for tumorigenesis, second a means to transfect functioning genes and third the ability to analyse nucleic acid base sequences. These techniques all came to fruition in the 1970s in the hands of tumour virologists working on the small oncogenic RNA viruses[1] which could induce morphological 'transformation' (ie immortalisation, loss of contact inhibition and a reduction in requirement for specialised nutrients) in mammalian or avian cells in vitro. Such transformed cells were tumorigenic on inoculation into syngeneic animals and the transforming ability of a given virus was shown to depend on the integrity of a specific portion of its genome, the oncogene. It was found that retroviral **oncogenes** have their origins in the transduction of cellular sequences and that somatic mutations in the original cellular genes (the **proto-oncogenes**) can contribute to tumorigenesis without the agency of any virus.[2–4] When sheared DNA from certain human tumours is precipitated onto a monolayer culture of mouse 3T3 or C127 cells in the presence of calcium phosphate, a few transformed colonies appear and these can be shown to have incorporated human oncogenes, usually of the *ras* family. Although this would appear to be a very simple and direct means of demonstrating oncogene activity, it depends upon the existence of quite abnormal cell lines, already on the brink of transformation. More widely applicable versions of the assay involve transfection of a putative oncogene in a construct which includes a powerful promoter, exposure of the target cells to exogenous growth factors or simultaneous transfection of two oncogenes that can act in synergy(Table 1).[2–6]

Transformation reversal

One implication of the type of experiment just described is that oncogenesis comes about through the positive influence of altered dominantly-acting genes. If that were a universal truth then fusion of a transformed with an untransformed cell would be expected to generate a hybrid with the transformed phenotype. In practice, however, such hybrids, as a rule, are untransformed. On prolonged culture they tend to shed chromosomes and transformed colonies emerge, from which the inference can be drawn that some of the shed chromosomes carried genes whose effect was to inhibit the expression of malignant characteristics.[5–8] This provided the basis for the concept of **tumour suppressor** genes and

Table 1　Oncogenes detected by transfection/transformation assays

Some c-oncogenes able to transform established cell lines (eg C127 or 3T3)	Associated human tumours
Ha - *ras*	Ca pancreas, colon, lung, melanoma, others
Ki - *ras*	AML, melanoma, thyroid
N - *ras*	G-U tract, thyroid, melanoma
dbl/mcf2	Diffuse B cell lymphoma/breast cancer
fos	Renal, colon, ovary, lung, others
int 1	Breast
met	Osteosarcoma
mos	Breast
myc	Breast, colon, Burkitt's lymphoma, lung, ovary, others
raf	Lung
ret	Thyroid
sis	Astrocytoma
trk	Thyroid

Combinations of oncogenes + other factors transforming primary cultures (eg rat embryo fibroblasts)

Ha - *ras*		c - *myc*
Ki - *ras*	+	N - *myc*
N - *ras*		L - *myc*
src	+	p53 (mutant)
Erb B1	+	EGF
fms	+	CSF - 1
Erb B2	+	Powerful promoter

the experimental principle has been extended to encompass reversal of the transformed phenotype by transfection of a small number of chromosomes (by microcell fusion), of a single chromosome, of sub-chromosomal fragments and ultimately of cloned genes (Table 2). There are obvious difficulties in selecting for *suppression* of growth in such a transfection experiment and in many instances what is demonstrated is partial, rather than complete, reversion of the transformed pheno-type. This, of course, serves to illustrate the involvement of multiple molecular events in oncogenesis. By definition, tumour suppressors, in contrast to oncogenes, contribute to the process when they are lost or functionally inactivated. It has also emerged, mainly from studies in familial cancers discussed elsewhere in this volume, that tumour sup-pressors tend to act in a recessive manner at the cellular level, whereas oncogenes are usually dominant or co-dominant. It is consistent with our understanding of these concepts that heritable cancers tend to be associated with germline transmission of a single inactivated copy of a tumour suppressor, conferring the risk rather than the certainty of disease. However, some revision of that general principle has been required in the light of recent molecular genetic and clinical findings. The p53 gene, for example, is now known to be a tumour suppressor in its normal 'wild type'configuration but mutant forms behave as oncogenes with varying degrees of 'dominant negative' effect and some of these can be inherited (see Lane, this issue). The APC gene, associated with familial polyposis, though by most criteria an authentic tumour suppressor, seems to confer a growth advantage on colonic epithelium when only one copy is inactivated (see Dunlop and Cunningham, this issue). By contrast, ret,which has strong credentials as an oncogene, has been implicated as the site of heritable mutations responsible for one of the multiple endocrine neoplasia syndromes, MEN 2.[14]

Table 2 Examples of the reversal of transformed phenotype by chromosome, sub-chromosomal fragment or gene transfer (data mainly from Refs 8–13)

DNA transferred	Target cell line
Chromosome 1	HT 1080 fibrosarcoma
Chromosome 1,6,9	Endometrial Ca
Chromosome 3	Renal cell Ca
Chromosome 5,17,18	Colorectal Ca
Chromosome 6	Melanoma
Chromosome 11	HeLa
Chromosome 17	Breast Ca, Neuroblastoma
Sub-chromosomal fragments (11p15)	Rhabdomyosarcoma
Rb 1 gene	Reinoblastoma, Osteosarcoma, Prostatic Ca
p53 (wild type)	Osteosarcoma
Krev 1	K-ras transformed 3T3
GAP	src-transformants
NM23-H1	Breast Ca (reduced metastases)

Blockade of apoptosis

As indicated above, the malignant phenotype, even in tissue culture, has several components. Attempts have been made to equate these with the contributions of different oncogenes and tumour suppressor genes. This carries the risk of oversimplification but one element that does appear to be separable from the rest is immortalisation. Whereas normal cells in vitro or in vivo have a finite life span and may be required to die prematurely in the interests of the whole organism (eg for tissue modelling or to accommodate the expansion of selected clones), cancer cells often ignore or fail to generate the signals that should trigger self-destruction (**apoptosis**).[15,16] The 3 oncogenes specifically implicated in different aspects of apoptosis are *bcl 2*, *myc* and p53. *bcl 2* is a potent blocker of the process. The effect can be demonstrated by inducing apoptosis (eg by exposing lymphocytes to steroid hormones or tumour cell lines to cytotoxic agents) and showing the relative resistance of cells transfected with the gene in an active configuration. *myc* is generally associated with immortalisation and where growth conditions are favourable the combined expression of *myc* plus *bcl 2* is highly tumorigenic. However, when cells enter a growth arrest phase due to absence of growth factors or the action of cytostatic drugs, *myc* becomes an inducer of apoptosis. Similarly, wild type p53 seems to be required not only to regulate cell division, for example after DNA damage, but also to direct those cells in which the damage cannot be repaired along the pathway to apoptosis. Some p53 mutants cannot perform this function and so permit genetically damaged cells to survive and proliferate.

Disruption of embryogenesis

Some candidate tumour suppressor genes have been identified by locating the sites of damage in early Drosophila embryos which show hyperplasia and disordered growth of the imaginal discs following mutagenesis. On transplantation into normal host embryos, the affected tissue continues to grow in an uncontrolled fashion.The target genes evidently contribute to normal intercellular communication and several that have been identified so far show evolutionary conservation, suggesting that corresponding genes may be relevant to tumour development in higher species, including man.[17]

Oncogenesis in transgenic animals

The ultimate test of an oncogene or tumour suppressor must be the production of an appropriate transgenic animal. This begs the question of which species represents the appropriate model for man. To date, almost all interpretable data have come from the mouse, initially using micro-injection into the nucleus of the fertilized ovum but, more recently, by in vitro site-directed mutagenesis of embryonic stem (ES) cells which are then introduced into the mouse embryo at the 8 cell blastocyst stage. Breeding from the resulting mosaic animals (usually recognised from a patchy coat colour pattern) will yield some progeny that carry the ES genotype in all their cells.[18] A cautionary note was sounded by the observation that mice homozygous for inactivating mutations of Rb suffer widespread and lethal developmental abnormalities while heterozygotes develop pituitary tumours which are not seen in members of human retinoblastoma families. In general, however, both oncogene and tumour suppressor gene mutations in the mouse germline result in patterns of tumour development that might have been predicted from their known involvement in human cancer. Animals heterozygous for an overexpressed mutant p53 appear healthy at birth but show a high incidence of epithelial tumours and sarcomas as young adults.[19] Mice heterozygous for a non-functional p53 have a moderate excess of spontaneous cancers and increased susceptibility to a chemical carcinogen but those homozygous for the non-expressing mutation, though they develop normally, show a very high incidence of lymphomas, sarcomas and other malignancies (sometimes multiple) by about 6 months.[20] As regards transgenic oncogenes, the most interesting experiments are those in which the construct used incorporates a tissue-specific promoter. Examples include the IgH enhancer for B lymphoid cells and the whey acidic protein (Wap) gene promoter for mammary epithelium. Individual oncogenes such as *ras* and *myc* tend to induce tumours in the targeted tissues but with a long latent period. In some instances, for example mice bearing *ras* coupled to the clastase 1 gene promoter (designed to target pancreatic acinar cells), no tumours have been observed. Cross-breeding to produce animals doubly transgenic for combinations of activated oncogenes generally leads to a much higher incidence of cancers with reduced latency but, even then, one or more additional somatic events seems to be required since only a few cells actually undergo the change to frank malignancy. Hyperplasia and cellular atypia are commonly seen as pre-malignant lesions in transgenic animals; thus one of the most valuable attributes of the experimental system is the opportunity it affords to correlate pathological and molecular phases in tumour evolution.[18,21–23] There are also naturally occurring syndromes of genetic cancer predisposition in mice that provide useful information on human counterparts. The 'Min' mouse, for example, is an instructive model for familial adenomatous polyposis.[24,25]

LOCALISING CANCER GENES AND MUTATIONS

While there are instances of oncogenes that were discovered through the application of one of the direct functional assays outlined above, an even more fruitful path has been accurate localisation of recurrent molecular lesions in particular types of tumour, followed by isolation and characterisation of a specific gene.

Cytogenetics

The chromosomes of malignant cells are notoriously hard to analyse and only in the case of leukaemias and lymphomas has this approach proved a major route towards the localisation of cancer genes. The **Philadel-**

phia chromosome (characteristic of CML), was, for many years, the only truly consistent aberration specifically associated with any human malignancy but after the advent of chromosome banding techniques and the development of modern classification systems for lymphomas, several others (mainly translocations) were recognised. In due course, these have become prime targets for gene mapping and several new oncogenes have been discovered at translocation breakpoints.[26,27] Some have been activated by juxtaposition with inappropriate promoters, particularly those of the immunoglobulin or T cell receptor genes. Other translocations have generated fusion oncogenes (Table 3).

Table 3 Some consistent visible chromosome aberrations in human tumours (data mainly from Refs 26 & 27).

Disease	Chromosome aberration	Genes implicated
CML	t(9;22)(q34;q11)	bcr-abl fusion
Burkitt's lymphoma	t(8;14)(q24;q32),t(2;8)(p12;q24), t(8;22)(q24;q11)	myc-Ig (H,K or L)
Follicular lymphoma	t(14;18)(q32;q21)	bcl 2-IgH
Lymphocytic lymphoma	t(11;14)(q13;q32)	PRAD 1-IgH
CLL	+12	?
CLL	del/t 13(q14)	?DBM
Null ALL	t(1;11)(p32;q23),t(11;19)(q23;p13)	MLL-various
Pre-B ALL	t(1;19)(q23;p13)	PBX-TCF fusion
Infant ALL	t(4;11)(q21;q23)	AF4 - MLL fusion
T-ALL	t(7q35),t(14q11)	TCRβ,TCRα, δ fusion) (eg TAL 1-TCRα, fusion)
AML	t(8;21)(q22;q22)	AML 1 - ETO fusion
APML	t(15;17)(q22;q12)	PML-RARA fusion
AMML (+eosinophils)	inv(16)(p13;q22)	CBFB-MYH 11 fusion
AMoL	t(11q23)	MLL-various
AML (+basophils)	t(6;9)(p23;q24)	DEK-CAN fusion
AML (+platelets)	inv(3)(q21;q26)	?EVI 1
Renal cancer	t/del 3p	?VHL
Small-cell lung cancer	del(3)(p14p23)	?
Pleomorphic salivary adenoma	t(3;8)(p21;q12)	?mos
Ewing's sarcoma	t(11;22)(q24;q12)	FLI 1-EWS
Retinoblastoma	t/del 13(q14)	Rb 1
Wilms' tumour	t/del 11(p13)	WT 1
Meningioma	-22	NF 2
Lipoma	t(12)(q13-14)	?
Uterine leiomyoma	+12/t(12;14)(q14-15;q23-24)	?

Comparable studies in solid tumours have generally yielded a plethora of inconclusive data but there have been some consistent findings that could yet lead to the identification of new oncogenes or tumour suppressors.[27] There have also been notable successes in relation to 2 familial cancer syndromes.[28] Localisation of the Rb locus resulted from the identification of constitutional 13q lesions in a few retinoblastoma patients and somatically acquired aberrations involving the same region in a number of tumours. The *apc* (Adenomatous Polyposis Coli) gene was correctly assigned to the long arm of chromosome 5 after a single case report describing APC (without a family history) in a patient with multiple developmental abnormalities who had a new constitutional deletion of 5q. However, efforts to find associations between other hereditary cancers and constitutional chromosome aberrations have been unsuccessful to date.

It is worth emphasising that acquired cytogenetic abnormalities are not exclusive to malignant cells. Uterine fibroids, benign ovarian tumours, fibro-adenomas of breast and many other innocent growths, even including atheromatous plaques, frequently show trisomies or other aberrations indicating clonal evolution, although the range of abnormalities tends to be much wider in cancers. In a few cultured tumour lines (much more rarely in direct preparations from tumours) metaphase cells show expanded blocks of chromatin termed **homogeneous-staining regions** (HSRs) which consist of multiple repeats of a single region that includes a proto-oncogene such as *n-myc* or a drug-resistance gene. The same phenomenon may present as hundreds or even thousands of copies of a tiny acentric **double minute** 'chromosome'.[29] Most oncogene amplifications, however, cannot be detected at the visible chromosome level.

Molecular cytogenetics

Many alterations in the genome of tumour cells can be demonstrated and localised by techniques that do not require direct inspection of the chromosomes. As more and more human DNA sequences are mapped opportunities are growing for regional assignment of amplifications and deletions by analysis of extracted DNA. One such approach involves comparing constitutional (usually blood) and tumour tissue from the same patient to detect allele imbalance at polymorphic loci. Microsatellite (dinucleotide or oligonucleotide repeat) sequences are particularly useful for this purpose since they can be amplified by PCR and hence require very little starting material. They are also extremely polymorphic so that most individuals are constitutionally heterozygous.[30] When the relative intensities of the two alleles differ markedly between blood and tumour we infer that there has been a somatic change involving the site to which the polymorphic sequence has been mapped.[31] By applying this principle to a series of near-contiguous markers, the extent of the chromosome region involved can be estimated and where the genome map density is high, that estimate can be very precise. Studies of this type are often presented in terms of 'Loss of Heterozygosity' (LOH) and it is implied that where two alleles are present in the constitutional DNA but only one can be seen in the tumour DNA, the underlying mechanism is a simple chromosomal deletion. This is true in some, but not in all instances. More complex events such as mitotic recombination can generate a localised region of homozygosity without any net loss of chromosome material.[32] Furthermore, duplication or regional amplification of one chromosome will generate imbalance in the intensity of alleles of polymorphic markers which might be misinterpreted as a deletion,with contaminating non-malignant cells contributing the fainter allele signal (Fig. 1). It is therefore important not only to ensure that the portions of tumour analysed contain as little normal tissue as possible, but also to recognise the range of structural changes that could give rise to any given abnormality found at the DNA level.

The status of **known** cancer gene sequences in tumour cells can also be examined by analysis of tumour and constitutional DNA. Where an oncogene is grossly amplified, this may well be evident from a Southern blot and lesser degrees of amplification can be demonstrated by differential PCR where the oncogene and a control sequence are amplified in the same reaction. The relative intensities of the two signals from tumour and normal DNA are then compared.[33] For these purposes, the sequences examined do not require to be polymorphic.

Even more specific information can be obtained by DNA analysis in those situations where oncogene activation depends upon a chromosome translocation generating a fusion gene. With primers from either side of the breakpoint, PCR amplification will only be possible where the translocation is present. That principle is now widely applied in confirming the diagnosis of chronic myeloid leukaemia (CML) (detecting the 9:22 translocation *bcr/abl* product) and of follicular lymphoma (detecting the 14:18 translocation *IgH/bcl2* product) among others. Because the PCR reaction is tumour genome specific, the procedure also lends itself to accurate and exquisitely sensitive measurement of tumour burden, for example in the detection of minimal residual disease after chemotherapy.[34]

A logical extension of the foregoing is to analyse tumour DNA in situ. Using, in the main, fluorescence-labelled probes, individual regions of the genome can be examined in interphase nuclei. Centromere-specific probes give a crude indication of the copy number of individual chromosomes while other sequences can be assessed both for copy number and for evidence of local amplification or deletion.[35-37] There are many novel developments of **FISH** (fluorescence in situ hybridisa-

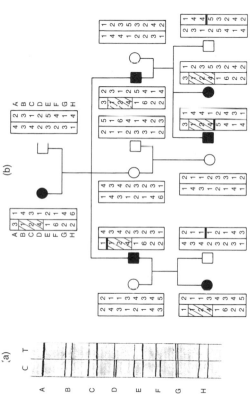

Fig. 1 Subchromosomal localisation of a cancer gene. (a) By allele imbalance. The diagram represents a comparison of alleles (revealed by Southern blotting) in constitutional and tumour-derived DNA (lanes C and T) at a series of polymorphic loci (A – H) which have been mapped, in the order given, to the same chromosome arm. Note that there is a much weaker signal from one allele in DNA from the tumour for loci C, D, E and F ('allele imbalance'). Locus A is uninformative because this particular patient is constitutionally homozygous for that marker, and so a weaker signal from one allele cannot easily be detected. When comparable data sets from several patients are combined, a small region where allele imbalance is present in any tumour (eg extending only from locus C to D) may be identified. This region contains the putative tumour suppressor gene. (b) By genetic linkage. In the illustrative cancer family tree, filled symbols are affected individuals. All of the family members have been typed for each of the polymorphic marker loci A – H and haplotypes (the groups of alleles carried on each of the homologous chromosomes) have been deduced. Inheritance of the cancer trait appears to be linked to this region defined by loci B,C,D (haplotype 1,2,4). Meiotic cross-overs (points marked by heavy horizontal lines) eliminate loci proximal to B or distal to D. This evidence therefore places the cancer gene within the hatched portion of the genetic map.

tion) technology which promise to be of great value in cancer research. One of these is chromosome 'painting' whereby a collection of probes is prepared that will hybridise to the entire length of a given chromosome but not to any part of other chromosomes (*see*, for example, P. Rabbitts this issue). When applied to metaphase spreads, this procedure will identify the components of any 'marker' chromosome of uncertain provenance and can highlight unsuspected rearrangements such as complex translocations that may involve small chromosome fragments. This is particularly useful for interpreting cytogenetic abnormalities in tumour cells where the quality of the metaphase preparations is often suboptimal for conventional banding pattern analysis. Painting also has a place in interphase cytogenetics. It can demonstrate monosomy, trisomy and, particularly where two or more different chromosomes are painted with distinct fluorochromes, it can be used to confirm the presence of translocations.[38]

A second important development is Comparative Genomic Hybridisation (CGH), the principle of which is very simple. Representative genomic DNA is prepared separately from tumor and normal tissue of the same patient. The DNAs are labelled, one with a green, the other with a red fluorochrome. In single-stranded form they are then mixed and hybridised to normal human metaphase preparations. The chromosomes are scanned with a sensitive CCD camera and the red/green fluorescence intensity ratio measured along the length of each one. Where there has been either a deletion or a localised amplification of DNA in the tumour, the red/green ratio will deviate from the norm. Thus CGH potentially provides the same sort of information as an allele imbalance study but it covers the entire genome in one sweep. At present the method has limited sensitivity, detecting deletions only if they extend for 10Mb or more. However, refinements are in train and the potential of the technique is clearly enormous.[39,40]

Genetic linkage (Fig. 1b)

For those genes associated with hereditary predisposition to some form of cancer, genetic linkage analysis in affected families provides an additional route to localisation and identification. The underlying concept depends on the process of crossing over between homologous chromosomes at meiosis which means that sequences, even on the same chromosome arm, will not be transmitted together over several generations unless they are physically very close together. Meiotic reassortment only becomes apparent, of course, if homologous sequences on the two parental chromosomes can be distinguished from each other, ie if they are polymorphic. Where one of the sequences in question is an unknown gene whose presence is denoted by the phenotype (in this instance, a hereditary cancer syndrome) the purpose of linkage analysis is to identify its close physical neighbours in the genome.[41] This involves testing a range of polymorphic markers until one is found that shows co-inheritance of the same allele with the disease in all (or almost all) affected members of any given cancer family. If the finding is confirmed in further families (though the association may be with a different allele, at the same locus, in each family) linkage between the cancer trait and the polymorphic marker is established. Linkage mapping then proceeds by testing other markers from the same chromosome arm and measuring the frequency of meiotic crossing over between each of them and the cancer trait. In this way a very accurate picture of the relative positions of a number of DNA sequences (including the putative cancer gene) can be built up as a prelude to physical mapping and gene isolation, as discussed below. The availability of growing numbers of accurately mapped polymorphic DNA probes has greatly increased the power of linkage mapping.

Positional cloning

With exceptions that are becoming increasingly rare, gene isolation proceeds from sub-chromosomal localisation (achieved by one or more of the above routes) to detailed molecular dissection of the region of interest until one or more 'gene-like' sequences are identified. These then become 'candidates' for the gene causing the disorder in question and are examined, both for any mutations that segregate with the disease in affected families and for a putative function that might plausibly account for the observed phenotype.

The entire human genome has already been subdivided into fragments varying in size from a few kilobases to more than a megabase. These are accessible in the form of 'genomic libraries'. For the purposes of constructing a physical map of a region believed to harbour a cancer gene, a start may be made by probing one of the large-fragment collections, such as a yeast artificial chromosome (YAC) or bacterial artificial chromosome (BAC) library, with some of the marker sequences believed to lie close to the gene of interest. YACs or BACs can also be tested with PCR primers for smaller markers such as microsatellites. When a group of large fragments has been assembled, each bearing one or more of the molecular tags that identifies the vicinity of the cancer gene, a series of cross-hybridisation experiments is undertaken to detect overlaps, to establish the relative positions of the various markers and ultimately to construct a contiguous series of cloned DNA segments that extends perhaps for tens of megabases.[42] The detail on such a 'contig' map is filled in by searching it for further polymorphic sequences that can be applied, in linkage and allele imbalance studies, to familial and sporadic tumours, thus localising the cancer gene even more precisely. When its position has been determined to within about a megabase, spanned by no more than 2 or 3 YACs, cloning the gene itself becomes a realistic goal (Fig. 2).

Occasionally a strong candidate gene mapping to the right region is already known. Thus p53, the retinoic acid alpha receptor and the *ret* oncogene had been mapped (to 17p, 17q and 10q) before their specific involvement in multiple cancers, acute promyelocytic leukaemia and multiple endocrine neoplasia type 2 respectively was suspected. More typically, however, the task resolves itself into finding and cataloguing a series of previously unknown genes, one of which can be incriminated. Since genes consist of DNA chemically indistinguishable from the non-coding 95% of the genome, it is not a trivial excercise. Three approaches are commonly applied. The first depends on the fact that many genes are flanked on the 5' side by a cluster of unmethylated CpG dinucleotides. These can be recognised and cleaved by the 'rare-cutting' restriction endonuclease *Not 1*, generating a large downstream segment likely to include at least part of the adjacent gene. The second exploits the fact that genes are more highly conserved in evolution than non-coding DNA and may therefore hybridise to DNA from other species in a so-called 'zoo' or 'Noah's ark', blot. The third involves a direct search for transcribable sequences, for example by screening messenger RNA (usually in the form of a cDNA library) from an appropriate tissue, with the labelled YAC clones.

These broad approaches, and variations on them, are undergoing constant refinement.[43] For example, automated direct sequencing of large tracts of DNA is now possible and advances in computer analysis of such data hold the promise of being able to identify open reading frames (ie transcribable sequences) without human intervention. There remains, of course, the problem of knowing (or guessing) which tissue is likely to be the best source of RNA (or cDNA) since, until the gene has been characterised, there is no certainty that it will be expressed at an appreciable level in any particular cell type.

Mutation analysis

Once a gene has been detected in the region of interest, its full extent and the intron/exon structure still have to be defined. The detailed mapping can be very time-consuming but a search for mutations may begin before the complete sequence of the gene has been determined. Both tumour tissue from sporadic cancers and constitutional tissue from affected members of cancer families provide DNA (or mRNA, from which the complementary DNA can be derived) for mutation analysis. The ultimate test is a direct comparison of the nucleotide sequence from

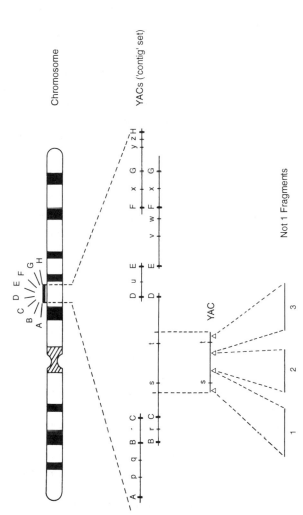

Fig. 2 Steps in positional cloning. When the gene has been mapped to a subchromosomal region bearing a number of marker DNA sequences (A – H), a YAC library is screened with these probes and an overlapping 'contig' set is assembled as shown. Each YAC in the set is then scanned for additional polymorphic markers, such as microsatellites (p – z). Further allele imbalance and/or genetic linkage studies with the expanded marker set should lead to improved localisation of the gene. In this example, s and t have been found to flank the gene so a further search of the YAC library is undertaken to find the smallest YAC bearing both these markers. This is then digested with *Not 1* and the individual fragments scanned for candidate genes.

a normal and a potentially mutant source but in most instances one of several less onerous screening procedures (Table 4) is tried first, followed by confirmatory sequencing of any portion of the gene that generates an abnormal result. It is, of course, necessary to examine a large panel of DNAs from unselected individuals to establish the range and population frequencies of polymorphic variants of the 'standard' sequence, otherwise these may be mistaken for pathological mutations. When substantial numbers of mutants have been characterised and shown to be associated with either sporadic or familial tumours, or both, a pattern may emerge identifying particular regions of the gene as vulnerable to carcinogenic mutations. Codons 12 and 61 of the *ras* oncogene family and the conserved exons 5–8 of p53 are examples. Such a finding simplifies larger scale screening to determine the extent of that gene's involvement in cancer.

The complete sequence of the gene may be derived from genomic or complementary DNA and is required to work out the corresponding amino acid sequence of the protein product. A search of the very extensive databases now available may suggest homology with other proteins belonging to one of the functional classes that includes many known cancer genes (*see below*).

EXPRESSION OF CANCER GENES IN TUMOUR TISSUE

Gene activity can be measured at the level of transcription (mRNA) or of translation (protein). The former approach has the advantage that once the nucleotide sequence is known, any gene can be assayed by the same techniques. These include Northern blotting, which measures RNA extracted from tissues, and in situ hybridisation which, as the term implies, identifies the transcript within the cells where it is produced. Specific proteins are generally recognised by immunological procedures, dependent on the availability of appropriate polyclonal or monoclonal antibodies. Like RNA, proteins can be detected in extracts (by Western blotting) or *in situ*.

Although the route from gene to product (DNA → RNA → Protein) is fixed, there is not always a simple quantitative relationship between the 3 molecular species. Messenger RNA is often short-lived and hence may be difficult to detect even though it is being produced continuously. The rate of translation (protein production) from a given amount of mRNA can vary enormously as can its half-life; many proteins persist long after the RNA transcription has ended and residual mRNA has been degraded.

Where a good antibody is available – and this is now the case for a growing number of oncogenes and tumour suppressors – identification of protein is likely to be the easier procedure. However, it must be

Table 4 Screening procedures to detect mutations in defined DNA sequence (data mainly from Ref 44)

Procedure	Principle
Single strand conformational polymorphism (SSCP) Heteroduplex gel mobility assay (HET)	Conformation determines mobility in electrophoretic gel
Denaturing gradient gel electrophoresis (DGGE) Constant denaturing gel electrophoresis (CDGE)	Minor mismatch between strands affects melting point of the duplex under denaturing conditions and hence mobility in gel
Chemical cleavage of mismatch (CCM, HOT) Bacterial mismatch-specific DNAse cleavage RNAse 'protection'	Cleavage of DNA or RNA at the point of mismatch with a complementary strand. Cleavage products are identified by gel electrophoresis and the point of mismatch predicted from their size
Allele-specific oligonucleotide (ASO) hybridisation	At high stringency, hybridisation (eg slot blot) between a mutable template sequenc and a panel of oligonucleotides complementary to known variants is spec for a single probe
Allele-specific amplification (ASA) or amplification resistance (ARMS)	PCR primers are designed with the 3′ base varying according to known point mutations in the template. Amplification will occur only where primer and template match at that position
Ligase assay	Contiguous oligonucleotides will ligate on a template strand only if there is complementarity at the 3′ end of the 5′ primer. As with ASA or ARMS, this method detects base-substitution at a predicted position

remembered that a large protein molecule comprises several antigens capable of reacting with a number of different antibodies, that changes in the conformation of a protein (as a result of mutations in the gene, for example) can affect antigenicity and that there may be antigenic cross reactivity with other proteins. Nevertheless the procedure can be exquisitely sensitive, thanks to the amplification provided by multi-layer techniques leading ultimately to a fluorescent or coloured signal that can often be localised to subcellular compartments.

Radiolabelled nucleotides remain the most sensitive probes for RNA so that the final step in detection is autoradiography. This limits the accuracy of localisation of the signal though distinction between positives and negatives is usually possible at the single cell level. Colourimetric and luminometric detection systems are under development and their performance is constantly improving. There can be definite advantages in being able to measure both mRNA and protein. For example, in studying p53 expression, several antibodies will distinguish between wild type and mutant gene product. Many mutant forms of the protein have a prolonged half-life and are therefore detected by antibodies even when transcription is not enhanced.

One great advantage of *in situ* procedures, for either mRNA or protein, in cancer genetics is that the expression of specific genes may be demonstrated in particular regions of a tumour. Thus, in breast cancer, stromelysin 3 (which appears to be associated with metastasis) is transcribed in stromal cells but not in the adjacent tumour epithelium.[45] The presumption that patterns of cancer gene expression will vary between tumour and normal cells and even between different components of the same tumour (non-invasive, invasive and metastatic regions, for example) has been exploited in a range of differential hybridisation protocols designed to isolate any message whose abundance varies greatly between two otherwise similar cell types. Stromelysin 3 was identified through such an approach as were *nm23* and *Krev2* which both show reduced expression in metastatic lesions.

MOLECULAR FUNCTIONS OF CANCER GENES

Cellular growth control involves a complex signal generation/receipt/transduction/response pathway (Fig. 3) which can be subverted at almost any point. Many of the elements of the pathway are known to be proto-oncogenes or tumour suppressors though our understanding of how mutations alter cell behaviour is still very superficial. In particular, our limited grasp of the scale and subtleties of interactions between cancer genes was admitted at the outset. Nevertheless some comment on the early forays into this crucial territory is necessary to avoid distortion through oversimplification. Among the specific examples of oncogene interaction that have been studied experimentally are the formation of dimeric transcription factors fos/jun and myc/max, the regulation of ras GTPase activity by gap and by Krev 2, the role of TGF beta as an inhibitor of Rb phosphorylation (and hence of *myc* induction) and, most recently, the finding that the tumour suppressor protein NM 23-H2 is a transcription factor for *c-myc*.[50] Interactions involving p53 have proved of particular interest and are discussed in the chapter by Lane (this issue). However, it is clear that these examples provide only glimpses of a molecular and physiological network, exploration of which will be the major goal of fundamental cancer research for the 21st century. As Figure 3 seeks to convey, the very use of the term 'cancer gene' can be misleading because once cellular homeostasis has been disturbed, by whatever mechanism, normal growth factors and receptors, normal cell adhesion molecules, normal protein kinases and normal transcription factors may be turned against the cell and contribute to carcinogenesis. A common consequence of oncogene activation is upregulation of growth factor production and of growth factor receptors, generating potential autocrine loops. Similarly, release of metalloproteinases and of angiogenesis factors is often increased.[23,47] Since these effects do not seem to be specific to any one oncogene nor even to a particular functional class, they are presumably secondary or tertiary consequences of the initial mutation. There is some question as to whether phenotypic characteristics of malignant change – and hence underlying molecular events – show some specificity for the cell types involved. Thus changes in cell adhesion molecules and in cytoskeletal organisation are more apparent in epithelial cells than in fibroblasts or other mesenchymal elements[51] while, at least until recently, soluble growth factors and cytokines seemed to play a more prominent role in the regulation of haemopoietic cells than of other tissues.[47] It is very likely that such apparent differences reflect the particular opportunities for experimental approaches to carcinogenesis offered by different cellular models rather than fundamental distinctions in the molecular routes to malignancy and that, as knowledge grows, all of the elements illustrated in Figure 3 will be seen to play a part in each case. The idea that oncogenic events tend to converge on one – or at most a few – common pathways is gaining ground and MAP (mitogen-activated protein) kinase could represent a nodal point.[49] It is consistent with this general concept that, as a cancer advances, mutations in oncogenes and tumour suppressors tend to accumulate but not usually in any predictable sequence.

The evidence that a cancer gene belongs to a given functional class (growth factor, receptor, protein kinase, G protein, transcription factor etc) can come from analysis of the amino-acid sequence, from subcellular localisation, from demonstration of its enzyme activity or its ability to bind to a hormone, growth factor, or cell-surface receptor or from the observation that it binds to DNA, recognising a particular nucleotide sequence.

Protein/DNA interactions

The DNA-binding cancer genes, comprise transcription factors and proteins that influence DNA stability. The fact of DNA/protein interaction can be shown in 'gel shift' assays whereby the mobility of cloned DNA fragments in an electrophoretic gel is compared before and after incubation with the protein under examination. A complex of DNA and protein moves more slowly in the electrophoretic field than DNA alone, so

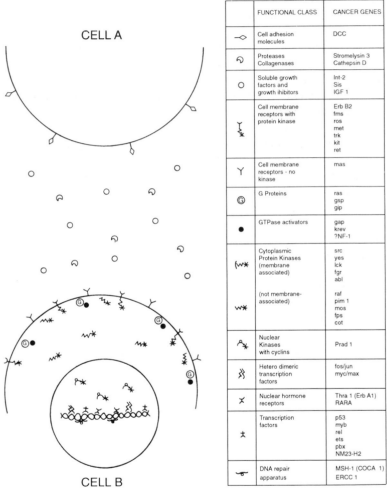

	FUNCTIONAL CLASS	CANCER GENES
—◦	Cell adhesion molecules	DCC
ᕫ	Proteases Collagenases	Stromelysin 3 Cathepsin D
O	Soluble growth factors and growth ihibitors	Int-2 Sis IGF 1
Y*	Cell membrane receptors with protein kinase	Erb B2 fms ros met trk kit ret
Y	Cell membrane receptors - no kinase	mas
Ⓖ	G Proteins	ras gsp gip
●	GTPase activators	gap krev ?NF-1
⋀⋇	Cytoplasmic Protein Kinases (membrane associated)	src yes lck fgr abl
⋀⋇	(not membrane-associated)	raf pim 1 mos fps cot
⌒⋇	Nuclear Kinases with cyclins	Prad 1
⟩⟩	Hetero dimeric transcription factors	fos/jun myc/max
⤬	Nuclear hormone receptors	Thra 1 (Erb A1) RARA
⟂	Transcription factors	p53 myb rel ets pbx NM23-H2
↝	DNA repair apparatus	MSH-1 (COCA 1) ERCC 1

Fig. 3 Some molecules and pathways involved in control of cell growth and differentiation: functional classes of some cancer genes (data mainly from Refs 6, 23 and 46–50).

scanning the pattern for a band that has shifted identifies the clone with specific affinity for that protein. In many instances regulatory proteins bind to DNA not only at specific sites relative to structural genes but also to particular sequence motifs which are often palindromic. The nature of the binding site can help to confirm the postulated function of a given protein and it can be determined by nuclease digestion of a DNA/protein mixture. Portions of the DNA strand to which protein is tightly bound are protected against digestion and when compared to protein-free DNA in a Maxam–Gilbert sequencing run, a gap in the sequence is created by the 'footprint' of the bound protein.[52] The influence of a bound protein on transcription of an adjacent gene can be assessed directly by inserting into a suitable expression vector an artificial construct of promoter region (including the protein binding site) coupled to a 'reporter' structural gene such as chloramphenicol acetyl transferase or luciferase. After transfection of a host cell, expression of the indicator product is measured in the presence or absence of the protein. A greater degree of sophistication can be built into the system, for example by testing mutant forms of the protein, by deleting various portions of the promoter complex or by introducing additional proteins to form an interactive regulatory system.[52–55]

Apart from transcription factors, proteins bind to specific DNA sequences for other purposes. The maintenance of DNA stability is clearly of the highest importance to the integrity of the organism and the association between heritable disorders of genome stability and cancer is well recognised (*see* Taylor, this issue). Two genes associated with Lynch type 2 cancer family syndrome (comprising hereditary clustering of colorectal, uterine and other cancers) have been discovered recently, partly through their homology with yeast replication mismatch suppressors. These encode DNA-binding proteins which identify and correct the slippage that can occur during DNA replication, particularly in tandem oligonucleotide repeats. A hallmark of inactivation at either locus (on chromosomes 2p and 3p) is the appearance of 'new' microsatellite alleles in tumour DNA.[56,57] DNA excision repair genes have also been cloned from man and other mammalian species and are being studied in transgenic mice. They too encode DNA-binding proteins[58] and it is likely that several more oncogenes or tumour suppressors, belonging to the general class of DNA stability genes will be identified in the coming years.

FUTURE DIRECTIONS

The long-term objective, a comprehensive understanding of the molecular basis of cancer, will ultimately be achieved through the dogged application of techniques such as those outlined above, as well as many that have yet to be developed. In the medium term, however, there are practical consequences of our partial knowledge. It is certain that molecular analysis will be applied increasingly to the diagnosis and classification of solid tumours by extension of the methods now widely used for leukaemias and lymphomas. They may help, for example to identify the subsets of apparently early breast or ovarian cancer that have a bad prognosis, so that these patients can be treated more aggressively from the outset. However, for the reasons discussed, it may be unrealistic to expect any single molecular screening test (such as level of *Erb B2* expression or presence of a p53 mutation) to serve this purpose. A more complete assessment of the overall oncogene and tumour suppressor gene status of the tumour is likely to be required. Hence there could be dangers in the development of simple 'kits' to detect mutant, overexpressed or inactivated genes. Applied in isolation, or out of context, these may confuse rather than clarify.

Inevitably, when cancer genes are discussed, the question of gene therapy arises. Where this means therapy designed to correct a specific cancer-inducing mutation, it seems impracticable; not because the lesions are almost always multiple (experimentally, correction of one molecular defect among many can reverse a transformed phenotype) but because no mechanism yet devised comes anywhere near the 100% level of transfection efficiency that would be required for a lasting anti-tumour effect. Anti-sense oligonucleotides and anti-oncogene monoclonal antibodies have proved to be dramatically illuminating tools for studies of cancer gene function in model systems[23,59] and may ultimately have a place in therapy but problems of cost and effective delivery to the target suggest that their first role may be in 'purging' autologous bone marrow or peripheral blood stem cells in the context of intensive chemotherapy and 'rescue' programmes. In a wider sense, however, gene therapy is the whole object of the excercise. Given that molecular events within the cell have biochemical consequences it must be possible to counteract or correct them at the biochemical (ie pharmacological) level. Current cancer chemotherapy aims to do just that but is guided largely by the traditional process of trial and error. A genuine understanding of the molecular basis of cancer will open up the possibility of designing drugs to reach very precise biochemical targets, simultaneously increasing effectiveness and reducing toxicity. For many forms of cancer, existing treatments already achieve a great deal so that even a modest gain in therapeutic index could lead to cure.

REFERENCES

1 Varmus H. Retroviruses. Science 1988; 235: 1427–1435.
2 Slamon DJ, de Kernion JB, Verma IM, Cline MJ. Expression of cellular oncogenes in human malignancies. Science 1984; 240: 256–262.
3 Bishop JM. Trends in oncogenes. Trends Genet 1985; 1: 245-259.
4 Bishop JM. The molecular genetics of cancer: 1988. Leukaemia 1988; 2: 199–208.
5 Weinberg RA. Oncogenes, anti-oncogenes and the molecular basis of multi-step carcinogenesis. Cancer Res 1989; 49: 3713–3721.
6 Bishop JM. Molecular themes in oncogenesis. Cell 1991; 64: 235–248.
7 Harris H. The analysis of malignancy by cell fusion: the position in 1988. Cancer Res 1988; 48: 3302–3306.
8 Stanbridge EJ. A brief review of the evidence of the genetic regulation of tumorigenic expression in somatic cell hybrids. IARC Sci Publ (Lyon) 1988; 92: 23–31.
9 Huxley C, Griske A. Transfer of yeast artificial chromosomes from yeast to mammalian cells. Bio Essays 1991; 13: 545–549.
10 Stanbridge EJ. Functional evidence for human tumour suppressor genes: chromosome and molecular genetic studies. Cancer Surveys 1992; 12: 5–24.
11 Koi M, Johnson LA, Little PFR et al. Tumor cell growth arrest caused by subchromosomal transferable DNA fragments from chromosome 11. Science 1993; 260: 361–364.
12 Leone A, Flatow U, Van Houtte K, Steeg PS. Transfection of human nm23-H1 into the human MDA-MB-435 breast carcinoma cell line: effects on tumor metastatic potential, colonisation and enzymatic activity. Oncogene 1993; 8: 2325–2333.
13 Casey G, Plummer S, Hoeltge H et al. Functional evidence for a breast cancer growth suppressor gene on chromosome 17. Hum Mol Genet 1993; 2: 1921–1927.
14 Mulligan LM, Kwok JBJ, Healey CS et al. Germ-line mutations of the RET proto-oncogene in multiple endocrine neoplasia type 2A. Nature 1993; 363: 458–460.
15 Wyllie AH. Apoptosis: the 1992 Frank Rose Memorial lecture. Br J Cancer 1993; 67: 205–208.
16 Martin SJ, Green DR, Cotter TG. Dicing with death: dissecting the components of the apoptosis machinery. Trends Biochem Sci 1994; 18: 26–30.
17 Woods DF, Bryant PJ. Genetic control of cell interactions in developing drosophila epithelia. Annu Rev Genet 1992; 26: 305–350.
18 Hanahan S. Transgenic mice as probes into complex systems. Science 1989; 246: 1265–1275.
19 Lavigueur A, Maltby V, Mock D et al. High incidence of lung, bone and lymphoid tumours in transgenic mice overexpressing mutant alleles of the p53 oncogene. Mol Cell Biol 1989; 9: 3982–3991.
20 Harvey M, McArthur MJ, Montgomery CA et al. Spontaneous and carcinogen – induced tumorigenesis in p53 – deficient mice. Nature Genet 1993; 5: 225–229.
21 Adams JM, Cory S. Oncogene co-operation in leukaemogenesis. Cancer Surv 1992; 15: 119–141.
22 Groner B, Schonenberger C-A, Andres AC. Targeted expression of the *ras* and *myc* oncogenes in transgenic mice. Trends Genet 1987; 3: 306–308.
23 Hunter T. Co-operation between oncogenes. Cell 1991; 64: 249–270.
24 Moser AR, Pitot HC, Dove WF. A dominant mutation that predisposes to multiple intestinal neoplasia in the mouse. Science 1990; 247: 322–324.
25 Dietrich WF, Lander ES, Smith JS et al. Genetic identification of *Mom-1*, a major modifier locus affecting *Min* – induced intestinal neoplasia in the mouse. Cell 1993; 75: 631–639.
26 Rowley JD. The clinical applications of new DNA diagnostic technology on the management of cancer patients. JAMA 1993; 270: 2331–2337.
27 Heim S, Mitelman F. Primary chromosome abnormalities in human neoplasia. Adv Cancer Res 1989; 52: 1–43.
28 Editorial. Molecular mechanisms in familial and sporadic cancers. Lancet 1988; i: 92–93.

29 Schwab M, Amler LC. Amplification of cellular oncogenes: a predictor of clinical outcome in human cancers. Genes Chromo Cancer 1990; 1: 181–194.
30 Weber JL. Human DNA polymorphisms based on length variations in simple-sequence tandem repeats. Genome Anal 1990; 1: 159–181.
31 Devilee P, van Vliet M, van Sloun P et al Allelotype of human breast carcinoma: a second major site for loss of heterozygosity is on chromosome 6q. Oncogene 1991; 6: 1705–1711.
32 Cavenee WK, Dryja TP, Philips RA et al Expression of recessive alleles by chromosomal mechanisms in retinoblastoma. Nature 1983; 305: 779–784.
33 Frye RA, Benz CC, Liu E. Detection of amplified oncogenes by differential polymerase chain reaction. Oncogene 1989; 4: 1153–1157.
34 Beishuizen A, Hahlen K, van Wering ER, van Dongen JJM. Detection of minimal residual disease in childhood leukaemia with the polymerase chain reaction. N Engl J Med 1991; 324: 772–773.
35 Matsumura K, Kallioniemi A, Kallioniemi O et al. Deletion of chromosome 17p loci in breast cancer cells detected by fluorescence in situ hybridisation. Cancer Res 1992; 52: 3474–3477.
36 Heppel-Parton AC, Albertson DG, Fishpool R, Rabbitts PH. Multicolour fluorescence in situ hybridisation to order small, single copy probes on metaphase chromosomes. Cytogenet Cell Genet 1994; 66: 42–47.
37 Shibasaki Y. High resolution mapping of the MYCN proto-oncogene at human chromosome 2p24.3 by fluorescence in situ hybridisation. Cytogenet Cell Genet 1994; 66: 75–76.
38 Trask BJ. Fluorescence in situ hybridisation: applications in cytogenetics and gene mapping. Trends Genet 1991; 7: 149–154.
39 Kallioniemi A, Kallioniemi O-P, Sudar D et al. Comparative genomic hybridisation for molecular cytogenetic analysis of solid tumours. Science 1992; 258: 818–821.
40 Kallioniemi A, Kallioniemi O-P, Piper J et al. Chromosomal mapping of amplified DNA sequences in breast cancer by comparative genomic hybridisation. Proc Natl Acad Sci USA 1994; 91: 2156–2160.
41 Yates JRW, Connor JM. Genetic Linkage. Br J Hosp Med 1986: 133–136.
42 Evans GA. Combinatoric strategies for genome mapping. BioEssays 1991; 13: 39–44.
43 Hochgeschwender U, Brennan MB. Identifying genes within the genome: new ways for finding a needle in a haystack. BioEssays 1991; 13: 139–144.
44 Dianzani I, Camaschella C, Ponzone A, Cotton RGH. Dilemmas and progress in mutation detection. Trends Genet 1993; 9: 403–405.
45 Basset P, Bellocq JP, Wolf C et al. A novel metalloproteinase gene specifically expressed in stromal cells of breast carcinomas. Nature 1990; 748: 699–704.
46 Nigg EA. Mechanisms of signal transduction to the cell nucleus. Adv Cancer Res 1990; 55: 271–309.
47 Cross M, Dexter TM. Growth factors in development, transformation and tumorigenesis. Cell 1991; 64: 271–280.
48 Pawson T. Signal transduction in the control of cell growth and development. Trends Genet 1991; 7: 343–346.
49 Leevers SJ, Marshall CJ. MAP kinase regulation – the oncogene connection. Trends Cell Biol 1992; 2: 283–286.
50 Postel EH, Berberich SJ, Flint SJ, Ferrone CA. Human c-myc transcription factor PuF identified as nm23-H2 nucleoside diphosphate kinase, a candidate suppressor of tumour metastasis. Science 1993; 261: 478–480.
51 Schoenenberger C-A, Matlin KS. Cell polarity and epithelial oncogenesis. Trends Cell Biol 1991; 1: 87–92.
52 Latchman DS. Eukaryotic Transcription Factors. London: Academic Press, 1991.
53 Stabel S, Jones N. Regulation of transcription. In: PJ Parker, M Katan eds. 'Molecular Biology of Oncogenes and Cell Control Mechanisms. Chichester: Ellis Horwood, 1990 pp 121–144.
54 Fields S, Jang SK. Presence of a potent transcription activating sequence in the p53 protein. Science 1990; 249: 1046–1049.

55 Raycroft L, Wu H, Lozano G. Transcriptional activation by wild-type but not transforming mutants of the p53 anti-oncogene. Science 1990; 249: 1049–1051.
56 Aaltonen L A, Peltomaki P, Leach FS et al. Clues to the pathogenesis of familial colorectal cancer. Science 1993; 260: 812–816.
57 Lindblom A, Tannergard P, Werelius B, Nordenskjold M. Genetic mapping of a second locus predisposing to hereditary non-poyposis colon cancer. Nature Genet 1993; 5: 279–282.
58 McWhir J, Selfridge J, Harrison DJ, Squires S, Melton DW. Mice with DNA repair gene (ERCC-1) deficiency have elevated levels of p53, liver nuclear abnormalities and die before weaning. Nature Genetics 1993; 5: 217–224.
59 O'Brien SG, Kirkland MA. Antisense oligodeoxynucleotides in malignant disease. Cancer Top 1993; 9: 86–87.

British Medical Bulletin (1994) Vol. 50, No. 3, pp. 560–581
© The British Council 1994

Viruses and human cancer

K H Vousden
P J Farrell
Ludwig Institute for Cancer Research, St Mary's Hospital Medical School, London, UK

Epstein-Barr virus (EBV), hepatitis B virus (HBV), HTLV-I and some human papillomaviruses (HPVs) appear to contribute to the development of a large proportion of certain human cancers. Although the epidemiological evidence linking infection with these viruses to malignancies is generally convincing, only for the HPVs have experimental systems indicated a clear role for some of the HPV encoded genes in tumour cell growth. In these cases, molecular analysis is revealing the mechanisms by which the virally encoded oncogenes function to perturb the normal regulation of cell growth. For HTLV-I, EBV and HBV the mechanism by which the viruses contribute to tumour cell growth is obscure, even though much has been learned about cell transformation in culture by these viruses. A detailed understanding of the mechanism of oncogenesis will be required to design therapeutic drugs for the treatment of these cancers. Prophylactic vaccination resulting in prevention of infection may be an effective approach to reduce the incidence of some of these common cancers.

Viral infection is thought to contribute to the development of a few types of human cancer. Some of these cancers are very common, and this leads to the conclusion that up to 20% of all cancer worldwide may have a viral aetiology. One obvious explanation for the unusual geographic distribution of some cancers is that an infectious agent endemic only in those areas is contributing to the disease. Consistent with this, there is a close relationship between infection with hepatitis B virus and a high incidence of primary hepatocellular carcinoma. A similar close relationship exists between adult T cell leukaemia and human T cell leukaemia virus type I infection. Cervical carcinoma is linked worldwide to human papillomavirus. The two cancers linked to Epstein-Barr virus also have regions of exceptionally high incidence,

Burkitt's lymphoma in central Africa and nasopharyngeal carcinoma (NPC) in southern China, but these geographic constraints must be due to other factors since Epstein-Barr virus (EBV) infection is very common worldwide.

There are 2 general strategies by which these viruses are thought to contribute to carcinogenesis. In some cases expression of certain viral genes bypasses the need for one or more of the steps that would normally be involved in multistep carcinogenesis. The other general mechanism seems to involve the virus stabilising or promoting the growth of a cell population in which oncogenic genetic change may then occur. For each of the 4 human tumour viruses the basic virology will be described and then the likely role of the virus in development of its associated cancer will be considered.

EPSTEIN-BARR VIRUS

EBV infection is extremely common in humans. About 90% of the world's population are thought to be infected and carry this member of the herpes virus family for life. The virus infects B lymphocytes and certain epithelial cells. The receptor for infection of lymphocytes is CD21 but the mechanism of infection of epithelial cells is uncertain. The usual consequence of infection of human B lymphocytes in culture is immortalisation of the lymphocyte resulting in a lymphoblastoid cell line (LCL), with EBV remaining latent (non-productive) in the lymphocyte (reviewed in[1,2]). In this situation, 11 of the approximately 85 viral genes are expressed and these are thought to initiate and maintain the immortalised state. Construction of EBV mutants has permitted testing which of these genes are essential for immortalisation and this has focussed attention on the viral nuclear proteins EBNA-1, 2, 3A, 3C, LP and the viral membrane protein LMP1. All of these 6 proteins are essential for EBV immortalisation of lymphocytes[3-7] and their continued expression is a standard feature of LCLs. The other viral genes expressed in LCLs are the EBER small RNAs, the nuclear protein EBNA-3B and the membrane proteins TP1, 2 (LMP 2A, B) but these are not essential for immortalisation. The organisation of the immortalising genes of EBV is shown in Figure 1. The splicing and gene structures have been simplified for clarity in Figure 1 but the full details can be found in reference 8.

The clearest causal role for EBV in human disease is in infectious mononucleosis, the symptoms of which represent the course of the immune response to an EBV primary infection which has been delayed into adolescence or adulthood.[9] The EBV infects B lymphocytes but the mononucleosis is mainly of T lymphocytes which are responding to the EBV infected cells. Most people are infected with EBV in the

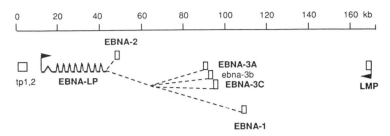

Fig. 1 EBV immortalising genes. The viral proteins expressed in B lymphocytes immortalised by EBV are shown, with those essential for immortalisation titled in upper case. The EBNA genes are transcribed from a single large alternatively spliced transcription unit, the splicing being shown by dotted lines. The splicing of several of the genes has been simplified for clarity in this large scale diagram; for the details see reference 8.

first few years of life and no significant disease is associated with the normal infection. Infectious mononucleosis is found only in Western countries where hygiene standards can result in the delayed infection. EBV is shed into the saliva and transmission is normally via kissing or shared eating utensils.

Functions of EBV immortalisation genes

The EBNA-1 protein is thought to be expressed in all latent infections of EBV. It is a sequence-specific DNA binding protein (consensus binding site GGPuTAGCATATGCTAPyCC) and plays a key role in the maintenance replication of the EBV episome.[10] The origin of replication, ori P, is composed of two sets of repeats of the EBNA-1 binding site and the high affinity binding of EBNA-1 and consequent EBNA-1 mediated looping of the DNA between the two sets of repeats is essential to direct the cell replication machinery to replicate the EBV episome. No other EBV protein is required for this. EBNA-1 exists as a dimer in solution and binds DNA in this form, but when bound to DNA a conformation change permits further aggregation of the EBNA-1 dimers. Binding of EBNA-1 to the multiple sites at ori P also reveals a transcription enhancer function of ori P that activates the nearby Cp promoter[11] and possibly some other EBV promoters. The C terminal part of EBNA-1 mediates dimerisation and DNA binding.[12] Much of the N terminal half of the protein is composed of a long gly-ala repeat which appears to be dispensable for all of the protein functions identified so far.

EBNA-2 acts as a gene regulator, transactivating both EBV and cell gene expression.[10] In EBV infection of B lymphocytes, EBNA-2 and

EBNA-LP are the first EBV genes to be expressed, within 12 to 24 h
of infection, depending on the method used to isolate the lymphocytes.
At this time after infection, cyclin D2 is the first cell gene whose transcription is known to be activated[13] but subsequently EBNA-2 activates
cell genes such as CD23 and the EBV genes LMP1 and TP1 and 2.[10]
The functions of EBNA-3A and 3C are obscure at present, although
complementation of an EBNA-3C deletion in the Raji strain of EBV
with wild type EBNA-3C results in a modified expression of LMP1.[14]
The mechanism of action of EBNA-LP is also unknown but deletion
of part of the EBNA-LP gene seems to greatly reduce the efficiency of
immortalisation and to render the outgrowth of infected lymphocytes
dependent on a feeder cell layer.[6,15] EBNA-LP has been reported to
bind the tumour suppressor proteins Rb and p53 in vitro.[16] LMP1 is the
only gene of EBV which has been found to transform cells in culture.
It will convert Balb/3T3 cells[17] or Rat 1 cells[18] to a transformed phenotype and prevents the differentiation of keratinocytes in raft culture
systems,[19] possibly relevant to NPC.

EBV in human cancer

The cancers classically linked to EBV are Burkitt's lymphoma (BL)[2]
and nasopharyngeal carcinoma.[9,20] These are both very rare tumours
in Europe and the USA but have a much higher incidence in certain
geographic areas, BL in the malarial parts of Africa and New Guinea,
NPC in South East Asia. More recently some other cancers have been
linked with EBV. Thus EBV is found in immunoblastic B lymphoma in
immunosuppressed people (including AIDS patients)[9] certain rare T cell
lymphomas[21] and the Reed-Sternberg cells of many cases of Hodgkin's
lymphoma.[22] Apart from the immunoblastic lymphomas, which are often essentially like LCLs that have escaped immune surveillance, in no
case has a clear mechanism for EBV contributing to the development
of the cancer been established. The number of virus infected cells in
any normal individual is very small (less than 0.1% of circulating B
lymphocytes are infected) so the fact that 100% of the tumour cells
carry EBV in the EBV associated cancers is an impressive association,
although it does not necessarily indicate a causal role for the virus in the
tumour. In NPC all of the tumours are of the EBV positive type. In BL
the EBV positive tumours account for the excess of cases in the high
incidence (endemic) areas over the worldwide background (sporadic)
level of BL, where the tumour cells do not usually have EBV. The
endemic areas in Africa and New Guinea appear to be those regions
where malaria is hyperendemic.

The common feature of all the BL tumours is the translocation of
the c-*myc* proto-oncogene to one of the immunoglobulin loci, but the

way in which this translocation arises is different between endemic and sporadic BL.[23] In the sporadic BLs the breakpoint in the immunoglobulin gene is normally at the switch region, consistent with this type of translocation arising in the lymph node germinal centre where isotype switching occurs. In endemic BLs, however, the breakpoint on the immunoglobulin gene is usually at the J region or sometimes in the V or D regions, which would be consistent with the translocation occuring as a result of an error in VDJ joining, which normally occurs in the bone marrow. So it seems that in the endemic areas in people with chronic malaria, cells with this type of translocation escape immune surveillance and other constraints and can become BL cells. Clonality of the cells and the EBV in them indicates that the virus infects early in the process and may well be in the cell when malignant transformation occurs. Very little is known about EBV in the bone marrow except that it is present because it can be transmitted by the bone marrow in a transplant.[24]

It might be expected that a contribution of EBV to BL and NPC would be readily explained by some of the immortalisation genes of EBV combining with oncogenic cell mutations to cause the malignant conversion. In fact most of these genes are not expressed in the tumour cells and the BL cell phenotype (as revealed by B cell suface markers)[25] is quite different from the LCL cells in which EBV is clearly causing the cell growth. In BL only EBNA-1 and the EBER RNAs are expressed[25] and in NPC only EBNA-1, the EBER RNAs and in 50% of cases the LMP1 protein are detected.[26,27] This pattern of usually only EBNA-1 protein expression has been rationalised as being the minimum necessary to maintain the virus replication in the face of cytotoxic T cell mediated immune surveillance directed against epitopes derived from the other immortalisation genes. It is not, however, consistent with complementation of oncogenic cell changes by EBV unless EBNA-1 is the complementing gene. Since no cell gene or process has yet been found to be transregulated by EBNA-1 this possibility is difficult to evaluate. It is tempting to speculate that early in the development of the BL more of the immortalising genes might be expressed, perhaps LMP1 preventing apoptotic death[28] of the cells with aberrant c-*myc* expression[29] as a result of translocation. It is noteworthy, however, that the tumour cells from EBV positive BLs always retain the episomal EBV genome, suggesting that it is contributing to cell growth.

HUMAN PAPILLOMAVIRUSES

Human papillomaviruses (HPVs) comprise a large group of epitheliotropic viruses which infect a variety of cutaneous and mucosal epithelia. Infection with most HPV types gives rise to benign, self limiting hyperproliferations which usually regress spontaneously. Several HPV types, however, cause lesions with malignant potential and genital HPV infection is associated with the development of an extremely common cancer, carcinoma of the uterine cervix. In world-wide terms, this is the second most common female malignancy and represents the most common cancer in developing countries.[30] Not all genital HPV types show this malignant potential, and two groups of viruses can be identified, the 'high risk' HPV types (most commonly HPV16 and 18) which are found in almost all cervical cancers and the 'low risk' HPV types, like HPV6 and 11, which give rise to benign genital condyloma.[31] Understanding the differences between these two groups of viruses has been one of the challenges of this field of research.

Epidemiology of cervical cancer

Cervical cancer was identified as a sexually transmitted disease over a century ago and considerable effort has been made to identify an infectious agent with a causative role in the development of this malignancy. Herpes viruses were once under suspicion but for the past 20 years it has become increasingly evident that the high risk genital HPV types are involved in the genesis of most of these cancers.[32] Whilst over 90% of cervical cancers and high grade pre-malignancies show evidence of HPV infection, amongst women with normal cervical cytology detection of the virus is much lower, ranging from around 25% in young women first becoming sexually active to under 5% in groups of older women.[33] It is now apparent that infection with viruses like HPV16 gives rise to a cervical intraepithelial neoplasia, a lesion long recognised as having malignant potential,[34] although clearly not all infections with high risk HPV types result in the appearance of a cancer. The complicated interplay of genetic and epigenetic factors governing regression or progression of an HPV induced lesion are still poorly understood, but it seems likely that the immune and hormonal status of the infected women play very important roles in governing the outcome of infection. HPV infection therefore represents one of the multiple events necessary for the full malignant conversion of a normal cell.

The HPV genome

Unlike other viruses which play a role in the development of human cancers, the mechanisms by which HPV may contribute to the onco-genic process are rather well understood. Analysis of the activity of the virally encoded proteins in tissue culture systems rapidly revealed the presence of virally encoded oncogenes, the molecular activities of which are now being unravelled. All HPVs show a similar genome organisation, shown in Figure 2, encoding 8 major open reading frames from a circular double stranded DNA genome of around 7.9kb in length.[35] Like HBV, no efficient in vitro system is available to culture HPV virions and as a consequence little is known about the natural life cycle of the virus. Activities for most of the ORFs have been identified, however, and the viral genome is broadly divided into the late ORFs, L1 and L2, which encode the viral structural proteins, and the early region encompassing E1–E7. Of these, E4 encodes the most abundant viral protein found in cells in a productive infection and the ability of this protein to interfere with the normal cytoskeletal structures of the infected keratinocyte suggests that this is in fact another late protein, possibly allowing maturation or release of virus particles.[36] The E1 ORF encodes proteins important for viral replication, the E2 ORF encodes the major viral transcriptional control proteins.[37] Both E1 and E2 proteins bind specific DNA sequences within the non-coding or upstream regulatory region (URR), where the major promoters and origin of replication are located, and interactions between the E1 and E2 proteins have been shown to result in the participation of both proteins in transcription and replication control. The 3 other open reading frames, E5, E6 and E7, encode proteins with transforming properties and it is possible that they all play a role in malignant progression of the infected cell.

HPV oncoproteins

The E5 ORF encodes a small hydrophobic protein which is found predominantly in the cell membranes. The E5 protein exhibits a mitogenic activity which is related to its ability to inhibit down regulation and enhance the activity of cell surface receptors, such as the EGF receptor.[38] This activity certainly increases the sensitivity of the infected cell to endogenous growth factors and may contribute to the inappropriate cell division seen in HPV induced lesions. Interestingly, this mitogenic activity is displayed by the E5 proteins encoded by both high and low risk HPV types and the observation that the E5 region of the virus is frequently not expressed in cervical malignancies diminishes, although does not rule out, a role for E5 in the oncogenic process.

The major transforming proteins encoded by the high risk HPV types are E6 and E7.[39] Expression of E6 and E7 in primary human genital epithelial cells can lead to the production of an immortal cell line which show subtle abnormalities in differentiation to resemble very closely the in vivo lesion identified as cervical intraepithelial neoplasia.[40] The E6 and E7 proteins encoded by the low risk HPV types fail to show this activity in cells. Like HBV, the HPV genome often becomes integrated into host chromosomes during progression to malignancy, although dur-

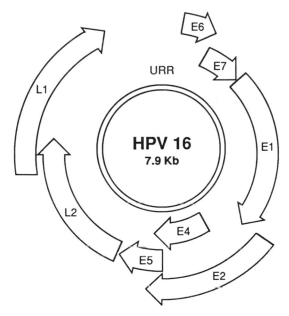

Fig. 2 Genetic structure of HPV16, showing the circular double stranded DNA genome of 7.9kb. The major open reading frames and the non-coding region are indicated. All papillomaviruses show the same basic genome organisation and express similar proteins from ORFs transcribed from only one DNA strand.

ing a normal productive viral infection the viral genome is maintained episomally in the nucleus of the infected cell. There is no apparent specificity for site of viral integration and much of the viral genome is often lost or fails to be expressed. Interestingly, the E6/E7 region is almost always conserved and expressed in cells containing integrated viral sequences, and studies indicating that inhibition of E6 and E7 expression reverts the transformed phenotype of HPV containing cervical carcinoma cell lines strongly support a role for these two viral proteins in both the development and maintenance of the malignancy.

Mechanisms of E6 and E7 function

The mechanisms by which E6 and E7 contribute to oncogenesis appear to be related to their ability to form complexes with, and inactivate the normal function of several cell proteins.[41] E7 has been shown to form a complex with a family of cell proteins related to the retinoblastoma gene product, Rb, and interaction with E7 can interfere with complexes which normally form between these proteins and cellular transcription factors.[42,43] The *Rb* gene itself was originally identified as a target for mutation in several types of human cancers and belongs to the diverse family of tumour suppressor genes.[44] These genes encode proteins whose normal function is to negatively regulate cell growth and whose loss is associated with malignant development. The significance of these interactions to HPV mediated oncogenesis is therefore clear; expression of E7 results in the loss of normal tumour suppressor protein function and provides one step in the oncogenic process. E6 also interacts with a tumour suppressor protein, p53, and has been shown to target the p53 protein for rapid degradation.[45] E6 expressing cells are therefore unable to express significant levels of p53 protein and this results in the loss of normal p53 functions within these cells. The ability of the high risk HPV types to interfere with normal p53 function is particularly significant for oncogenic activity since alterations of the p53 gene are the most common genetic event detected so far in almost all types of human cancers.[46] Expression of E6 and E7 in a cervical cell would therefore be predicted to have the same net effect as somatic Rb and p53 mutations, a hypothesis strongly supported by the unusual lack of p53 mutations in HPV associated cervical cancers.[47]

HEPATITIS B VIRUS

The prevalence of infection with human hepatitis viruses, members of the hepadna virus family, shows strong geographical variation, with an unusually high incidence in tropical Africa and South East Asia. The epidemiological evidence linking chronic infection caused by hepatitis B (HBV) with the development of hepatocellular carcinoma is quite clear[48,49] and chronic HBV infection is a major risk factor for development of this cancer.[50] High incidence of liver cancer is detected in those regions with a high prevalence of viral infection; in East Asian countries hepatocellular carcinomas occur at rates of around 20 per 100 000 per annum, compared to rates in Northern Europe and North America of only 3 per 100 000 per annum.[30] Interestingly, there is also a sex bias with respect to the eventual outcome of chronic HBV infection and in the high incidence areas hepatocellular carcinoma rates are 3–4 times higher in men than women. There are estimated to be at least 300 million HBV carriers worldwide; and studies estimating the lifetime risk of developing hepatocellular carcinoma in chronically infected males as 50%,[48] serve to emphasize the considerable health risks associated with these viruses.

The HBV genome

HBV, the most common of the malignancy associated hepatitis viruses, is also the best understood. The small HBV particle is approximately 42nm in diameter with a 27nm core.[51] The genome, shown in Figure

3, consists of a circular DNA molecule which is only partially double stranded; the long or L(-) strand is approximately 3200 base pairs in length whereas the short or S(+) strand is variable. The circular nature of the molecule is maintained by base pairing between the 2 strands at their 5' ends, regions which contain two DNA repeats, DR1 and DR2. Replication of HBV proceeds via an RNA pregenome. After entering the hepatocyte, the virus undergoes DNA repair so that the S(+) strand is completed. The L(-) DNA strand is then transcribed into RNA and this is used as a template for reverse transcription to form the full length L(-) DNA strand. The S(+) strand is then formed by elongation from the 3' end at the DR1 site. The HBV genome contains 4 major open reading frames, the largest P ORF overlapping the other 3 ORF's, S, C and X. The P ORF, which extends over 80% of the viral genome, is thought to be translated from the RNA pregenome. The P gene encodes the reverse transcriptase activity[52] and appears to be necessary for several activities required for viral replication. The S ORF is divided into 3 regions which comprise the S gene preceded by the pre-S2 and pre-S1 regions and initiation of transcription from 3 distinct internal initiation codons within this region give rise to the 3 viral envelope proteins.[53] The C ORF codes for the core protein and the HBeAg, which may be truncated and secreted or expressed on the surface of the infected hepatocyte and is a major target for the immune system. The product of the X region functions as a transcriptional regulator. The identification of a glucocorticoid responsive element in the HBV genome may partially explain the sex difference in rates of infection and disease development.[54]

Natural history of HBV infection

Despite the overwhelming evidence that infection with HBV carries a strong risk of subsequent development of hepatocellular carcinoma, the exact mechanisms by which these viruses contribute to malignant progression remain to be elucidated. The outcome of HBV infection can be extremely variable and in adults infection usually ends in complete recovery. Perinatal infection, however, results in chronic disease in almost all infected children. In the Asian population initial HBV infection usually occurs very early in life and can be followed by the presence of HBV antigens in the infected individual. Recently, 3 distinct phases during the course of this infection have been identified.[55] During the first period, the length of which may be extremely variable but is broadly around 20 years, viral replication is accompanied by the presence of high serum concentrations of HBeAg. After these years of chronic infection, levels of HBeAg decline and this loss is paralleled by a rise in the HBe antibody (HBeAb) titre and the production of

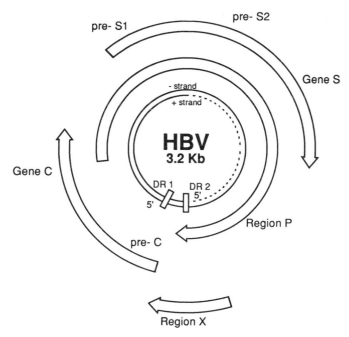

Fig. 3 Genetic structure of HBV, showing the 3.2kb DNA genome which is partially double, partially single stranded. The position of the four open reading frames is indicated, as is the position of the two direct repeats.

a cell mediated immune response against the HBV specific antigens. Although the reasons for this development of an immune response are not clear, the result is the killing of HBV infected liver cells, clearance of the virus from the infected individual and the development of active hepatitis or cirrhosis. Infectivity markedly declines during this phase since the cells actively producing virus are killed and virus production is eventually lost. This second phase is also rather protracted, again lasting many years. The consequence of the immune response is not, however, necessarily complete loss of HBV. In some cases expression of the HBV surface antigen, HBsAg, persists following integration of the HBV genome into the host chromosomes. Since cells containing integrated HBV sequences no longer make virus particles, they are no longer targets for the immune response and integration therefore allows life-long persistence of the viral genome and subsequent development of hepatocellular carcinomas, which almost all show evidence of integrated HBV.[56] As with HPV and the development of cervical cancer, interaction of the HBV genome is thought to play a role in subsequent malignant progression, although the random nature of the integration sites makes it unlikely to be through a mechanism of activation of cellular proto-oncogenes.[57] HBV sequences have been found to be integrated at some interesting points in the human genome, however, and may result in the deregulation of expression of genes such as *myc*, cyclin A or retinoic acid receptor β. Integration of HBV sequences probably occurs and accumulates throughout the phase of replication, so it is possible that the probability of hepatocellular carcinoma development is related to the length of this phase.

The mechanisms by which HBV contributes to hepatocellular carcinoma

The contribution of HBV infection to eventual malignant progression has been thought by some to result simply from the effect of necrosis and subsequent liver regeneration which is the hallmark of chronic hepatitis.[58] There is, however, increasing evidence that the virus itself also encodes gene products which may also participate in oncogenic progression. At present the strongest candidate for a virally encoded oncogene is the X gene, although a possible transcriptional function for the preS/S region of integrated HBV has also been described,[59] an activity which could be envisaged as contributing to oncogenesis. The X gene encodes a 154 amino acid protein which shows no clear similarity to other known proteins but is conserved amongst other hepadna viruses. Transgenic mice expressing the X gene from its own transcriptional regulatory region were shown to develop specifically liver cancers, with male mice developing disease and dying sooner than female animals.[60] The X protein is a very general activator of transcription with both HBV and a large number of cellular promoters as targets. Recent studies have shown that the X protein functions by an unusual mechanism to activate transcription indirectly, by activating protein kinase C and Raf-1 kinase, two key proteins in the process of signal transduction. Expression of X therefore results in a signalling cascade which nevertheless remains dependent on growth factor stimulation.[61,62] This activity fails to account for all the previously described functions of the protein, which suggested that X might directly form a part of the transcription complex. This is an extremely interesting observation, however, and suggests that protein X might mimic the function of tumour promoters such as phorbol esters. The inappropriate activation of signal transduction in the hepatocyte might provide a larger dividing population for the acquisition of other oncogenic genetic alterations or allow the outgrowth of genetically damaged cells, a contribution which might be similar to that of recurrent liver damage and regeneration.

Aflatoxin B1 as a co-carcinogen

A tumour promoting function of HBV is entirely consistent with the long latency preceding the development of hepatocellular carcinoma and it is clear that this cancer, like others, arises following the accumulation of several genetic lesions. The environmental carcinogen aflotoxin B1 is linked to the development of hepatocellular carcinoma[63] and at least one target for the action of this mutagen appears to be the tumour suppressor gene p53. Liver cancers arising in regions of high aflotoxin B1 exposure, like many other human cancers, show evidence of p53 point mutation. The resultant loss of wild type p53 function and expression of mutant p53 proteins therefore appear to contribute to the development of these hepatocellular carcinomas, with the specific type of mutation that is found in these tumours strongly indicating that the damage was caused by aflatoxin B1.[64,65] Strong synergy is seen between HBV infection and aflatoxin B1 exposure in the development of hepatocellular carcinoma and it is possible that the combination of mutagenic event and cell proliferation stimulus allows this, and maybe other, oncogenic mutations to become fixed in the genome. Activation of expression of other cell genes by the HBV X protein could also play a role in this process and further possible mechanisms of cooperation are suggested by the recent report describing an association between the p53 and HBV X proteins.[66] The biological consequences of such an interaction remain unknown, although inactivation of p53 by complex formation with X (similar to that seen following HPV E6/p53 interactions) might substitute for somatic p53 mutations in some cases and could explain the low incidence of p53 mutations seen in hepatocellular carcinomas from regions of low aflotoxin B1 exposure.[67]

HUMAN T CELL LEUKAEMIA VIRUS (HTLV-I)

The epidemiological evidence linking HTLV-I to adult T cell leukaemia (ATL) is very strong. HTLV-I infection prevalence is very low in most of the world, for example only 0.025% of the normal population of the USA carry the virus, but in Southern Japan, the Caribbean islands, some parts of Africa and South America the incidence is much higher, reaching 30% in parts of Japan.[68,69] ATL is restricted to the same areas as the virus. Although HTLV-I infection usually appears to be necessary for the development of ATL, the lifetime chance of an HTLV-I infected person developing ATL is only about 2%, so the majority of cases of HTLV-I infection are asymptomatic. A few cases of ATL-like disease lacking HTLV-I have also been reported. The other quite different disease linked to HTLV-I, called tropical spastic paraparesis (TSP) or HTLV-I associated myelopathy (HAM), is also found in all the HTLV-I endemic areas. HTLV-I is frequently transmitted from infected mothers to their babies via virus infected lymphocytes present in the milk in breast feeding. In adults male to female sexual transmission is the most common route, infected lymphocytes being present in the semen.

HTLV-I infects mainly CD4 lymphocytes in vivo. About 1–2% of peripheral lymphocytes are infected in a typical asymptomatic virus carrier but up to 10% of peripheral lymphocytes are infected in TSP patients.[70] This contrasts greatly with EBV where the number of infected B lymphocytes is very low in asymptomatic infected people. HTLV-I is a retrovirus and in the infected lymphocyte HTLV-I is found as proviral DNA integrated in the cell chromosomes. There is no unique or highly preferred site of integration in the cell DNA and there is no evidence for a virus insertion mechanism for ATL. In addition to the usual *gag*, *pol*, and *env* retroviral genes, HTLV-I contains additional genes at the 3' end of the genome in the X region.[68] These are not captured cell genes but represent additional viral genes and give rise to p40[tax], p27[rex], p21[X III] and the recently described rof, tof and orf-2 proteins.[71] The genetic structure of HTLV-I is shown in Figure 4. The splicing that permits the use of the multiple reading frames in the X region has been simplified slightly for clarity.

T cell transformation by HTLV-I

Most retroviruses will only infect growing cells, but HTLV-I has the capacity to infect and immortalise resting T cells, rendering it unnecessary to add IL-2 to the medium to maintain their growth. Infection by cell-free HTLV-I virus particles is usually of very low efficiency and the normal mode of infection is through cell contact in coculture. A heat inactivated virus preparation was found to cause the appearence of activation markers and transiently cause the cells to divide[72] but it may be cell components which are responsible for the initial activation.[73] Cells transformed in vitro express several HTLV-I genes and may replicate virus at a low level. The *tax* gene product is an activator of expression of the HTLV-I LTR and of many cell genes[74] working at least in part via the ATF family of transcription factors[75,76] and the NF-kB transcription factor.[77,78] The ATF mechanism seems to be mediated by *tax* stabilising the dimerisation of the factor.[79] Among the cell genes modulated, *tax* is able to up regulate the promoters of both IL-2 and the IL-2 receptor. *Rex*, which is required for accumulation of the mRNA for the viral structural proteins,[80] also stabilises the IL-2 receptor mRNA. This suggested an autocrine growth loop in which endogenously produced IL-2 might maintain the growth of the culture.[81] Consistent with this, infection of bulk populations of peripheral human T lymphocytes results in continuous growth of the T cell population independent of added IL-2 and a monoclonal antibody to IL-2 receptor p55 chain can

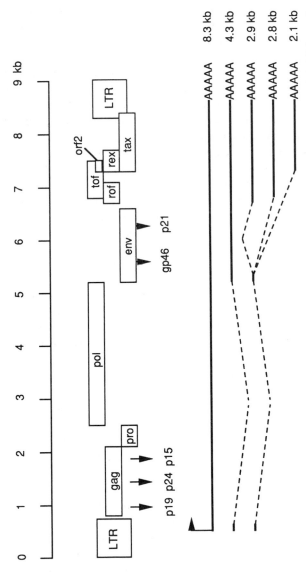

Fig. 4 Genetic structure of HTLV-I. The open reading frames encoding the proteins of HTLV-I are shown beneath a scale in kilobases. Some of the proteins are cleaved proteolytically to give the final products shown. The mRNAs are illustrated below, splicing being shown by dotted lines. The most abundant mRNAs are the 8.3, 4.3 and 2.1 kb RNAs, the 2.8 and 2.9 kb structures have only been demonstrated by PCR so far. For clarity the details of the splicing have been slightly simplified. A complete description has been published.[88]

inhibit the cell growth. The realisation that the simple autocrine model is not an accurate explanation of HTLV-I immortalisation came from cloning the infected immortalised cells. The cloned cells continue to grow permanently in the absence of added IL-2 and they usually have elevated expression of the p55 chain of the IL-2 receptor. But they do not secrete IL-2 into the growth medium and they do not express the mRNA for IL-2.[82,83] It is possible that in the bulk cultures a T cell interaction mediated by the infected cells is causing the proliferation of non-infected T cells by a mechanism involving IL-2, resulting in the sensitivity of the growth of the whole culture to the IL-2 receptor antibodies, but the HTLV-I immortalisation is working by a different mechanism. Perhaps in the immortalised cells the IL-2 receptor has become activated independent of its ligand or control has been subverted further down the pathway. Sensitivity of the growth of the cloned HTLV-I transformed cells to rapamycin but resistance to FK506 and cyclosporin A provides a clue to the control pathways involved[83] and it is clear from HTLV-I mutants that the X region encoding *tax* and *rex* is required for immortalisation[84] but the precise mechanism remains unknown.

HTLV-I and adult T cell leukaemia

A long period, typically 20–30 years, elapses between infection with HTLV-I and development of ATL and only a small percentage of HTLV-I carriers will develop ATL during their lifetimes. It is presumed that in this period cell mutations accumulate which may eventually combine to give the malignant ATL phenotype. Several intermediate premalignant stages are recognised prior to the development of ATL and these are distinguished by the degree of raised lymphocyte count, the clonality or oligoclonality of HTLV-I integration site in the lymphocytes and clinical features such as skin lesions. Good clinical descriptions of these stages can be found in.[68] It is not certain that the stages necessarily constitute a linear progression towards disease but this seems likely. In pre-ATL a monoclonal provirus integration site and raised lymphocyte counts are found, but in about half of these patients the raised lymphocyte count will regress spontaneously and patients often have several episodes of smouldering ATL over many years prior to development of acute ATL. Several chromosome translocations have been reported in ATL cells but no translocation common to all cases has yet been identified. In acute ATL, many problems develop in the immune system and complications frequently develop from opportunistic infections.

In contrast to HTLV-I immortalised T lymphocytes which express several HTLV-I transcripts and can replicate virus, in freshly isolated ATL cells there is very low or no detectable transcription of the provirus.[85,86] After culturing for several weeks, virus gene expression is activated and replication can occur. This repressed state of the virus may help to avoid immune surveillance of the ATL cells based on recognition of viral antigens but it seems to exclude an HTLV-I gene product complementing oncogenic cell mutations in the malignant growth of the final ATL cell. A role for HTLV-I in the tumour development presumably comes earlier in the process, perhaps by expanding the pool of T cells and promoting survival of T cells containing some oncogenic mutations. The repressed form of viral gene expression in the tumour cells is reminiscent of EBV in BL cells and the same problems of alteration of the tumour cells when they are brought into culture occur in ATL as in BL research. The most likely role for HTLV-I in the development of ATL is in promoting over many years the expanded pool of replicating lymphocytes being controlled by immune surveillance in smouldering ATL. This would increase the possibility of a cell acquiring the mutations necessary to cause it to become a malignant ATL cell. Whether the viral genome is playing a direct role in the final tumour is very uncertain.

PREVENTION OF DISEASE

The ultimate goal following the identification of a human tumour virus, prevention of infection and eventual eradication of the disease, is closer to reality for HBV than the other viruses discussed in this chapter. Immunisation of young children has proved extremely effective in preventing infection[87] and many countries in the regions of high incidence of infections are now routinely vaccinating infants. Whether or not this will result in a reduction in the incidence of liver cancers remains an exciting prospect for future studies.

Prophylactic immunisation to prevent infection with EBV, HTLV-I and HPV is under study but there is no evidence so far for the efficacy of such vaccines. Therapeutic immunisation directed against the virus-associated cancers is also being considered. An alternative approach is the development of drugs to specifically target the activities of the viral oncoproteins, although the molecular mechanisms by which these proteins function are so far only understood in sufficient detail for the HPVs to allow any progress in this direction. Interesting possibilities for this would be agents that could prevent the functions of the E6 or E7 proteins. Agents that could reactivate EBV or HTLV-I expression might render tumour cells susceptible to immune surveillance and provide a novel therapeutic strategy. In virus positive cases of these cancers, the virus provides an excellent tumour cell marker and might thus be used for various forms of immune or gene therapeutic targetting.

ACKNOWLEDGEMENTS

We would like to thank Tim Harrison, Alan Farthing and Martin Allday for their helpful comments. We are also grateful to Matthew Brimmel for help with the artwork.

REFERENCES

1 Keiff E, Liebowitz D. Epstein-Barr virus. In: Fields B, Knipe D, eds.Virology 2nd edn. 1990: pp 1889–1920.
2 Farrell PJ, Sinclair AJ. Burkitt's lymphoma. SGM Symposia 1994; 51: 101–121.
3 Cohen JI, Wang F, Mannick J, Kieff E. Epstein-Barr virus nuclear protein 2 is a key determinant of lymphocyte transformation. Proc Natl Acad Sci USA 1989; 86: 9558–9562.
4 Hammerschmidt W, Sugden B. Genetic analysis of immortalizing functions of Epstein-Barr virus in human B lymphocytes. Nature 1989; 340: 393–397.
5 Tomkinson B, Robertson E, Kieff E. Epstein-Barr virus nuclear proteins EBNA-3A and EBNA-3C are essential for B-Lymphocyte growth transformation. J Virol 1993; 67: 2014–2054.
6 Mannick JB, Cohen JI, Birkenbach M, Marchini A, Kieff E. The Epstein-Barr virus nuclear protein encoded by the leader of the EBNA RNAs is important in B-lymphocyte transformation. J Virol 1991; 65: 6826–6837.
7 Kaye KM, Izumi KM, Kieff E. Epstein-Barr virus latent membrane protein I is essential for B lymphocyte growth transformation. Proc Natl Acad Sci USA 1993; 90: 9150–9154.
8 Farrell PJ. Epstein-Barr virus. In: O'Brien SJ ed. Genetic Maps, 6th edn., Vol. 1. 1993; pp 120–133.
9 Miller G. Epstein-Barr virus; biology, pathogenesis and medical aspects. In: Fields BN, Knipe DM eds. Virology, 2nd edn. New York: Raven Press 1990; pp 1921–1958.
10 Sinclair AJ, Farrell PJ. Epstein-Barr virus transcription factors. Cell Growth and Differentiation 1992; 3: 557–563.
11 Sugden B, Warren N. A promoter of Epstein-Barr virus that can function during latent viral infection can be transactivated by EBNA-1, a viral protein required for viral DNA replication during latent infection. J Virol 1989; 63: 2644–2649.
12 Chen M-R, Middeldorp JA, Hayward SD. Separation of the complex DNA binding domain of EBNA-1 into DNA recognition and dimerization domains of novel structure. J Virol 1993; 67: 4875–4885.
13 Sinclair AJ, Palmero I, Peters G, Farrell PJ. 1994. EBNA-2 and EBNA-LP cooperate to cause G0 to G1 transition during immortalisation of resting human B Lymphocytes by Epstein-Barr virus. EMBO J 1994 (In press).
14 Allday MJ, Crawford DH, Thomas JA. Epstein-Barr virus (EBV) nuclear antigen 6 induces expression of the EBV latent membrane protein and an activated phenotype in Raji cells. J Gen Virol 1993; 74: 361–369.
15 Allan GJ, Inman GJ, Parker BD, Rowe DT, Farrell PJ. Cell growth effects of Epstein-Barr virus leader protein. J Gen Virol 1992; 73: 1547–1551.
16 Szekely L, Selivanova G, Hagnusson KP, Klein G, Wiman KG. EBNA-5, an EBV encoded nuclear antigen, binds to the RB and p53 proteins. Proc Natl Acad Sci USA 1993; 90: 5455–5459.
17 Baichwal VR, Sugden B. The multiple membrane-spanning segments of the BNLF-1 oncogene from Epstein-Barr virus are required for transformation. Oncogene 1989; 4: 67–74.
18 Wang D, Liebowitz D, Kieff E. An EBV membrane protein expressed in immortalized lymphocytes transforms established rodent cell lines. Cell 1985; 43: 831–840.
19 Dawson CW, Rickinson AB, Young LS. Epstein-Barr virus latent membrane protein inhibits human epithelial cell differentiation. Nature 1990; 344: 777–780.
20 Van Hasselt CA, Gibb AG. Nasopharyngeal carcinoma 1991. Chinese University Press, Hong Kong.

21 Harabuchi Y, Yamanaka N, Kataura A, et al. Epstein-Barr virus in patients with lethal midline granuloma. Lancet 1990; 335: 128–130.

22 Herbst H, Steinbrecher E, Niedobitek G, Young LS, Brooks L, Muller-Lantzsch N, Stein H. Distribution and phenotype of Epstein-Barr virus harboring cells in Hodgkin's disease. Blood 1992; 80: 484–491.

23 Shiramizu B, Barriga F, Neequaye J, et al. Patterns of chromosomal breakpoint locations in Burkitt's lymphoma: relevance to geography and Epstein-Barr virus association. Blood 1991; 77: 1516–1526.

24 Gratama JW, Oosterveer MAP, Zwaan FE, Lepoutre J, Klein G, Ernberg I. Eradication of Epstein-Barr virus by allogeneic bone marrow transplantation: implications for sites of viral latency. Proc Natl Acad Sci USA 1988; 85: 8693–8696.

25 Rowe M, Rowe DT, Gregory CD, Young LS, Farrell PJ, Rupani H, Rickinson AB. Differences in B cell growth phenotype reflect novel patterns of Epstein-Barr virus latent gene expression in Burkitt's lymphoma cells. EMBO J 1987; 6: 2743–2751.

26 Fahraeus R, Fu HL, Ernberg I, et al. Expression of Epstein-Barr virus genome in nasopharyngeal carcinoma. Int J Cancer 1988; 42: 329–338.

27 Young LS, Dawson CW, Clark D et al. Epstein-Barr virus gene expression in nasopharyngeal carcinoma. J Gen Virol 1988; 69: 1051–1065.

28 Henderson S, Rowe M, Gregory C et al. Induction of bcl-2 expression by Epstein-Barr virus latent membrane protein 1 protects infected B cells from programmed cell death. Cell 1991; 65: 1107–1115.

29 Evan G I, Wyllie AH, Gilbert CS et al. Induction of apoptosis in fibroblasts by c-myc protein. Cell 1992; 69: 119–128.

30 Parkin DM, Laara E, Muir CS. Estimates of the worldwide frequency of sixteen major cancers in 1980. Int J Cancer 1988; 41: 184–197.

31 Vousden KH: Human papillomaviruses and cervical cancer. Cancer cells 1989; 1: 43–49.

32 zur Hausen H. Human papillomaviruses in the pathogenesis of anogenital cancer. Virology 1991; 184: 9–13.

33 Schiffman MH, Bauer HM, Hoover RN et al. Epidemiological evidence showing that human papillomavirus infection causes most cervical intraepithelial neoplasia. J Natl Cancer Inst 1993; 85: 958–964.

34 Koutsky LA, Holmes KK, Critchlow CW et al. A cohort study of the risk of cervical intraepithelial neoplasia grade 2 or 3 in relation to papillomavirus infection. N Engl J Med 1992; 327: 1272–1278.

35 Spalholz BA, Howley PM. Papillomavirus-host cell interactions. In: Klein G (ed). Advances in viral oncology 8: tumorigenic DNA viruses. New York: Raven Press, 1989: pp 27–53.

36 Doorbar J, Ely S, Sterling J, McLean C, Crawford L. Specific interaction between HPV-16 E1-E4 and cytokeratins results in collapse of the epithelial cell intermediate filament network. Nature 1991; 352: 824–827.

37 Lambert PF. Papillomavirus DNA replication. J Virol 1991; 65: 3417–3420.

38 Straight SW, Hinckle PM, Jerews RJ, McCance DM. The E5 oncoprotein of human papillomavirus type 16 transforms fibroblasts and effects the downregulation of the epidermal growth factor receptor in keratinocytes. J Virol 1993; 67: 4521–4532.

39 Vousden KH. Human papillomavirus transforming genes. Semin Virol 1991; 2: 307–317.

40 Hudson JB, Bedell MA, McCance DJ, Laimins LA. Immortalisation and altered differentiation of human keratinocytes in vitro by the E6 and E7 open reading frames of human papillomavirus type 18. J Virol 1990; 64: 519–526.

41 Vousden KH. Interactions of human papillomavirus transforming proteins with the products of tumor supresor genes. FASEB J 1993; 7: 872–879.

42 Chellappan S, Kraus V, Kroger B, Munger K, Howley PM, Phelps WC, Nevins JR. Adenovirus E1A, simian virus 40 tumor antigen, and human papillomavirus E7 protein share the capacity to disrupt the interaction between transcription factor E2F and the retinoblastoma gene product. Proc Natl Acad Sci USA 1992; 89: 4549–4553.

43 Dyson N, Howley PM, Münger K, Harlow E. The human papilloma virus-16 E7 oncoprotein is able to bind to the retinoblastoma gene product. Science 1989; 243: 934–937.

44 Hamel PA, Phillips RA, Muncaster M, Gallie BL. Speculations on the role of RB1 in tissue specific differentiation, tumor initiation and tumor progression. FASEB J 1993; 7: 846–854.

45 Scheffner M, Werness BA, Huibregtse JM, Levine AJ, Howley PM. The E6 oncoprotein encoded by human papillomavirus types 16 and 18 promotes the degradation of p53. Cell 1990; 63: 1129–1136.

46 Hollstein M, Sidransky D, Vogelstein B, Harris CC. p53 mutations in human cancers. Science 1991; 253: 49–53.

47 Crook T, Wrede D, Tidy JA, Mason WP, Evans DJ, Vousden KH. Clonal p53 mutation in primary cervical cancer: association with human-papillomavirus- negative tumours. Lancet 1992; 339: 1070–1073.

48 Beasley RP, Lin CC, Hwang LT, Chein CS. Hepatocellular carcinoma and hepatitis B virus. Lancet 1981; ii: 1129–1133.

49 Blumberg BS, London WT. Hepatitis B virus. Pathogenesis and prevention of primary cancer of the liver. Cancer 1982; 50: 2657–2665.

50 Beasley RP, Hwang LY. Overview on the epidemiology of hepatocellular carcinoma. Viral Hepatitis and Liver Disease. New York: Grune & Stratton 1991: pp 532–535.

51 Robinson W. Hepadnaviridae and their replication. Virology 1990; 2: 2137–2169.

52 Bartenschlager R, Schaller H. The amino-terminal domain of the hepadnaviral P-gene encodes the terminal protein (genome-linked protein) believed to prime reverse transcription. EMBO J 1988; 7: 4185–4192.

53 Ganem D. Assembly of hepadnaviral virions and subviral particles. Microbiology 1991; 168: 61–83.

54 Tur-Kasta R, Burk RD, Shaul Y, Shafritz DA. Hepatitis B virus DNA contains a glucocorticoid-responsive element. Proc Natl Acad Sci USA 1986; 83: 1627–1631.

55 Chen DS. From hepatitis to hepatoma: Lessons from Type B viral hepatitis. Science 1993; 262: 369–370.

56 Tiollais P, Pourcel C, Dejean A. The hepatitis B virus. Nature 1985; 317: 489–495.

57 Nagaya T, Nakamura T, Tokino T, Tsurimoto T et al. The mode of hepatitis B virus DNA integration in chromosomes of human hepatocellular carcinoma. Genes 1987; 1: 773–782.

58 Smuckler EA, Ferrell L, Clawson GA. Proliferative hepatocellular lesions, benign and malignant. In: Vyas GN, Dienstag JL, Hoofnagle JH, eds. Viral Hepatitis and Liver Disease. New York: Grune & Stratton, 1984: pp 201–207.

59 Kekule AS, Lauer U, Meyer M, Caselmann WH, Hofschneider PH, Koshy R.The preS2/S region of integrated hepatitis B virus DNA encodes a transcriptional transactivator. Nature 1990; 343: 457–461.

60 Kim CM, Koike K, Saito I, Miyamura T, Jay G. HBx gene of hepatitis B virus induces liver cancer in transgenic mice. Nature 1991; 351: 317–320.

61 Cross JC, Wen P, Rutter WJ. Transactivation by hepatitis B virus X protein is promiscuous and dependent on mitogen-activated cellular serine/threonone kinases. Proc Natl Acad Sci USA 1993; 90: 8078–8082.

62 Kekule AS, Lauer U, Weiss L, Luber B, Hofschneider. Hepatitis B virus transactivator HBx uses a tumour promoter signalling pathway. Nature 1993; 361: 742–745.

63 Harris C. Hepatocellular carcinogenesis: recent advances and speculations. Cancer Cells 1990; 2(5): 146–148.

64 Bressac B, Kew M, Wands J, Ozturk M. Selective G to T mutations of p53 gene in hepatocellular carcinoma from Southern Africa. Nature 1991; 350: 429–431.

65 Hsu IC, Metcalf RA, Sun T, Welsh JA, Wangs NJ, Harris CC. Mutational hotspot in the p53 gene in human hepatocellular carcinomas. Nature 1991; 350: 427–428.

66 Feitelson MA, Zhu M, Duan LX, London WT. Hepatitis B x antigen and p53 are associated in vitro and in liver tissues from patients with primary hepatocellular carcinoma.Oncogene 1993; 8: 1109–1117.

67 Buetow KH, Sheffield VC, Zhu M et al. Proc Natl Acad Sci USA 1992; 89: 9622–9626.

68 Cann AJ, Chen ISY. Human T-cell leukemia virus types I and II. In: Fields BN, Knipe DM, eds. Virology, 2nd edn. New York: Raven Press 1990; pp 1501–1527.

69 Hollsberg P, Hafler DA. Pathogenesis of diseases induced by human lymphotropic virus type I infection. N Engl J Med 1993; 328: 1173–1182.

70 Bangham CRM. Human T cell leukaemia virus type I and neurological disease. Curr Opin Neurobiol 1993; 3: 773–778.

71 Ciminale V, Pavlakis GN, Derse D, Cunningham CP, Felber BK. Complex splicing in the human T cell leukemia virus (HTLV) family of retroviruses: novel mRNAs and proteins produced by HTLV type I. J Virol 1992; 66: 1737–1745.

72 Gazzolo L, Duc Dodon MD. Direct activation of resting T lymphocytes by human T lymphotropic virus type I. Nature 1987; 326: 714–717.

73 Kimata JT, Palker TJ, Ratner L. The mitogenic activity of human T-cell leukemia virus type I is T-cell associated and requires the CD2/LF3A activation pathway. J Virol 1993; 67: 3134–3141.

74 Lindholm PF, Kashanchi F, Brady JN. Transcriptional regulation in the human retrovirus HTLV-I. Semin Virol. 1993; 4: 53–60.

75 Xu YL, Adya N, Siores E, Gao Q, Giam CZ. Cellular factors involved in transcription and tax mediated transactivation directed by the TGACGT motif in human T cell leukemia virus type I promoter. J Biol Chem 1990; 265: 20285–20292.

76 Fujisawa JI, Toita M, Yoshida M. A unique enhancer element for the transactivator (p40^{tax}) of human T-cell leukemia virus type I that is distinct from cyclic AMP and 12-O-tetradecanoylphorbol 13-acetate responsive elements. J Virol 1989; 63: 3234–3239.

77 Duyao MP, Kessler DJ, Spicer DB, Sonenshein GE. Transactivation of the c-myc gene by HTLV-I tax is mediated by NF-kB. Curr Top Microbiol Immunol 1992; 182: 421–424.

78 Lilienbaum A, Paulin D. Activation of the human vimentin gene by the tax human T-cell leukemia virus I. Mechanisms of regulation by the NF-kB transcription factor. J Biol Chem 1993; 268: 2180–2188.

79 Wagner S, Green MR. HTLV-I tax protein stimulation of DNA binding of bZIP proteins by enhancing dimerization. Science 993; 262: 395–399.

80 Ahmed YF, Gilmartin GM, Hanly SM, Nevins JR, Greene WC. The HTLV-I rex response element mediates a novel form of mRNA polyadenylation. Cell 1991; 64: 727–737.

81 Tendler CL, Greenberg SJ, Blattner WA, et al. Transactivation of interleukin 2 and its receptor induces immune activation in human T-cell lymphotropic virus type I-associated myelopathy: pathogenic implications and a rationale for immunotherapy. Proc Natl Acad Sci USA 1990; 87: 5218–5222.

82 Arya SK, Wong-Staal F, Gallo RC. T-cell growth factor gene: lack of expression in human T-cell leukemia-lymphoma virus infected cells. Science 1984; 223: 1086–1087.

83 Hollsberg P, Wucherpfennig KW, Ausubel LJ, Calvo V, Bierer BE, Hafler DA. Characterization of HTLV-I in vivo infected T cell clones; IL-2 independent growth of non-transformed T cells. J Immunol 1992; 148: 3256–3263.

84 Chen ISY, Slamon DJ, Rosenblatt JD, Shah NP, Quan SG, Wachsman W. The x gene is essential for HTLV replication. Science 1985; 229: 54–58.

85 Kinoshita T, Shimoyama M, Tobibai K, et al. Detection of mRNA for tax1/rex1 gene of human T cell leukemia virus type I in fresh peripheral blood mononuclear cells of adult T cell leukemia patients and viral carriers by using the polymerase chain reaction. Proc Natl Acad Sci USA 1989; 86: 5620–5624.

86 Franchini GF, Wong-Staal F, Gallo R. Human T cell leukemia virus (HTLV-I) transcripts in fresh and cultured cells of patients with adult T cell leukemia. Proc Natl Acad Sci USA 1984; 81: 6207–6211.

87 Tsen YJ, Chang MH, Hsu HY, Lee CY, Sung JL, Chen DS. Seroprevalence of hepatitis B virus infection in children in Taipei, five years after a mass hepatitis B vaccination program. J Med Virol 1991; 34: 96–99.

88 Wain-Hobson S. HTLV-I. In: O'Brien SJ, ed. Genetic Maps, 6th edn. 1993: pp 190.

British Medical Bulletin (1994) Vol. 50, No. 3, pp. 582–599
© The British Council 1994

p53 and human cancers

D P Lane

Cancer Research Campaign Laboratories, Department of Biochemistry, University of Dundee, Dundee, UK

Mutations in the p53 gene are one of the commonest specific genetic changes found in human cancer. The p53 gene is not required for normal development but lack of p53 function confers an enormously elevated risk of developing cancer, thus it seems truly to act as a tumour suppressor gene. The p53 protein is normally present in minute amounts in cells but when cells are exposed to genotoxic stimuli p53 levels rise rapidly and initiate a programme of cell death, probably by means of transcriptional regulation. This response is lost in many tumour cells as they have either inactivated their p53 genes by mutation or blocked the activity of p53 through the production of proteins that bind to it and neutralise it. Mutant p53 proteins accumulate to high levels in many cancer cells and the p53 protein and the p53 response to DNA damage represent key points for therapeutic intervention.

The p53 tumour suppressor gene is located on chromosome 17 p and encodes a 393 amino acid nuclear phosphoprotein. Mutations in this gene are one of the commonest somatic genetic changes found in human cancer.[1] They have been found in a very wide range of tumour types including the most common solid tumours – such as breast, lung and bowel cancer. It has been estimated that as many as 3×10^6 cancers per annum will contain mutations in this gene.[2] The p53 gene appears to act as a real tumour suppressor gene since its function is not essential for the viability of the organism but acts to profoundly suppress the rate of development of cancer.[3] A powerful current model of p53 function proposes that it acts as 'the guardian of the genome' sensing damage or potential damage to the DNA and invoking a protective response either by blocking the cell cycle or by inducing apoptosis (programmed cell death) in the affected cell.[4,5] Loss of this gene function allows the propagation of cells with genetic damage and this is a key step in the development of neoplasia.

The inheritance of a germ line mutation in the p53 gene confers a greatly elevated life time risk of developing cancer and is frequently the genetic basis of the rare Li-Fraumeni syndrome of inherited cancer susceptibility.[6] The spectrum of both germ line and somatic mutations found in the p53 gene is unusual when compared to other tumour suppressor genes since the vast majority of the p53 mutations are missense mutations that are localised in the central 190 amino acids of the protein. This suggests that these mutant proteins retain important biological activities that confer selective advantage for the tumour cells. These mutant proteins are often produced in large amounts specifically in tumour cells suggesting that elevated levels of the protein may be a useful marker of malignancy and a target for therapy.

p53 'GUARDIAN OF THE GENOME'

In the last 2 years a compelling model for the function of the p53 protein has emerged. This model suggests that the p53 protein acts to protect the organism from genetic damage. This damage may be caused directly by external factors, for example by exposure to DNA damaging drugs or radiation; or it may be caused internally, perhaps by mitotic failures resulting from aberrations in cell cycle control of the type associated with the action of dominant transforming oncogenes. The basis on which this model was originally proposed was: (a) the finding that wild type p53 when introduced by DNA transfection into tumour cells that either failed to make p53 at all or made only mutant forms of the protein arrested their growth and caused death by apoptosis;[7-10] and (b) the finding that while p53 levels in normal cells are very low, exposure of cells to DNA damaging agents induces a dramatic increase in p53 protein level.[11-14]

Putting these two concepts together it was first shown that the G1 growth arrest response to ionising radiation of cells in culture was dependent on the presence of a wild type p53 gene and was accompanied by increase in p53 protein level.[15] More recently this work has been greatly extended by the analysis of the response to DNA damaging agents of mice in which both copies of the p53 gene have been inactivated 'p53 knock out mice'.[16,17] Normally when murine thymocytes are exposed to DNA damaging agents (such as ionising radiation or topoisomerase 2 inhibitors) either in vivo or in vitro, the p53 protein accumulates in the nuclei of the exposed cells and the cells die by apoptosis. In contrast, when the thymocytes of the p53 knock out mice are irradiated, no apoptotic response is seen. The difference in sensitivity is enormous since apoptosis is induced efficiently by doses as low as 1

Gy in normal mice but even 20 Gy fail to induce apoptosis in the p53 knock out cells. Another key finding was that the apoptotic response to other stimuli was unaffected by the absence of p53. Thus, the knock out cells showed a vigorous apoptotic response to treatment with calcium ionophore or glucocorticoid. Also of interest was the observation that their 'spontaneous' rate of apoptosis was not p53 dependent. Cells derived from heterozygous mice that had only one copy of the p53 gene showed some degree of enhanced resistance to radiation induced apoptosis. In other words, it was possible to see a clear gene dosage effect. This suggests that the control and regulation of the p53 response to DNA damage must be very finely balanced. This gene dosage effect has important implications, particularly in models of tumour progression, since it means that mutation of only one allele of the p53 gene would affect the response characteristics of the mutant cell, and might perhaps predispose to subsequent inactivation of the remaining allele. The results with thymocytes have now been extended to the intestinal epithelial cells of the large and small intestine.[18] In normal mice 4 h after exposure of the animal to 8 Gy whole body irradiation a characteristic and striking apoptotic response is seen in the stem cell zone of the crypts of the small intestine. Using newly developed antibodies to murine p53 that are effective on paraffin embedded sections it could be seen that p53 protein accumulated selectively in exactly the same zone. Consistent with this was the complete absence of an apoptotic response to radiation in the cells of the p53 knock out mice. This study suggests that the p53 response to radiation and the apoptotic response it induces is under tight control and that in the small bowel at least it is the stem cells that are especially sensitive. The p53 dependent apoptotic response to DNA damage can clearly be seen to protect the organism against the survival of stem cells that have sustained genetic damage from external sources. The effectiveness of this response could be ablated by any agent that reduced the induction of the response or by gene products such as the bcl-2 gene that act to inhibit apoptosis.[19]

Striking evidence that this same response may limit the activity of dominant oncogenes has come from examination of the role of p53 in transformation by viral oncogenes.[20,21] The adenovirus E1a gene is a potent transforming oncogene that can act in concert with an activated ras gene to transform primary rodent cells. Cells into which just the E1a gene has been introduced enter cell cycle but accumulate high levels of wild type p53 and cannot be readily established in culture. Close examination shows that these cells are dying at a high rate by apoptosis. This apoptotic response to the action of a dominant transforming oncogene is p53 dependent, so that E1a will efficiently transform cells if the p53 pathway is ablated either by blocking the terminal stages of apoptosis or by inactivating p53 function, for example with viral oncoproteins that bind p53. In this context it is not surprising but is nevertheless of great importance that the ability of many anti-cancer drugs to kill tumour cells may proceed through a p53 dependent apoptotic pathway. The abrogation of this pathway by mutations in p53 may confer a generalised resistance to the common drug therapies.[22]

PROPERTIES OF THE WILD TYPE p53 PROTEIN

The complete three-dimensional structure of the p53 protein has not yet been reported but a great deal has been learnt about its basic properties from extensive analysis of the protein. The recombinant protein and domains of the protein have been expressed and purified from bacterial, yeast and insect cell based expression systems.[23,24] In addition, a large collection of monoclonal antibodies directed at different defined sites (epitopes) within the protein have been characterised.[25,26]

The p53 protein binds specifically to double stranded DNA, and a core recognition motif has been defined.[27] This motif has been found within the non-coding regions of certain genes whose transcription rate is enhanced in the presence of p53.[28] The protein has at its N terminus a highly charged region that can interact with the cellular transcription machine, directing it to promoter sequences located near to p53 binding sites in the DNA.[29,30] Thus the normal p53 protein has all the features of a specific transcription factor. The protein may have other activities as well since it can act to promote the reannealing of complementary strands of DNA, thus neutralising the effectiveness of DNA unwinding proteins (DNA helicases) and inhibiting replication.[31] The p53 protein can also act in a non sequence specific manner to suppress transcription from a wide variety of promoters.[32] At the cellular level the normal p53 protein acts to suppress transformation by a wide variety of oncogenes[7,33] and is a potent inducer of both cell cycle arrest and programmed cell death (apoptosis)[34] in a wide variety of cell types. It can act to suppress genetic instability, as indicated by the rate of detection of gene amplification in cells without wild type p53.[35,36] While, as discussed below, the p53 protein can be split into at least 3 domains that retain independent function it is clear that in the complete protein these 3 domains act co-ordinately and each can affect and regulate the function of the other.

The DNA binding domain

Partial proteolysis of the complete p53 protein has shown that the sequence specific DNA binding activity is the property of a separate independently folding structural domain that occupies the central region of the molecule from amino acids 101–290 (Figure).[37–39] Comparison of the predicted amino acid sequences of the p53 protein from mammals, birds, fish and amphibians shows that this central domain of p53 has been highly conserved in evolution and is therefore probably essential for function.[40,41] Indeed *Xenopus* p53 binds double stranded DNA (dsDNA) with a similar sequence specificity to the human protein. In addition to containing the sequence specific DNA binding activity of p53, this central domain also contains the binding site for the SV40 virus large T protein, which can form specific molecular complexes with p53. The T antigen binding activity has also been highly conserved in evolution, suggesting that there may be conserved cellular proteins that bind this domain. In support of this, 3 host proteins that bind the central region of p53 and whose binding is inhibited by T antigen have been discovered but not yet identified.[42] The central domain of p53 contains many conserved cysteine and histidine residues and it has been reported that the domain has the capacity to bind zinc.[37,43] Treatment of wild type p53 with sulfhydryl modifying agents such as N-ethyl-maleimide or diamine completely eliminates the DNA binding function of the protein.[44,45] This suggests that a reactive cysteine is required for p53 to bind DNA.

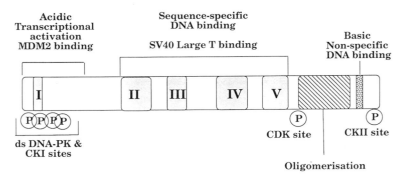

Figure Functional domains of p53.

The conformation of the central region of the p53 molecule seems to be relatively unstable and may shift between two states. In one conformation the domain can bind specifically to the consensus DNA sequence and to T antigen while in the other conformation these activities are absent. This conformational change can be readily detected using monoclonal antibodies.[46] The PAb240 antibody recognizes the linear peptide sequence RHSVV present in the centre of the DNA binding

domain.[47] This peptide is sequestered from the antibody in the DNA binding conformation but is exposed in the inactive conformation. In contrast the antibodies PAb246 (mouse specific) and PAb1620 (mouse and human p53 reactive) are able to bind only the DNA binding competent conformation of this domain and indeed the PAb246 antibody can block the binding of p53 to dsDNA.[48] There is some evidence to suggest that binding zinc may stabilise the DNA binding conformation of p53.[43] As discussed below most of the point mutations found in p53 in human tumours affect this central domain of the protein. Typically they abolish the sequence specific binding of p53 to dsDNA and alter the conformation of the protein into the state in which the PAb240 epitope is exposed.

The N terminus of p53

The N terminal region of p53 is readily proteolysed and is in general much less conserved in evolution than the DNA binding domain. It contains the binding sites for the adenovirus Elb protein[49] and the host encoded mdm2 protein.[50] It can act as a transcriptional transactivation domain when fused to the DNA binding domain of another protein[29,30] (for example that of the yeast GAL4 protein; Fig.), and like other domains of this type which are present in other transcription factors, this domain appears to be highly charged. If it acts as a transcription transactivation domain it is assumed that this region of p53 will presumably interact with components of the core transcription machinery.

The N terminus of p53 contains a number of specific phosphorylation sites.[51] Of particular interest are sites that are recognised by the recently described dsDNA dependent protein kinase. This enzyme requires DNA ends for activity and may therefore be activated in cells that have sustained DNA damage.[52] The p53 protein has a very short half life in normal mammalian cells and, while the mechanism of this degradation is not understood, the N terminus of p53 may be involved since deletion of the N terminal 42 amino acids of p53 seems to greatly increase the stability of the protein.[53] Many of the monoclonal antibodies to p53 that have been isolated react with epitopes within this N terminal region of the molecule. They include the PAb1801, PAb242, PAb248 and D0-1, D0-2 and D0-7 antibodies. This region of p53 is also recognised by the anti-p53 antibodies present in the sera of some cancer patients.[54]

The C terminus of p53

The C terminus of p53 also appears to be an independent protein domain[37] (Fig.). It is responsible for the oligomerisation of p53, and current work suggests that p53 assembles through this domain to form stable tetramers. Cross linking experiments show that the C terminus

alone will assemble into dimers and tetramers.[55] The C terminus alone can act as a transforming oncogene to complement an activated *ras* gene in the transformation of primary rodent fibroblasts.[56,57] This activity has been localised to amino acids 320–360 of p53, making it one of the smallest oncogenic proteins known. Since this small domain of p53 will form oligomers with the wild type p53 protein it is reasonable to suggest that the transforming activity of the C terminal 'mini protein' is due to this activity.

Oligomerisation with the mini protein inactivates the transcription and DNA binding activity of wild type p53 protein. The C terminus contains multiple phosphorylation sites that are substrates for at least 3 kinases. These are a CK11 site at amino acid 392,[58] an as yet unidentified site for protein kinase C, and a site recognised by a member of the cdc2/cyclin kinase family at amino acid 315.[51,59] The C terminus also includes the sequences that target p53 for transport to the cell nucleus. The strongest of these sites is at amino acids 315–320 but other regions may also be involved. The last 28 amino acids of p53 act as a site of negative regulation of sequence specific DNA binding function of p53 and may also encode a non-specific DNA binding site.[23,38,44]

MUTATIONS OF THE p53 GENE IN HUMAN CANCERS

A large database has been created of the types of p53 mutation found in human tumours and the human germline. Over 2580 mutations have been studied yielding a wealth of information about both the potential nature of the mutagens involved in human neoplasia and the selective pressures placed on the p53 locus. Most are point missense mutations clustered in the central conserved DNA binding domain of the protein. Many different amino acids within this domain have been altered in individual tumours, and distinct hot spot mutations in certain tumour types. The spectrum of mutations found must depend both on the functional properties of the mutant protein (ie neutral mutations that do not affect function will not be scored); and within that constraint, on the effect of the relevant mutagens on the target DNA.[2] Thus the mutations found in p53 in skin tumours that arise in sun exposed skins are consistent with the types of mutations found in DNA after exposure to UV light.[60] These mutations are principally the consequence of the formation of pyrimidine dimers that characteristically produce tandem base changes, eg CC>TT. and are not produced by other mutagens. The mutations found in p53 in hepatocellular carcinomas from individuals exposed to aflatoxin in the diet are very different from those found in individuals who have the same tumour type but have not been exposed to that particular specific mutagen.[61,62] The aflatoxin-exposed individuals have a very high rate of a particular point mutation: a G:C > T:A

transversion at codon 249 AGG>AGT), replacing arginine with serine. This mutation is not particularly common in hepatocellular carcinomas of non exposed individuals. Since aflatoxin exposure is a great risk factor for the development of hepatocellular carcinoma, these results provide a direct connection between the environmental mutagen and the target gene in an important human cancer. This approach has in theory great potential to help in the identification of environmental carcinogens and risk factors, though it is clearly dependent on the specificity of each mutagen for particular sites within p53. More intense study of the types of p53 mutation found in populations exposed to known agents that dramatically increase risk might be very revealing. For example, a recent report identified a striking selectivity for a particular p53 mutation in the lung cancers of uranium miners exposed to high levels of radon in their lungs.[63]

The spectrum of mutations found in the p53 protein must also tell us about the selective pressure placed on the altered gene during the development of neoplasia. At a simple level, p53 clearly functions as a suppressor gene since complete ablation of its activity (as found in the p53 null mice) confers a profound predisposition to neoplasia. In most human tumours both copies of the normal p53 gene are inactivated. Commonly one allele is completely deleted; however, the other allele is often retained but mutated in a way that inactivates its normal function. One would expect, as indeed is found at other suppressor loci, that mutations that completely inactivated p53 such as deletions, promoter mutations, splice site mutations and premature stop codons would be very frequent, while point missense mutations would be rare. This is not the case, however, as the spectrum of mutations in the retained allele is in fact strongly biased in favour of point missense mutations. These mutations are clustered in the centre of the molecule and lead to the production of altered protein. This mutational spectrum is more consistent with the expressed mutant protein having some positive selective role to play in tumour progression, an idea consistent with and supported by the frequently very high levels of mutant p53 protein found in tumours.

What function might be selecting for this type of mutation? To answer this question we need to examine the biochemical and biological properties of mutant p53 proteins. Mutant p53 proteins are inactive as positive transcription factors acting at the wild type p53 consensus binding site.[27,64-66] The basis of this inactivity seems to be 2-fold. First, mutations in the central region of the molecule either reduce greatly or completely inactivate the ability of p53 to bind with sequence specificity to the consensus dsDNA binding site. This may occur either because key contact residues that interact with the DNA are altered, or in many cases because the conformation of the central region of the molecule

is altered. Indeed many of the mutant proteins appear to be temperature sensitive for sequence specific DNA binding, at least in vitro.[67] Secondly, there seems to be an effect of the DNA binding domain on the activity of the transcription transactivation domain. When full length wild type p53 protein is fused to the DNA binding domain of the Gal4 promoter, the hybrid protein acts as a potent transcription factor for genes containing Gal4 DNA binding sites. However, several point mutations in the p53 DNA binding domain block the activity of the hybrid protein. Since these proteins do not contain any mutations in the transactivating domain itself (which has been localised to the N terminal 42 amino acids of p53) we must assume that the block is due to an effect of the central region of the molecule on the activity of the N terminus. This idea is supported by the finding that a mutation at amino acid 273, which is known to occur commonly in human tumours and which has a relatively modest effect on the conformation of the central domain of the protein, does not affect the ability of the protein to act as a transcription factor when fused to Gal4. The mutation does, however, abolish the ability of p53 itself to suppress growth and to activate transcription from a p53 specific DNA binding element.[30] The ability of p53 to bind DNA seems therefore to have been strongly selected against in the mutations found in human cancer.

What functions are retained or gained by the mutant proteins? The most compelling is the ability of the mutant p53 proteins to promote cell transformation and tumourgenicity. This property has been measured by the ability of mutant, but not wild type, p53 proteins to complement other oncogenes in the transformation of cells in culture. Mutant p53 will cooperate efficiently with activated *ras* genes to transform primary rat cells and this has provided a powerful assay of mutant p53 function. The ability of mutant p53s to act in this manner is abolished by deletion of the C terminus of the molecule, and indeed (as discussed above) the isolated C terminus of the protein alone can act as a dominant transforming oncogene. This strongly suggests that the primary selection for the point mutations in p53 is the ability of such mutants to act as dominant negative mutants that act to neutralise the function of any wild type p53 molecules present in the cell. Support for this idea has come from an examination of the genetic changes associated with tumour progression in mice that contain either two copies of the p53 gene or a single copy of the gene. When two copies are present, point mutations are frequent, as they are in human tumours. In mice that are heterozygous at the p53 locus, however, the remaining wild type allele is often inactivated by complete loss of the gene rather than a point mutation. Is this dominant negative function of mutant p53 its only activity of importance in human cancer? Probably not, since when

the mutant p53 protein is expressed in cells that lack p53 completely, it can enhance their tumorgenicity;[68,69] and mutant p53, again in a null background, can promote the transcription of certain genes including the gene for multi drug resistance.[70] However, although these effects can be detected, it is difficult to assess their importance. A critical experiment will be to examine the growth response of p53 null cells to the levels of expression of a mutant p53 gene introduced under the control of a tightly regulated promoter.

Are p53 mutations dominant or recessive?

Transfection of a wild type p53 gene into many human tumour cells that are expressing an endogenous mutant p53 gene will suppress their growth. In this case the wild type phenotype is dominant. In contrast, transfection of a mutant p53 gene will, in cooperation with an activated *ras* gene, transform primary rodent cells that contain two wild type copies of the endogenous gene. In this case the mutant phenotype is dominant. These laboratory models suggest that the relative levels of expression of the wild type and mutant protein may have a decisive effect on gene function. The acute sensitivity of the p53 system to protein levels is underscored by the detectable differences in apoptotic phenotype of p53 heterozygous mice, compared to homozygous null or homozygous wild type mice. This issue is of great importance when considering the behaviour of Li-Fraumeni cells or tumour cells in which only one allele of p53 is mutant while the other allele is maintained. The analysis of tumours suggests that the mutant allele is not completely dominant, otherwise one would not expect to see the selection for loss of the remaining wild type allele that is such a common feature of human solid tumours. This idea is also supported by the relatively low cancer incidence and the cancer spectrum in Li-Fraumeni families compared to the heterozygous and homozygous p53 null mice. The tumour spectrum in the heterozygous mice closely reflects that seen in the Li-Fraumeni families; but that of the null mice, with its very early incidence and dominance of lymphoma (specifically thymoma), does not.[71] Loss of the wild type allele is seen in tumours in Li-Fraumeni individuals, again suggesting that the wild type allele is functioning even in the presence of a 'dominant negative' mutant allele. Given the dramatic increase in p53 protein seen after DNA damage it is tempting to speculate that there may be an inducible dominant negative phenotype in the Li-Fraumeni families, such that only under conditions of sufficient genetic stress is enough mutant protein produced to inactivate the product of the wild type allele.

REGULATION OF p53 PROTEIN FUNCTION

As discussed above, the p53 protein has an enormously powerful biological effect. It can kill cells. This function clearly must be tightly controlled so that it is only invoked under precisely the correct conditions. The principal stimulus to the p53 response so far identified is DNA damage. The response to that stimulus must be tightly regulated by the cell in which the damage occurs. The response will be defined by the growth state of the cell, its exposure to extracellular and intracellular survival factors, and its state of differentiation.

The biochemical activity of p53 is known to be controlled by its stability, by its association with other proteins and by covalent modification. The viral proteins SV40 large T antigen,[72] adenovirus E1b 55K protein,[73] and human papilloma virus E6[74] have all been clearly shown to bind to p53 and to inactivate its function as a specific transcription factor.[75,76] This seems to happen either by blockading the DNA binding domain of the protein or by blocking the transcription transactivation domain. Similarly, the cellular protein MDM2 has been shown to bind at or near the transcriptional activation domain and to block its function,[50] though it has been reported to interfere with DNA binding as well. In addition to these mechanisms of inactivation, the HPV E6 protein also acts to promote the rapid breakdown of p53 by specifically targeting its destruction through the ubiquitin pathway.[77]

Recent biochemical studies of the p53 protein have highlighted an internal allosteric regulatory pathway.[78-80] The wild type protein can exist in a latent non DNA binding form, which can be activated by modifications to the extreme C terminus (the last 30 amino acids) of the molecule remote from the DNA binding domain. The extreme C terminus encodes a negative regulatory domain since its simple removal activates the protein constitutively. This kind of self regulation is an increasingly common theme, being important for example in the regulation of protein kinases such as c-src. The C terminus can be modified by phosphorylation at the penultimate amino acid, and this induces a conformational change that activates the DNA binding function of the protein. This effect can also be achieved by the binding of antibody molecules within the C terminal regulatory domain.[78]

Finally, a critical control pathway regulates the stability of the p53 protein such that it is stable in the environment of a cell that has DNA damage, but is otherwise very unstable. The mechanism by which DNA damage is detected and transduced to the p53 degradation pathway is not yet understood.

EXPRESSION OF p53 PROTEIN IN HUMAN TUMOURS AND NORMAL TISSUE

Analysis of p53 mRNA levels suggest that the gene is expressed in all tissues of the body throughout development. Particularly high levels are seen in early embryonic development and in the testis of the adult.[81] As yet little work using *in situ* hybridisation has been reported, and so the local distribution of mRNA within tissues is not yet known. In contrast to this picture of ubiquitous expression seen at the mRNA level, attempts to detect the p53 protein in normal tissues using sensitive immunochemical methods have proved uniformly negative except recently in the case of testicular tissue, where low levels of p53 specific staining have been seen. The explanation for this discrepancy appears to lie in the very short half life of p53 protein in normal tissues. Thus the protein is being constantly produced but then very rapidly broken down so that its steady state level remains very low. Exposure to DNA damaging agents such as UV light or ionising radiation results in a dramatic local increase in p53 protein levels that is readily detected immunohistochemically.[82] The response differs between different tissues and cell locations, as is clearly seen in the intestinal epithelial cells of mice exposed to ionising radiation.[18] Dose dependency and cellular variation is also a feature of the p53 accumulation response noted in in vitro systems.[13] In contrast to this simple picture, striking accumulation of p53 protein is a common feature of many different human neoplasias. For example, it is found in about 50–60% of malignant lung cancers.[83] The effect can be compelling, with the cancer cells intensely stained in a background of unstained normal stroma.[84,85] In several tumour types, those tumours that express high levels of p53 show a significantly poorer survival than those that do not and, in some larger analyses, p53 staining has been shown to be an independent prognostic indicator.[86]

In most cases, tumours that accumulate high levels of p53 turn out to have lost one allele of the gene and are expressing only an allele bearing a point mutation.[83,87,88] So it is mutant p53 protein that is being detected by immunohistochemistry. The tight association between mutation and the accumulation of p53 leads to the simple hypothesis that the mutations are selected for the property of making the protein metabolically stable. Support for this idea comes from some tissue culture studies that suggest that the mutant or non DNA binding form of p53 has a longer half life than protein in the wild type conformation, in cells that are expressing molecules in both conformations. More recently, a number of examples have accumulated that suggest that this simple hypothesis is not completely correct. In model systems, several mutant p53 proteins are unstable in normal cells, like the wild type protein, but may accumulate in cells exposed to DNA damage.[89] Similarly, wild type protein does accumulate to levels readily detectable by immunohistochemistry following exposure of normal tissue to DNA damaging agents.[90] Likewise, the mutant p53 proteins made in the normal cells of Li-Fraumeni patients are unstable; but the same mutant proteins accumulate to high levels in tumour cells in these patients. Therefore mutation is neither sufficient nor necessary to result in p53 levels that can be detected immunohistochemically. This suggests that the environment of the tumour cell is related to that of the irradiated cell, perhaps due to strand breaks that occur in the segregation of aberrant chromosomes.[91] If wild type p53 is present and functioning in such a cell it will kill it or arrest it until the p53 stabilising signal is switched off. In the absence of wild type p53, the signal cannot be switched off, the defect is uncorrected, and the cellular environment results in the continued accumulation of the defective p53 protein. Such a model may better explain the variations seen in p53 expression in different lesions and the association with poor prognosis.

How does p53 work as a tumour suppressor?

The mechanism by which p53 acts as a tumour suppressor gene is understood in broad outline, namely that in response to genetic error p53 initiates a protective cell cycle arrest and apoptotic response. What is now of key interest is to determine how that response is effected. We have already discussed the mechanisms by which p53 activity is increased in cells in which genetic damage has taken place. The critical question then becomes how does p53 exert its suppressor function. The most persuasive current model is that p53 acts as a specific transcription factor to promote the expression of genes that will initiate the cell cycle arrest and cell death pathway. The rise in p53 levels associated with the DNA damage response or the action of transforming oncogenes like *myc* and *ras*[91] or EIa[21] leads to an increase in p53 specific transcription readily measured using reporter gene constructs. Among the cellular genes that have been identified that respond to p53 are the MDM2 gene discussed above[92] and the gadd 45 gene,[93] a gene first identified because of its enhanced expression associated with growth arrest and DNA damage.

Very recently, however, a particularly exciting p53 responsive gene has been identified.[28] This gene was the major p53 induced transcript detected in a system where increased levels of p53 protein and growth arrest were induced by a wild type p53 gene which had been placed under the regulated control of a hormone response element. The transcript encoded a protein called WAF-1, a 21 kD molecular weight protein which simultaneously and independently had been identified as a potent inhibitor of cyclin/cdc2 protein kinase which has a function in cell cycle control. At once this observation links p53 responsive genes directly to inhibition of the cell cycle. The WAF-1 gene itself is able to suppress cell growth though not quite as efficiently as wild type p53. Elevated levels of WAF-1 may be postulated to induce apoptosis as well as growth arrest since inappropriate regulation of the cell cycle is probably a good inducer of the apoptotic response. While the WAF-1 model is at the moment very attractive it is unlikely to be the whole answer to the activity of p53 as a suppressor. Other target genes may also be important and specific suppression of gene expression may play a part since deletion of the N terminal transactivation domain of p53 renders it only partially defective in inducing growth arrest.[53] Finally, it is still possible to speculate that the high levels of p53 may arrest growth by other means than transcriptional regulation. Inhibition of DNA helicase or the blocking of the binding of DNA polymerase to initiator proteins have both been proposed on the basis of the activity of p53 in viral DNA replication models. Determining the precise mechanism of suppression is clearly vital for the design of any therapeutics intended to restore p53 function to tumour cells.

FUTURE PROSPECTS

A number of separate features of the p53 system discussed above make it an attractive one for the development of novel treatments for human cancer. These include the frequency of p53 mutations in common cancers, the potent apoptosis inducing function of the wild type protein in tumour cells and the accumulation of potentially latently active mutant protein in many tumours. A wide variety of approaches are undergoing trial. These include attempts to: restore p53 function to tumour cells either by gene therapy or by the action of small molecules that will activate the latent transcriptional activity of some point mutant p53 proteins; find agents that will liberate p53 from inactivating partner proteins such as MDM2 in sarcomas and HPV E6 in HPV positive ano-genital neoplasias; to exploit mutant p53 as a tumour specific antigen. Cytotoxic T cells have been isolated that recognise mutant but not wild type p53 peptides when presented by Class 1 MHC molecules.[94] It is to be hoped that these approaches will be successful so that our increased understanding of gene function in cancer will bring benefit to the patient.

REFERENCES

1 Hollstein M, Sidransky D, Vogelstein B, Harris C. p53 mutations in human cancer. Science 1991; 253: 49–53.

2 Greenblatt MS, Bennett WP, Hollstein M, Harris C. Mutations in the p53 tumor suppressor gene: Clues to cancer etiology and molecular pathogensis. Cancer Res 1994 (In press).

3 Donehower LA, Harvey M, Slagle BL et al. Mice deficient for p53 are developmentally normal but susceptible to spontaneous tumours. Nature 1992; 356: 215–221.

4 Lane DP. p53, guardian of the genome. Nature 1992; 358: 15–16.

5 Lane DP. Cancer. A death in the life of p53. Nature 1993; 362: 786–787.

6 Malkin D. p53 and the Li-Fraumeni syndrome. Cancer Genet Cytogenet 1993; 66: 83–92.

7 Finlay CA, Hinds PW, Levine AJ. The p53 proto-oncogene can act as a suppressor of transformation. Cell 1989; 57: 1083–1093.

8 Casey G, Lohsueh M, Lopez ME, Vogelstein B, Stanbridge EJ. Growth suppression of human breast cancer cells by the introduction of a wild-type p53 gene. Oncogene 1991; 6: 1791.

9 Baker SJ, Markowitz S, Fearon ER, Willson JKV, Vogelstein B. Suppression of human colorectal carcinoma cell growth by wild-type p53. Science 1990; 249: 912–915.

10 Mercer WE, Shields MT, Lin D, Appella E, Ullrich SJ. Growth suppression induced by wild-type p53 protein is accompanied by selective down-regulation of proliferating-cell nuclear antigen expression. Proc Natl Acad Sci USA 1991; 88: 1958–1962.

11 Maltzman W, Czyzyk L. UV irradiation stimulates levels of p53 cellular tumor antigen in nontransformed mouse cells. Mol Cell Biol 1984; 4: 1689–1694.

12 Kastan MB, Onyekwere O, Sidransky D, Vogelstein B, Craig RW. Participation of p53 protein in the cellular response to DNA damage. Cancer Res 1991; 51: 6304–6311.

13 Lu X, Lane DP. Differential induction of transcriptionally active p53 following UV or ionising radiation; Defects in chromosome instability syndromes. Cell 1993; 75: 765–778.

14 Fritsche M, Haessler C, Brandner G. Induction of nuclear accumulation of the tumor-suppressor protein p53 by DNA-damaging agents. Oncogene 1993; 8: 307–318.

15 Kuerbitz SJ, Plunkett BS, Walsh WV, Kastan MB. Wild-type p53 is a cell cycle checkpoint determinant following irradiation. Proc Natl Acad Sci USA 1992; 89: 7491–7495.

16 Clarke AR, Purdie CA, Harrison DJ et al. Thymocyte apoptosis induced by p53-dependent and independent pathways. Nature 1993; 362: 849–852.

17 Lowe SW, Schmitt EM, Smith SW, Osborne BA, Jacks T. p53 is required for radiation-induced apoptosis in mouse thymocytes. Nature 1993; 362: 847–849.

18 Merritt AJ, Potten CS, Kemp CJ et al. The role of p53 in spontaneous and radiation-induced apoptosis in the gastrointestinal tract of normal and p53 deficient mice. Cancer Res 1994; 54: 614–617.

19 Vaux DL, Cory S, Adams JM. bcl-2 gene promotes haemopoietic cell survival and co-operates with c-myc to immortalise pre-B cells. Nature 1988; 335: 440–442.

20 Lowe SW, Ruley HE. Stabilization of the p53 tumor suppressor is induced by adenovirus 5 E1A and accompanies apoptosis. Genes Dev 1993; 7: 535–545.

21 Debbas M, White E. Wild-type p53 mediates apoptosis by E1A, which is inhibited by E1B. Genes Dev 1993; 7: 546–554.

22 Lowe SW, Ruley HE, Jacks T, Housman DE. p53 dependent apoptosis modulates the cytotoxicity of anti-cancer agents. Cell 1993; 74: 957–967.

23 Hupp TR, Meek DW, Midgley CA, Lane DP. Regulation of the specific DNA binding function of p53. Cell 1992; 71: 875–886.

24 Friedman PN, Chen X, Bargonetti J, Prives C. The p53 protein is an unusually shaped tetramer that binds directly to DNA. Proc Natl Acad Sci USA 1993; 90: 3319–3323.

25 Yewdell JW, Gannon JV, Lane DP. Monoclonal antibody analysis of p53 expression in normal and transformed cells. J Virol 1986; 59: 444–452.

26 Gannon JV, Greaves R, Iggo R, Lane DP. Activating mutations in p53 produce a common conformational effect. A monoclonal antibody specific for the mutant form. EMBO J 1990; 9: 1595–1602.

27 El-Deiry WS, Kern SE, Pietenpol JA, Kinzler KW, Vogelstein B. Definition of a consensus binding site for p53. Nature Genet 1992; 1: 45–49.

28 El-Deiry WS, Tokino T, Velculescu VE et al. WAF1, a potential mediator of p53 tumor suppression. Cell 1993; 75: 1–20.

29 Fields S, Jang SJ. Presence of a potent transcription activating sequence in the p53 protein. Science 1990; 249: 1046–1049.

30 Raycroft L, Wu HY, Lozano G. Transcriptional activation by wild type but not transforming mutants of the p53 anti-oncogene. Science 1990; 249: 1049–1051.

31 Oberosler P, Hloch P, Ramsperger U, Stahl H. p53-catalyzed annealing of complementary single-stranded nucleic acids. EMBO J 1993; 12: 2389–2396.

32 Ragimov N, Krauskopf A, Navot N, Rotter V, Oren M, Aloni Y. Wild-type but not mutant p53 can repress transcription initiation in vitro by interfering with the binding of basal transcription factors to the TATA motif. Oncogene 1993; 8: 1183–1193.

33 Michalovitz D, Halvey O, Oren M. Conditional inhibition of transformation and of cell proliferation by a temperature-sensitive mutant of p53. Cell 1990; 62: 671–680.

34 Yonish RE, Resnitzky D, Lotem J, Sachs L, Kimchi A, Oren M. Wild-type p53 induces apoptosis of myeloid leukaemic cells that is inhibited by interleukin-6. Nature 1991; 353: 345–347.

35 Livingstone LR, White A, Sprouse J, Livanos E, Jacks T, Tlsty TD. Altered cell cycle arrest and gene amplification potential accompany loss of wild type p53. Cell 1992; 70: 923–935.

36 Yin Y, Tainsky MA, Bischoff FZ, Strong LC, Wahl GM. Wild-type p53 restores cell cycle control and inhibits gene amplification in cells with mutant p53 alleles. Cell 1992; 70: 937–948.

37 Pavletich NP, Chambers KA, Pabo C. The DNA binding domain of p53 contains the four conserved regions and major mutation hot spots. Genes Dev 1993; 7: 2556–2564.

38 Wang Y, Reed M, Wang P et al. p53 domains: identification and characterization of two autonomous DNA binding regions. Genes Dev 1993; 7: 2575–2586.

39 Bargonetti J, Manfredi JJ, Chen X, Marshak D, Prives C. A proteolytic fragment from the central region of p53 has marked sequence specific DNA binding activity when generated from wild type but not from oncogenic mutant p53 protein. Genes Dev 1993; 7: 2565–2574.

40 Soussi T, Caron dFC, Sturzbecher HW, Ullrich S, Jenkins J, May P. Evolutionary conservation of the biochemical properties of p53: specific interaction of Xenopus laevis p53 with simian virus 40 large T antigen and mammalian heat shock proteins 70. J Virol 1989; 63: 3894–3901.

41 Soussi T, Caron de Fromentel C, May P. Structural aspects of the p53 protein in relation to gene evolution. Oncogene 1990; 5: 945–952.

42 Maxwell SA, Roth JA. Binding of cellular proteins to a conformational domain of tumor suppressor protein p53. Oncogene 1993; 8: 3421–3426.

43 Hainaut P, Milner J. A structural role for metal ions in the 'wild-type' conformation of the tumor suppressor protein p53. Cancer Res 1993; 53: 1739–1742.

44 Hupp TR, Meek DW, Midgley CA, Lane DP. Activation of the cryptic DNA binding function of mutant forms of p53. Nucleic Acids Res 1993; 21: 3167–3174.

45 Hainaut P, Milner J. Redox modulation of p53 conformation and sequence specific DNA binding function in vitro. Cancer Res 1993; 53: 4469–4473.

46 Gannon JV, Greaves R, Iggo R, Lane DP. Activating mutations in p53 produce a common conformational effect. A monoclonal antibody specific for the mutant form. EMBO J 1990; 9: 1595–1602.

47 Stephen CW, Lane DP. Mutant conformation of p53: precise epitope mapping using a filamentous phage epitope library. J Mol Biol 1992; 225: 577–583.

48 Halazonetis TD, Davis LJ, Kandil AN. Wild-type p53 adopts a 'mutant-like' conformation when bound to DNA. EMBO J 1993; 12: 1021–1028.

49 Kao CC, Yew PR, Berk AJ. Domains required for in vitro association between the Cellular p53 and the adenovirus 2 E1B 55K proteins. Virology 1990; 179: 806–814.

50 Oliner JD, Pietenpol JA, Thiagalingam S, Gyuris J, Kinzler KW, Vogelstein B. Oncoprotein MDM2 conceals the activation domain of tumour suppressor p53. Nature 1993; 362: 857–860.

51 Meek DW, Street AJ. Nuclear protein phosphorylation and growth control. Biochem J 1992; 287: 1–15.

52 Anderson CW, Lees MS. The nuclear serine/threonine protein kinase DNA-PK. Crit Rev Eukaryot Gene Expr 1992; 2: 283–314.

53 Unger T, Mietz JA, Scheffner M, Yee CL, Howley PM. Functional domains of wild-type and mutant p53 proteins involved in transcriptional regulation, transdominant inhibition, and transformation suppression. Mol Cell Biol 1993; 13: 5186–5194.

54 Schlichtholz B, Legros Y, Gillet D et al. The immune response to p53 in breast cancer patients is directed against immunodominant epitopes unrelated to the mutational hot spot. Cancer Res 1992; 52: 6380–6384.

55 Sturzbecher H-W, Brain R, Addison C et al. A C-terminal α-helix plus basic regions motif is the major structural determinant of p53 tetramerization. Oncogene 1992; 7: 1513–1523.

56 Shaulian E, Zauberman A, Ginsberg D, Oren M. Identification of a minimal transforming domain of p53: negative dominance through abrogation of sequence-specific DNA binding. Mol Cell Biol 1992; 12: 5581–5592.

57 Reed M, Wang Y, Mayr G, Anderson ME, Schwedes JF, Tegtmeyer P. p53 domains: suppression, transformation, and transactivation. Gene Expr 1993; 3: 95–107.

58 Meek DW, Simon S, Kikkawa U, Eckhart W. The p53 tumour suppressor protein is phosphorylated at serine 389 by casein kinase II. EMBO J 1990; 9: 3253–3260.

59 Bischoff JR, Friedman PN, Marshak DR, Prives C, Beach D. Human p53 is phosphorylated by p60-cdc2 and cyclin B-cdc2. Proc Natl Acad Sci USA 1990; 87: 4766–4770.

60 Brash DE, Rudolph JA, Simon JA et al. A role for sunlight in skin cancer: UV-induced p53 mutations in squamous cell carcinoma. Proc Natl Acad Sci USA 1991; 88: 10124–10128.

61 Hsu IC, Metcalf RA, Sun T, Welsh Ja, Wang NJ, Harris CC. Mutational hotspot in the p53 gene in human hepatocellular carcinomas. Nature 1991; 350: 427–428.

62 Bressac B, Kew M, Wands J, Ozturk M. Selective G to T mutations of p53 gene in hepatocellular carcinoma from southern Africa. Nature 1991; 350: 429–431.

63 Taylor JA, Watson MA, Devereux TR, Michels RY, Saccomanno G, Anderson M. p53 mutation hotspot in radon-associated lung cancer. Lancet 1994 Jan 8; 343 (8889): 86-87 Section A.

64 Vogelstein B, Kinzler KW. p53 function and dysfunction. Cell 1992; 70: 523–526.

65 Kern SE, Pietenpol JA, Thiagalingam S, Seymour A, Kinzler KW, Vogelstein B. Oncogenic forms of p53 inhibit p53 regulated gene expression. Science 1992; 256: 827–830.

66 Scharer E, Iggo R. Mammalian p53 can function as a transcription factor in yeast. Nucl Acids Res 1992; 20: 1539–1545.

67 Medcalf EA, Takahashi'T, Chiba I, Minna J, Milner J. Temperature-sensitive mutants of p53 associated with human carcinoma of the lung. Oncogene 1992; 7: 71–76.

68 Wolf D, Harris N, Goldfinger N, Rotter V. Reconstitution of p53 expression in nonproducer Ab-MuLV-transformed cell line by transfection of a functional p53 gene. Cell 1985; 38: 119–126.

69 Dittmer D, Pati S, Zambetti G et al. Gain of function mutations in p53. Nature Genet 1993; 4: 42–46.

70 Zastawny RL, Salvino R, Chen J, Benchimol S, Ling V. The core promoter region of the P-glycoprotein gene is sufficient to confer differential responsiveness to wild-type and mutant p53. Oncogene 1993; 8: 1529–1535.

71 Harvey M, McArthur MJ, Montgomery CA, Butel JS, Bradley A, Donehower LA. Spontaneous and carcinogen induced tumorigenesis in p53 -deficient mice. Nature Genet 1993; 5: 225–229.

72 Lane DP, Crawford LV. T-antigen is bound to host protein in SV40-transformed cells. Nature 1979; 278: 261–263.

73 Sarnow P, Ho YS, Williams J, Levine AJ. Adenovirus E1b-58kd tumor antigen and SV40 large tumor antigen are physically associated with the same 54Kd cellular protein in transformed cells. Cell 1982; 28: 387–394.

74 Werness BA, Levine AJ, Howley PM. Association of human papillomavirus types 16 and 18 E6 proteins with p53. Science 1990; 248: 76–79.

75 Mietz JA, Unger T, Huibregtse JM, Howley PM. The transcriptional transactivation function of wild-type p53 is inhibited by SV40 large T-antigen and by HPV-16 E6 oncoprotein. EMBO J 1992; 11: 5013–5020.

76 Berk AJ, Yew PR. Inhibition of p53 transactivation required for transformation by adenovirus early1B protein. Nature 1992; 357: 82–85.

77 Scheffner M, Werness BA, Hulbregtse JM, Levine AJ, Howley PM. The E6 oncoprotein encoded by human papillomavirus types 16 and 18 promotes the degradation of p53. Cell 1990; 63: 1129–1136.

78 Hupp TR, Meek DW, Midgley CA, Lane DP. Regulation of the specific DNA binding function of p53. Cell 1992; 71: 875–886.

79 Hupp TR, Meek DM, Midgley CA, Lane DP. Activation of the cryptic DNA binding function of mutant forms of p53. Nucl Acids Res 1993; 21: 3167–3174.

80 Halazonetis TD, Kandi AN. Coformational shifts propagate from the oligomerisation domain of p53 to its tetrameric DNA binding domain and restore DNA binding to select p53 mutants. EMBO J 1993; 12: 5057–5064.

81 Almon E, Goldfinger N, Kapon A, Schwartz D, Levine AJ, Rotter V. Testicular tissue-specific expression of the p53 suppressor gene. Dev Biol 1993; 156: 107–116.

82 Hall PA, McKee PH, Menage HD, Dover R, Lane DP. High levels of p53 protein in UV-irradiated normal human skin. Oncogene 1993; 8: 203–207.

83 Iggo R, Gatter K, Bartek J, Lane D, Harris AL. Increased expression of mutant forms of p53 oncogene in primary lung cancer. Lancet 1990; 335: 675–679.

84 Bartek J, Bartkova J, Vojtesek B et al. Aberrant expression of the p53 oncoprotein is a common feature of a wide spectrum of human malignancies. Oncogene 1991; 6: 1699–1703.

85 Midgley CA, Fisher CJ, Bartek J, Vojtesek B, Lane DP, Barnes DM. Analysis of p53 expression in human tumours: an antibody raised against human p53 expressed in E.coli. J Cell Sci 1992; 101: 183–189.

86 Thor AD, Yandell DW. Prognostic significance of p53 overexpression in node-negative breast carcinoma: preliminary studies support cautious optimism. J Natl Cancer Inst 1993; 85: 176–177.

87 Davidoff AM, Humphrey PA, Igelhart JD, Marks JR. Genetic basis for p53 overexpression in human breast cancer. Proc Natl Acad Sci USA 1991; 88: 5006–5010.

88 Marks JR, Davidoff AM, Kerns BJ et al. Overexpression and mutation of p53 in epithelial ovarian cancer. Cancer Res 1991; 51: 2979–2984.

89 Vojtesek B, Lane DP. Regulation of p53 protein expression in human breast cancer cell lines. J Cell Sci 1993, 105: 607–612.

90 Hall PA, McKee PH, Menage HLP, Dover R, Lane DP. High levels of p53 proteins in UV-irradiated normal human skin. Oncogene 1993; 8: 203–207.

91 Lu X, Park SH, Thompson TC, Lane DP. ras-Induced hyperplasia occurs with mutation of p53, but an activated ras and myc together can induce carcinoma without p53 mutation. Cell 1992; 70: 153–161.

92 Wu X, Bayle JH, Olson D, Levine AJ. The p53-mdm-2 autoregulatory feedback loop. Genes Dev 1993; 7: 1126–1132.

93 Kastan MB, Zhan Q, el DW et al. A mammalian cell cycle checkpoint pathway utilizing p53 and GADD45 is defective in ataxia-telangiectasia. Cell 1992; 71: 587–597.

94 Yanuck M, Carbone DP, Pendleton CD et al. A mutant p53 tumor suppressor protein is a target for peptide-induced CD8+ cytotoxic T-cells. Cancer Res 1993; 53: 3257–3261.

British Medical Bulletin (1994) Vol. 50, No. 3, pp. 600–623
© The British Council 1994

Genetics of paediatric solid tumours

J K Cowell
ICRF Oncology Group, Institute of Child Health, London, UK

The average child in the UK stands a 1:600 chance of developing a malignancy by the time they are 16 years of age,[1] which compares with the 1 in 5 adults who die of cancer. The tumours children develop are very different from those seen in adult life. Histologically they resemble their relatively undifferentiated, fetal counterparts rather than the fully differentiated structures seen at, or soon after birth. The genetic events responsible for initiating children's tumours, therefore, must occur during embryonic life and prevent normal differentiation. These cells are frozen in the undifferentiated state and the malignant phenotype eventually arises as a result of secondary changes. The acquisition of secondary events occurs at varying rates and accounts for the variation in the time of presentation of the tumour. Unlike the adult situation environmental factors have not been identified as common causes of genetic damage in children's tumours.

The 'two-hit' hypothesis[2] presented a unifying hypothesis for the development of children's cancers (also now applied to many adult tumours). With modification,[3] this theory suggests that mutation of both copies of a single gene are sufficient for the initiation of tumorigenesis. In hereditary cases the first (germline) mutation is present constitutionally and the second is a random event in a somatic cell. In non-hereditary cases a cell must acquire both mutations as the result of sequential sporadic events in the same cell during development. The possibility of this occurring by chance is small so these tumours are usually characterised by a single focus (in contrast to hereditary tumours, which are often multifocal), and a later age of onset than hereditary tumours. Because, in hereditary cases, not all of the cells carrying the predisposing mutation develop into tumours, the initial mutation must be recessive at the cellular level; hence these genes have been described as 'tumour suppressor genes' or 'recessive oncogenes'. In fact, since their normal function is to ensure that differentiation and signal transduction occurs in the appropriate cell type, tumours cannot establish. The second, sporadic event can be either an independent mutation or a duplication of the first mutation with loss of the normal gene. This second mechanism was demonstrated in patients who were constitutionally heterozygous for DNA markers around the predisposition locus. The tumours in these patients became homozygous at these loci.[4,5] This 'loss of heterozygosity' (LOH) could occur through a variety of mechanisms including whole chromosome loss, mitotic recombination or non-disjunction. It is now generally accepted that LOH 'exposes' a recessive mutation as a result of loss of the normal allele. In fact, LOH analysis has proved a powerful way of identifying chromosome loci which may be involved in tumorigenesis in a variety of different tumours. However, this approach will not identify all genes which may be implicated in tumorigenesis, since certain parts of the genome appear to carry genes which, if mutated, give cells a growth advantage without the need for loss of the remaining allele.

Genetic linkage analysis of human hereditary cancer on the other hand allows unequivocal identification of the chromosomal location of genes which predispose to tumorigenesis. The first tumour suppressor gene to be isolated was that predisposing to the childrens eye cancer, retinoblastoma (Rb). The study of this gene has established many of the precedents for the analysis and the cloning of other tumour suppressor genes and, as such, the Rb gene is held as the paradigm for a recessive oncogene.

RETINOBLASTOMA GENETICS

As the name implies, Rb is a tumour of retinal cells and, with only rare exceptions, affects children under the age of 5 years – the majority of tumours occurring before they are 2 years old. Individuals can present with Rb at birth, suggesting that the tumours have been growing since early fetal life. This view is supported by the histopathology of the tumour which demonstrates a relatively undifferentiated, embryonic-like organisation, implying an arrest in development of a retinal precursor cell.

Approximately 10% of patients have a prior family history where the tumour phenotype segregates as an autosomal dominant trait. The remaining 90% of retinblastomas occur apparently sporadically.[6] However, 40–50% of these apparently sporadic cases are bilaterally affected which indicates that they carry 'new' germ line mutations. Pedigree analysis shows that, in 10% of cases, individuals who inherit the mutant gene do not develop a tumour – so called 'incomplete penetrance' – so it is clearly only a predisposition to tumorigenesis, rather than the tumour itself, that is inherited. Since only one additional mutation is required in any of the susceptible retinal cells – and the chances of this are high – hereditary Rb is characterised by the presence of multiple tumours in both eyes. However, we know empirically that approximately 10–15% of families have unilaterally affected individuals and, therefore, some unilaterally affected, sporadic cases will carry a predisposing mutation although it is difficult to identify which ones. In our experience this group probably represents less than 5%. In some families, apparently unaffected individuals have been seen to have retinal scars which resemble successfully treated tumours. These have been described as benign tumours – retinomas – or as regressed tumours.

ISOLATION OF THE RB1 GENE

Approximately 3% of Rb patients carry constitutional heterozygous 13q14.3 deletions and show mental retardation and/or other developmental abnormalities and dysmorphic features.[7] Linkage analysis demonstrated that the gene responsible for the familial form of Rb was also in 13q14[8] and LOH was observed in approximately 70% of sporadic tumours[5] for the same region. The isolation of the RB gene followed conventional reverse genetics procedures.[9] The cDNA, 4.7 kb long, identifies structurally abnormal mRNAs in approximately 20% of Rb tumours.[9,10] The RB1 gene spans approximately 200 kb of genomic DNA and consists of 27 exons encoding 928 amino acids. Constitutional reciprocal translocations predisposing to Rb were shown to interrupt the RB1 gene.[11] The tissue distribution of expression of RB1, however, was slightly surprising, expression being relatively high in all tissues examined.[9] This was unexpected since the hypothesis was that this gene controls important aspects of the developing fetal retina. Reintroduction of RB1 into cell lines deficient for its function appears to be able to reverse the malignant phenotype further demonstrating the recessive nature of this gene.

Only 20% of tumours showed gross structural abnormalities of RB1, so clearly the majority of mutations were more subtle. Once the structure of the gene was established, and the sequence surrounding the 27 exons determined,[12] an exon-by-exon survey of the gene using PCR amplification was possible. Mutations can be divided into 3 broad classes; those affecting correct splicing of the gene (presumably resulting in exon deletions), small deletions and insertions (which invariably generate a premature stop codon downstream) and point mutations which generate stop codons directly.[13] Whatever the type of mutation, however, premature stop codons invariably resulted. It was also possible, in many cases, to show homozygous mutations in tumour cells;

confirming predictions suggested by the LOH studies. In other tumours two independent mutations were found in the two alleles of RB1. It appears that errors in DNA replication are responsible in the majority of cases.[13]

Although the number of mutations reported in Rb patients is still quite small,[13-16] there do not appear to be any 'hot-spots' within RB1. The most common type of point mutations are C → T transitions, 70% of which convert CGA-arginine codons to TGA-stop codons. We have since shown that, approximately 20% of hereditary cases of Rb carry C → T mutations in one of the 14 CGA[arg] codons which are present in the gene. Missense mutations appear to be less common, and to be associated with a 'low penetrance' phenotype.[17] It is tempting to speculate that the substitution of a single amino acid merely compromises the function of the protein and, unless the second mutation in the tumour precursor cell causes loss of RB1 function, duplication of the 'weak' mutation allows a sufficient functional Rb protein (pRB) to be produced, to avoid tumorigenesis. Sakai et al[18] also investigated low penetrance families and found mutations in recognition sequences for different transcription factors in the RB1 promoter region. Again the suggestion is that, as a result of these mutations, there is a quantitative decrease in transcription rather than complete inactivity of the gene. Sufficient pRB is produced that any phenotypic consequences are mild.

Patients carrying constitutional Rb gene mutations are at significant risk for the development of second, non-ocular tumours later in life.[19] These are usually osteosarcomas and soft tissue sarcomas. Both of these tumours have been shown to lose heterozygosity for markers on chromosome 13. The same classes of tumours also show frequent structural and transcriptional abnormalities of RB1, suggesting that it plays a role in the development of the malignant phenotype in these cells. Structural abnormalities are also commonly found in RB1 in breast cancer[20] and small cell lung carcinoma[21] tumour DNA. Other tumours show less frequent involvement.[22] RB1 mutations in these tissues may contribute to tumour progression rather than initiation since, in many cases, the frequency of tumours with RB1 mutations is relatively low.

CLINICAL APPLICATION OF THE IDENTIFICATION OF RB1

Tumours which are detected early are usually more easily treated than those which present late (although in retinoblastoma, exactly where the tumour arises in the eye is also important). Tumours left to develop in the eye will eventually metastasise, often down the optic nerve, and prognosis is very poor indeed. Since early diagnosis offers a better prognosis, all 'at risk' individuals are screened regularly during the first years of life.

The autosomal dominant mode of inheritance of predisposition to retinoblastoma makes genetic linkage analysis relatively straightforward. Studies in these families can identify unequivocally, which individuals are at risk of tumour development and which are not.[23] In virtually all families, carriers of the mutant gene can be identified. It is equally important to identify those who do not carry the mutant allele, since they and their children will not have to undergo repeated ophthalmological examination. Prediction by linkage analysis has also proved important in families where incomplete penetrance is observed.[24] More recently it has been possible to offer prenatal screening using chorionic villus sampling[25] and, so far, this has proved to be a very successful screening programme. For those patients with no family history of tumours direct sequence analysis of the gene will be required before genetic counselling is possible.

THE FUNCTION OF THE RB1 GENE

The fact that Rb tumours are relatively undifferentiated, histopathologically, suggests an arrest in development of a retinal precursor cell at an early stage. Therefore by inference it might appear that RB1 controls 'directly or indirectly' the transition from this immature precursor cell to a photoreceptor cell. However, analysis of the structure of the gene does not reveal any 'tell-tale' motifs implicating it as a regulator of transcription.

The first clues to the function of pRB came from the demonstration that it could bind to the 'early' proteins from certain dominantly transforming DNA tumour viruses, such as E1a from adenovirus, large-T-antigen (LT) from SV40 and the E7 protein from human papilloma virus.[26] All of the viral transforming proteins share conserved regions which are necessary for their transforming function. Mutations in these conserved regions, which prevent cellular transformation, also prevent binding to pRB. In resting cells, pRB is unphosphorylated, but as the cell moves into S-phase of the cell cycle, pRB becomes phosphorylated until the end of mitosis where it is dephosphorylated again.[27] This observation led to the suggestion that the unphosphorylated form of pRB promotes cell quiescence. LT binds specifically to the underphosphorylated form of pRB and LT-pRB complexes are found only in G1 when the underphosphorylated form of pRB is present. Therefore it appears that, by sequestering pRB from the cell during G1 the viral transforming proteins allow the cell to enter S-phase. The association of the viral early genes with pRB is almost certainly an *in vitro* phenomenon, since it is unlikely that fetal retinal cells have been infected with these viruses. Rather, this model system points to associations of pRB with other naturally occurring proteins; and indeed, it has emerged that pRB participates in the establishment of protein complexes which associate and dissociate during the cell cycle. The whole system appears to be regulated by the biochemical modification of the participants in these complexes, which determines their availability to join the complex.[28]

The E1a protein is thought to transform cells by altering the activity of cellular transcription factors. One such protein is E2F, which has been shown to be involved as a transcription regulator of several cellular genes.[29] Ordinarily E2F is complexed with specific cellular proteins which effectively suppress its function. E1a, however, can dissociate E2F from its protein complexes, releasing free E2F. To exert its transcriptional regulation E2F must form a stable complex with other proteins in order to bind to specific DNA sequences in the promotor regions of the genes it controls. The conserved regions of E1a facilitate E2F binding; the same regions are also responsible for binding pRB. It was not surprising, therefore, to find that pRB also forms complexes with E2F and that E1a can dissociate them. The E2F/pRB complex ordinarily dissociates near the G1 S boundary, before S phase, releasing free E2F. It is thought that this process involves other cell-cycle specific proteins, such as cyclins and kinases, which alter the phosphorylation status of pRB. The suggestion is that pRB can control the transcriptional activities of E2F by binding to it. Dissociation of this complex allows free E2F to activate responsive cellular promotors which contribute to the release of cells from their proliferative suppression.

The RB-1 gene is involved in a number of interactions in complex pathways leading to transcription regulation in the nucleus, the specifics of which have been described by Horowitz.[28] Several genes, such as *fos* and *myc*, which are supressed soon after the decision for a cell to divide, appear to be down-regulated by pRB; which may also mediate the effects of transforming growth factor-β in downregulating *myc*. Presumably, by blocking expression of these genes the cells are kept firmly in G0. Evidence is emerging to suggest that the effects of RB1 on transcription control may be cell-type dependent and its function in a given cell type may depend on the modulation of levels of other cell-specific transcription factors. If this is the case then this might also provide a mechanism for pRB in the regulation of differentiation in fetal retinal cells.

TRANSGENIC MOUSE STUDIES

Although mice do not naturally develop Rb it was a realistic expectation that disrupting the RB1 gene in mouse embryos would predispose them to Rb. Mice constitutionally heterozygous for an RB1 mutation, however, did not develop tumours in their lifetime. This was against Knudson's prediction since a random mutational event in the homologous normal gene would have been suspected to initiate tumorigenesis. Homozygous RB1 null (RB–/RB–) mice developed apparently normally up to 11 days, but died in utero 13–14 days of gestation. These mice did not have Rb or retinal defects, but instead showed abnormal development of the mid-brain and haematopoietic system. The homozygous RB–/RB– mice could be rescued by introducing the normal RB1 gene.[30] Clearly the RB1 gene is very important for normal development of mice but loss of RB1 function in mice does not appear to predispose to Rb. Remarkably, RB1 does not appear to be important for normal early development and is not crucial for normal cell division during this period in mice. When heterozygous mice were followed for longer periods they were shown to develop adenocarcinomas of the pituitary which is not one of the second tumours often seen in hereditary cases of Rb in man. These tumours showed loss of the normal RB1 allele. A more detailed examination of this system is required before these observations are fully understood.

RB SUMMARY

The RB1 gene has proved to be the model tumour suppressor gene. Inactivation of this gene alone leads to the development of a highly specific type of cancer and its less frequent involvement in other tumours explains the increased risk that mutant gene carriers have of these malignancies. Reintroduction of a wild-type gene into cells deficient for its function apparently reverses the malignant phenotype. Hereditary cases carry inactivating mutations and their tumours either become homozygous for these initial mutations or experience a different inactivating mutation in the homologous gene. This analysis allows prenatal identification of mutant gene carriers and makes risk assessment for hereditary cases straightforward.

The other children's cancers, however, do not conform precisely to the same marker.

WILMS' TUMOUR

Wilms' tumour (WT) is a malignancy of the developing kidney affecting approximately 1:10 000 children.[31] Although most Wilms' tumours are sporadic there is a low incidence (1%) of familial cases with an apparently autosomal dominant mode of inheritance and incomplete penetrance.[32] Based on an epidemiological study of age of onset and frequency of bilateral tumours in the population, Knudson and Strong[32] suggested that WT conformed to the two-hit hypothesis which they had already advanced for Rb. Individuals with aniridia (congenital absence of irises) are at significantly increased risk for the development of Wilms' tumours.[33] This observation was extended by Riccardi and coworkers, who showed that Wilms-aniridia (WA) patients often also had abnormal gonadal development (G) and mental retardation (R): the WAGR syndrome.[34,35] The vast majority of WAGR patients carry a constitutional heterozygous chromosome deletion involving chromosome region 11p13 suggesting that genes critical for the normal development of the iris, kidney and gonads are located there. Less than 1% of all WT patients have WAGR, however, and of those carrying 11p deletions only 50% of them develop tumours.[36] Presumably the second critical mutation is not acquired in these cases, thus demonstrating the recessive nature of the WT predisposition gene.

LOSS OF HETEROZYGOSITY

LOH studies for 11p markers involving large numbers of tumours only demonstrated allele loss in 15–20% of sporadic unilateral WT.[37–39] In the majority of these cases, although LOH was seen at 11p13, allele loss extended to include the distal region of 11p15. In some tumours LOH occurred exclusively in 11p15 suggesting the possibility of another Wilms' tumour suppressor gene on chromosome 11p. Although WT is often considered to result from germline mutation[32] there are very few examples of families with affected individuals in more than one generation. In the few multiple-case families which have been described, no evidence for linkage to chromosome 11 markers could be found either at 11p13 or 11p15.[40–42] It appears, therefore, that there may be yet a third, familial, WT gene not on chromosome 11. Accepting that LOH might identify its location; Maw et al[43] undertook a systematic survey of most of the chromosome arms and found allele loss on 16q in 20% of cases. Despite this, Huff et al[44] were unable to demonstrate linkage to chromosome 16 markers.

ISOLATION OF THE CHROMOSOME 11p13 GENE: WT1

Although there seems perhaps to be several genes implicated in the development of Wilms' tumour, only the one in 11p13 , WT1, has been isolated.[45,46] The WT1 gene encodes a 3.2 kb transcript occupying approximately 50 kb of genomic DNA which contains 10 exons. Two alternative splice sites have been recognised, giving rise to 4 distinct mRNAs, the function of which is poorly understood.[47] The last 4 exons of the gene encode 4 distinct zinc finger motifs of the Cys_2-His_2 type, characteristic of DNA-binding proteins which regulate transcription. The first 6 exons code for a proline-glutamine rich region which is also typically associated with transcription regulators. The structure of this gene alone, therefore, strongly supports a role for WT1 in the orchestration of the normal development of the kidney. Invasion of the nephrogenic blastema by the ureteric bud after about

6 weeks of normal development results in an inductive interaction between these 2 structures which causes the condensation of the blastemal
cells around the advancing nephrogenic tube, resulting in their differentiation into nephrons. As the nephrogenic tube advances and invades
the mesonephros a wave of differentiation proceeds through the developing kidney. An apparently premalignant stage of WT is described as
nephroblastomatosis, characterised by the persistence of foci of stem
cells in the kidney. Wilms' tumour occurs more frequently in kidneys
showing evidence of 'nephroblastomatosis', which is found in the kidneys of 90% of cases with unilateral tumours and 100% of cases with
bilateral tumours.[48] The transition from nephroblastomatosis to WT is
not a common event, however, since approximately 1% of fetal biopsies
show nephroblastomatosis but only 1:10 000 children develop tumours.

WT1 is expressed predominantly in cells undergoing the transition
from mesenchyme to epithelium; that is, during the differentiation of
the metanephric blastema to the nephrons, the formation of the mesothelium from the mesenchymal lining of the coelom and the production of
the sex cords from the mesenchyme of the primitive gonad. Expression
is also seen in the glomerular epithelium of the related mesonephros.
In tumours, expression is found in the mesonephric glomeruli and cells
approximating to these structures. Tumours which are predominantly
blastemal, or show epithelial differentiation, have higher levels of expression compared with those which are predominantly mesenchymal.[49]
Thus, WT1 expression is only found in the malignant counterparts of
the cells which express it during normal development. The presence of
WT1 expression in the genital ridge, fetal gonad and mesoderm is consistent with the fact that these tissues are derived from embryologically
adjacent tissue in the developing embryo,[50] and the observation that
sporadic and syndrome-associated WT are accompanied by an increased
frequency of abnormalities involving the genitourinary system.[51]. Thus,
WT1 has pleiotropic effects on the development of different tissues.

MUTATIONS OF WT1

The first reports of mutations in WT were large deletions encompassing
the WT1 gene.[45,46] A low resolution search for structural rearrangements of WT1 in Wilms' tumours using Southern blot analysis met
with limited success, with fewer than 1% of tumours having detectable
changes.[52–55] All of the mutations found in Wilms' tumours resulted in
the generation of premature stop codons and were either homozygous
or hemizygous in the tumours. It was assumed that the majority of
mutations in WT1 would be more subtle. Large surveys of WT1 in
Wilms' tumours, however, failed to confirm this.[56,57] Curiously, there
are examples of heterozygous mutations in tumours. Therefore, it is

possible that a mutant WT1 protein could interfere with the function of the normal protein in a dominant-negative fashion, as suggested for p53. Another possibility is that a heterozygous mutation may interact with a mutation in another gene elsewhere in the genome. Haber et al[58] for example, reported a heterozygous deletion in WT1 which resulted in the loss of the third zinc finger. Although the tumour was heterozygous for the WT1 mutation it was homozygous for the rest of chromosome 11. This suggests that another recessive mutation has been exposed on chromosome 11 and that the WT1 mutation occurred as a later event. The majority of mutations, so far, affect the zinc finger (ZF) region of the gene. However, it may be that these regions have been the most extensively studied or, more likely, that disruption of the ZF function is more effective in destroying WT1 function. Curiously, tumours showing LOH for 11p did not carry mutations in WT1[59] suggesting that another tumour suppressor gene lies elsewhere on the chromosome.

The disappointingly few tumours showing deletions/mutations in WT1 cast some doubt about its central role in tumorigenesis, although it may be that its function is influenced by other genes (see below). This led to the question, does the remaining allele in the tumour cells from WAGR patients undergo mutational inactivation during tumorigenesis? In our own survey of 3 such tumours[60,61] all 3 showed inactivating mutations in the remaining allele. One was a C → T point mutation; the others were small duplications, all of which led to the production of a premature stop codon downstream. Brown et al[62] reported a large deletion in the remaining allele in a tumour from a WAGR patient, which also generated a stop codon. Presumably, therefore, inactivation of the WT1 gene is an important event in these tumours, at least, although this is not the general observation in sporadic Wilms' tumours.

MODE OF ACTION OF WT1

The WT1 zinc finger motif was shown to have approximately 50% sequence homology with that of the early growth response (EGR) family of transcriptional activators.[63] The products of these genes are required to initiate changes in the expression of specific target genes required for entry into the cell cycle, or for the initiation of the differentiated phenotype. The WT1 consensus binding recognition sequence, GCGGGGGCG is found in the promoter region of genes which are recognised by EGR genes.[63] Madden et al[64] showed that, in transfection assays, WT1 can suppress the activity of promoters which contain this motif, including IGF2[65] and PDGF.[66] Furthermore, WT1 mutations destroy the DNA binding capacity of WT1.[63,67] It is the proline-glutamine rich region in the 5′ part of WT1 (exons 1–6) which is responsible for repressing gene activity,[68] the zinc finger (ZF) motif serving only to bind DNA. Although the exact function of WT1 is not known, it is the only member of the EGR1 family of proteins which can suppress gene activity and one suggestion is that it does so as an antagonist, possibly by occupying the EGR1 site.[63,69] By inhibiting cell proliferation, a tissue specific programme of gene expression might be inherited which results in differentiation.

DENYS-DRASH SYNDROME

The observation that patients with 11p13 deletions also have abnormal genito-urinary (GU) development suggested that a gene important in the development of the gonads was located in this region. Denys-Drash syndrome (DDS) is a rare condition defined by the presence of characteristic kidney lesions, leading to progressive renal failure, and GU abnormalities which often manifest as male pseudohermaphroditism.[70,71] DDS patients are also predisposed to the development of WT. The nephropathy (mesangial sclerosis) may be associated with either genital abnormalities or WT; some have all 3 phenotypes.[72] Those DDS patients who develop WT usually have bilateral tumours, with an earlier age of onset than sporadic tumours, suggesting a genetic predisposition. The observation that one DDS patient also carried a constitutional 11p13 deletion[73] suggested that WT1 may be involved. Furthermore, in our study, one tumour from a DDS patient showed LOH for 11p.[39] In this tumour we found a homozygous mutation in WT1.[61] Pelletier and colleagues[55,67]showed that all DDS patients, in fact, carry constitutional mutations in WT1 which mostly involved 2 particular nucelotides in exons 8 and 9. Since then, mutations have been found in other exons[74,75] but the majority are still in exons 8 and 9.[76] The most common mutation, which occurs in over 50% of cases, converts an arginine amino acid to a tryptophan at position 394. Thus, DDS patients predominantly carry missense mutations, which is in contrast to those seen in WT. There has been much speculation as to how the amino acid changes seen in DDS cause the abnormal development of the kidney and gonads. The majority of mutations affect the zinc finger DNA binding domain of the WT1 protein which presumably affects its ability to regulate the expression of other genes. During development it is the cells which express this gene at the highest levels (glomerular epithelial cells) which are the precursors of the aberrant structures seen in the nephropathy which demonstrates the central role of WT1 in the differentiation in these cells.

It is clear that the WT1 mutations seen in DDS patients have a more profound effect than simply reducing gene expression as a result of inactivation. In WAGR patients, for example, the associated developmental abnormalities are generally less severe than those seen in DDS.

It has been suggested[67] that, as a result of mutation, the major disruption of the genital system is due to a gain of gene function which has a more profound effect than loss of function. Whether this gain of function allows the WT1 protein to bind to new sites, and affect transcription of other genes in the developmental pathway, is still not clear. WAGR patients clearly do not develop nephropathy and the associated GU abnormalites are usually cryptorchidism (undescended testes) or hypospadias (misplaced urethra). Thus, the renal system seems more tolerant to reduced WT1 expression during embryogenesis than the genital system. Loss of function, however, may play some role in the development of WT, since the majority of tumours from DDS patients undergo LOH.

Similarly, the expression of WT1 in cells in the developing gonads correlates well with the disordered differentiation in DDS patients. DDS patients have both Mullerian and Wolffian structures, implying that WT1 may play a key role in primary sex determination. The signals for the regression of the Mullerian ducts and development of the Wolffian structures are not present during development in DDS patients with 46XY karyotypes and their phenotypes range from streak gonads to the absence of Mullerian and Wolffian structures. Because individuals carrying the same mutation in WT1 have different phenotypes this possibly suggests that the gene product interacts with other differentiation factors which can modify the phenotype.

BECKWITH-WIEDEMANN SYNDROME

In 1963 Beckwith and Wiedemann independently described a rare congenital disorder, characterised by an excess growth of tissues and organs, which resulted in organomegaly, hemihypertrophy and a predisposition to the development of intra abdominal tumours.[77,78] The most common tumour was WT but adrenocortical carcinoma (ACC), embryonal rhabdomyosarcoma, hepatoblastoma and pancreatoblastoma were also common.[79] Interestingly, sporadic cases of these tumours showed LOH for 11p markers implicating the same genes responsible for WT in tumorigenesis in these tissues. In rhabdomyosarcoma the critical region for LOH was 11p15.5.[80] Although the majority of BWS cases are sporadic, up to 15% show evidence of an inherited predisposition with apparently autosomal dominant expression, low penetrance and variable expressivity.[81] Genetic linkage analysis demonstrated that the BWS locus is in 11p15.[82,83] On rare occasions,[84,85] BWS patients carried constitutional abnormalities involving the short arm of chromosome 11 which were frequently duplications of the 11p15 region which contains the growth promoting genes insulin and IGF2. However, as more reports emerged, it became clear that constitutional chromosome translocations were also found in BWS patients the breakpoints of which were always in 11p15. It appears, therefore, that an as yet unidentified gene in 11p15 is important for the BWS phenotype, but whether this is the same gene involved in the development of a variety of childrens cancers is not clear.

GENOMIC IMPRINTING

Gene function can be modified through mechanisms other than mutation. Genomic imprinting, which is described as a gamete-specific modification causing differential expression of the 2 alleles of a gene, can also be responsible.[86] In tumours showing LOH for 11p markers it was always the paternal chromosome which is retained[87] and in WAGR patients the deletion chromosome is always derived from the paternal germline.[54] Furthermore, 11p15 duplications in BWS patients were always paternal. The preferential loss of 11p alleles was also found in embryonic rhabdomyosarcoma[80] which is one of the tumour types seen associated with BWS. This is suggested to reflect tissue-specific imprinting of the 11p15.5 region. In the mouse the equivalent chromosome region to 11p15.5 also shows this phenomenon.[88,89] The assumption is that imprinting inactives one allele and then LOH removes the functioning allele, although there are complications with this simple interpretation.[90]

The insulin-like growth factors are the most potent mitogenic factors for kidney cells in culture. High levels of IGF2 have been demonstrated in the developing embryonic kidney[91] but only low levels are seen in the fully differentiated tissue. High IGF2 levels are also seen in WT which may simply reflect its undifferentiated, embryonic nature. Most of the IGF2 function is initiated by binding to the IGF1 receptor (IGF1R) which is a transmembrane tyrosine kinase. The promoter region of the IGF1R gene contains numerous potential binding sites for WT1. Werner et al[92] showed that the mRNA levels for the WT1 and IGF1R genes were inversely correlated, suggesting that WT1 may be a negative regulator of IGF1R. The suggestion is that, by mutating WT1, increased expression of IGF1R results which, in turn, promotes cell growth. By activating WT1 expression during normal kidney differentiation the growth potential of the cells will be reduced and differentiation ensues. How this mechanism might lead to tumorigenesis is not clear since the WT1 gene is apparently normal in the vast majority of WT[57,76] so IGF1R regulation should also be normal.

Two genes, H19 (whose function is not known) and IGF2, which map to the 11p15 region in humans, undergo reciprocal imprinting in mice with maternal expression of H19 and paternal expression of IGF2. The same was shown to be true for the homologous human genes.[93,94] When WTs which had not undergone LOH at 11p15 were analysed,

70% showed biallelic expression of one or both genes. This observation suggested that relaxation of imprinting is a new epigenetic mutational mechanism and that loss of imprinting is equivalent to the uniparental disomy seen in BWS where 2 doses of the IGF2 gene are expressed. Because transgenic mice lacking a functional paternal IGF2 gene are growth retarded, IGF2 has been proposed as a candidate for the BWS gene. The IGF2 gene, however, is unlikely to be the tumour suppresser gene located in 11p15, since it maps outside the region which can suppress malignancy[95] and is some distance from the breakpoints in the constitutional translocations predisposing some patients to BWS.

RELATIONSHIP WITH p53

When the WT1 gene was transfected into immortalised rat kidney cells, coprecipitation experiments identified a protein complex containing the gene products from the WT1 and p53 genes.[96] The presence of wild-type WT1 (but not mutant) appears to enhance transcriptional activation by p53, whereas wild-type p53 (but not mutant) appears to convert WT1 from being a transcriptional activator to being a transcriptional repressor. WT1 normally represses EGR and IGF2 genes, but in cells lacking p53 the EGR site could be activated by WT1. Transcriptional repression by WT1 appears to require interaction with other proteins including p53. We recently showed that the p53 gene was often stabilised in WT: a finding which usually indicates the presence of a mutant p53 gene.[97] This observation supports the suggestion that, in tumour cells lacking normal p53 function, WT1 is free to activate genes responsible for promoting cellular proliferation.

TRANSGENIC MICE

The importance of WT1 in normal development was demonstrated by generating mice deficient for WT1 function.[98] Mice with constitutional homozygous mutations died in utero after 13–15 days. Heterozygous mice, on the other hand, developed normally and did not develop tumours later in life. In the double mutant, although the Wolffian ducts were present, the ureteric bud did not develop. Although the metanephric blastema formed, there was evidence of increased apoptosis – although the surviving cells appeared normal. In in vitro assays, however, the blastema could not be induced to differentiate by the spinal cord which is usually the most potent inducer of differentiation. Thus, the kidneys fail to develop because of the absence of the ureteric bud. It appears, therefore, that ureteric outgrowth is dependent on a signal from the blastema and that WT1 is required for the generation of that signal. As suggested by the observations in DDS patients, the gonads failed to develop in mutant mice. Since death by renal failure usually only occurs at birth it seemed unlikely that this was the cause of death in the homozygous mutant mice. Post mortem analysis showed that there was also a failure of the heart to develop properly as well as the diaphragm and pleural tissues which are the most likely cause of death. These observations demonstrate that WT1 is important in maintaining the integrity of the mesothelium. The multiple developmental abnormalities seen in these mice reflect the tissues where WT1 is most prominently expressed.

WT SUMMARY

The cloning of the WT1 gene represented an early success for the positional cloning strategy of isolating genes which lie in defined chromosome regions. The fact that development of tumours does not always occur in patients carrying mutations in WT1 suggests this gene may not, after all, play a fundamental role in tumorigenesis. Rather, it appears that this gene is more likely involved in the control of fundamental events in embryonic development of a series of tissues and organs including the kidney and gonads. This suggestion was confirmed in transgenic mouse studies. However, as a result of the careful analysis of phenotypic abnormalities associated with WT predisposition, in combination with cytogenetic and genetic analysis, the presence of other genes important in tumour predisposition has been realised, and a few possible locations for these genes suggested.

NEUROBLASTOMA

Neuroblastoma (Nb) is the commonest single solid malignancy of childhood, accounting for 8% of all paediatric cancer. It is a tumour of the postganglionic sympathetic nervous system arising in the adrenal glands or the paraspinal ganglia of the sympathetic chain. Histologically it resembles fetal adrenal tissue and shares immunological markers with these early cells. Its clinical behaviour is curious as, on the one hand, it may show spontaneous resolution or differentiation into benign ganglioneuroma (especially in the dramatic stage 4S disease) and, on the other hand, it can be a highly malignant tumour, fatal in 80% of cases in spite of intensive multimodality treatment (stage 4 disease).

Knudson suggested that, as in retinoblastoma, 2 genetic hits with the loss of function of 2 critical alleles was important.[99] However, as in Wilms' tumour, the number of familial cases is small.[100] No complex phenotype is associated with Nb, but analysis of tumour karyotype shows frequent deletion of the short arm (1p) of chromosome 1.[101] This is only suggestive of a role for a 1p gene in predisposition, since abnormalities of tumour karyotype show the genetic events associated with progression as well as tumour initiation. Loss of heterozygosity studies also point to the short arm of chromosome 1 as the site of a critical gene in Nb with the frequency of loss of alleles in tumours varying from 28%[102] to 90%.[103] Other groups, however, have shown LOH on chromosome 14[104] and so the picture is not conclusive. There are also too few families with live, affected members suitable for linkage studies. Constitutional chromosome translocations have been reported in patients with Nb[105-107] and analysis of the breakpoints may well be the best chance of identifying the Nb tumour suppressor gene.

It is not only tumour suppressor genes that are important in paediatric malignancy. Dominantly acting oncogenes are also involved, and the role of Nmyc in Nb development has been well documented. Amplification of this oncogene, defined as greater than 3 copies per haploid genome (though often many hundred copies are present), is associated with rapid tumour progression and is a better predictor of bad outcome than surgical stage.[108] The amplified 'units' of Nmyc either insert themselves 'en bloc' into chromosomes forming homogeneously staining regions or exist independently in the nucleus as double minute chromosomes.[109] The function of the Nmyc gene product is unclear, though its nuclear location and ability to bind DNA suggest it may have a regulatory rather than a structural role. Preliminary evidence suggests that, if cells over-expressing Nmyc are treated with Nmyc 'antisense' RNA, the expression of Nmyc is blocked and the cells grow less quickly in tissue culture. Nmyc, therefore, seems to have an important effect on the control of cell division. Furthermore, treating Nb cells in tissue culture with retinoic acid causes Nmyc expression to fall and this fall precedes differentiation of the tumour cells to a more normal phenotype. This differentiation is not complete, as a sub-population of cells seem to 'escape' and start to divide rapidly. Nmyc expression in these cells returns to the high levels seen before retinoic acid treatment. Partial responses can also be obtained in vivo by treatment with retinoic acid and a clinical trial to evaluate its role in differentiating residual disease after therapy is underway.

40% of aggressive, metastatic neuroblastomas do not show Nmyc amplification; but alternative mechanisms may exist to raise the protein levels in the cell. A few tumours may overexpress Nmyc mRNA even though the copy number of the gene is normal.[108] One case has been recorded where the Nmyc protein product has increased stability, although gene copy number and mRNA expression levels are normal.[110] Despite these observations, the inescapable fact is that Nmyc is not inevitably involved in Nb and, hence, is more likely to be associated with disease progression than initiation of tumorigenesis.

RHABDOMYOSARCOMA

Rhabdomyosarcoma (RMS) is a malignant solid tumour arising from primitive mesenchyme that has shown some evidence of maturation into striated muscle. It is the most common soft tissue sarcoma in children less than 5 years of age and accounts for around 5% of cases of childhood cancer. Precise details of the histological classification of RMS are fiercely debated but it can be divided into 2 broad groups: alveolar (said to resemble normal lung parenchyma) which affects the trunk or extremities of older children, and embryonal (resembling immature muscle cells) which affects the head, neck and genitourinary systems of infants. The embryonal type is further subdivided into: (a) solid, growing within non-mucosal tissues; and (b) botryoid, which is more loosely arranged, covered with mucosa and often resembling a bunch of grapes when arising near a hollow viscus.

No constitutional chromosome translocations have been found in RMS patients[111] but alveolar RMS is characterised by a t(2:13)(q35:q14) translocation in tumour cells. Other translocations have been described, such as t(2:5) and t(2:8), where the invariable breakpoint is in 2q35 suggesting the critical gene lies here. However, other cases with alveolar RMS have been reported with t(1:13) or t(8:13) translocations and here 13q14 is the consistent breakpoint. Indeed these observations may have clinical relevance because, although tumours with t(1:13)(p36.1:q14) or t(8:13)(p21:q14) translocations have alveolar histology and extremity disease, they tend to occur in much younger children than those with the usual t(2:13) change.[112] Molecular analysis of the (2:13) rearrangement demonstrates that the PAX3 gene on chromosome 2 is interrupted by the translocation.[113] A chaemeric transcript is produced as a result of this rearrangement possibly producing a protein with novel properties. The PAX family of genes are implicated in the trancriptional control of genes important in development.[114] PAX3 is also implicated in the development of Waardenburg Syndrome which is characterised by deafness and pigmentary disturbances. Thus, inactivation of a single gene appears to be responsible for the generation of very different phenotypes suggesting it is the generation of a new transcript which is important.

Patients with BWS are at increased risk for the development of embryonal RMS as well as for two other embryonal tumours, hepatoblastoma and Wilms. All of these tumours occasionally show loss of heterozygosity for 11p15 markers. No RMS tumours have both LOH for 11p15 and (2:13) translocations, suggesting a different origin for the two histological subtypes. Rearrangements of these genes have not, as yet, been found in either constitutional or tumour DNA from BWS patients.

EWING'S SARCOMA AND PERIPHERAL NEURO-EPITHELIOMA

Ewings sarcoma (ES) is the second most common malignant bone tumour of childhood, accounting for about 1% of childhood malignancy. It affects mainly the axial skeleton. It occurs most frequently in the early to mid portion of the second decade of life and its most striking epidemiological feature is its extreme rarity in Africans and Chinese. Unlike many of the tumours noted above, ES has not been associated with any known congenital syndromes, though skeletal and genito-urinary malformations are occasionally seen. No constitutional chromosome abnormalities have been identified but a reciprocal translocation, t(11:22)(q24:q12), is consistently found in 83% of tumours.[115] The cell of origin of ES is unknown but the same translocation is seen in peripheral neuro-epithelioma (PN), a rare and aggressive malignancy of neural origin.[116] PN also arises in the extremities, chest and pelvis and, although the 2 tumours are structurally distinct, shares the ethnic distribution of ES.

The (11:22) breakpoint was cloned recently[117] and it was possible to show that the breakpoint on 22 was present in all tumours regardless of karyotype. Delattre et al[118] showed that the translocation generates a hybrid transcript from which the chimeric protein initiated from chromosome 22 is expressed. This rearrangement appears to deregulate the expression of human fli-1, which affects its ability to regulate other genes in the cell which, in turn, contributes to the development of the malignant phenotype.

REFERENCES

1   Draper GJ, Birch JM, Bithell JF et al. Childhood cancer in Britain: incidence, survival and mortality. Studies on Medical and Population Subjects. London: HMSO, 1982: 37.
2   Knudson AG. Mutation and cancer: statistical study of retinoblastoma. Proc Natl Acad Sci USA 1971; 68: 820–823.
3   Comings DE. A general theory of carcinogenesis. Proc Natl Acad Sci USA 1973; 70: 3324–3328.
4   Godbout R, Dryja TP, Squire J, Gallie BL, Phillips RA. Somatic inactivation of genes on chromosome 13 is a common event in retinoblastoma. Nature 1983; 304: 451–453.
5   Cavenee WK, Dryja TP, Phillips RA et al. Expression of recessive alleles by chromosomal mechanisms in retinoblastoma. Nature 1983; 305: 779–784.
6   Vogel F. Genetics of retinoblastoma. Hum Genet 1979; 52: 1–54.
7   Cowell JK, Hungerford J, Rutland P, Jay M. Genetic and cytogenetic analysis of patients showing reduced esterase-D levels and mental retardation from a survey of 500 individuals with retinoblastoma. Ophthalmic Paediatr Genet 1989; 10: 117–127.
8   Sparkes RS, Murphree AL, Lingua RW et al. Gene for hereditary retinoblastoma assigned to human chromosome 13 by linkage to esterase-D. Science 1983; 219: 971–973.
9   Friend SH, Bernards R, Rogelj S et al. A human DNA segment with properties of the gene that predisposes to retinoblastoma and osteosarcoma. Nature 1986; 323: 643–646.

10   Goddard AD, Balakier H, Canton M et al. Infrequent genomic rearrangement and normal expression of the putative RB1 gene in retinoblastoma tumours. Mol Cell Biol 1988; 8: 2082–2088.

11   Mitchell CD, Cowell JK. Predisposition to retinoblastoma due to a translocation within the 4.7R locus. Oncogene 1989; 4: 253–257.

12   McGee TL, Yandell DW, Dryja TP. Structure and partial genomic sequence of the human retinoblastoma susceptibility gene. Gene 1989; 80: 119–128.

13   Hogg A, Bia B, Onadim Z, Cowell JK. Molecular mechanisms of oncogenic mutations in tumours from patients with bilateral and unilateral retinoblastoma. Proc Natl Acad Sci USA 1993; 90: 7351–7355.

14   Yandell DW, Campbell TA, Dayton SH et al. Oncogenic point mutations in the human retinoblastoma gene: their application to genetic counselling. N Engl J Med 1989; 321: 1689–1695.

15   Dunn JM, Phillips RA, Zhu X, Becker A, Gallie BL. Mutations in the RB1 gene and their effects on transcription. Mol Cell Biol 1989; 9: 4596–4604.

16   Blanquet V, Turleau C, Gross M-S, Goossens M, Besmond C. Identification of germline mutations in the RB1 gene by denaturant gradient gel electrophoresis and polymerase chain reaction direct sequencing. Hum Mol Genet 1993; 2(7): 975–979.

17   Onadim Z, Hogg A, Baird PN, Cowell JK. Oncogenic point mutations in exon 20 of the RB1 gene in families showing incomplete penetrance and mild expression of the retinoblastoma phenotype. Proc Natl Acad Sci USA 1992; 89: 6177–6181.

18   Sakai T, Ohtani N, McGee TL, Robbins PD, Dryja TP. Oncogenic germ-line mutations in Sp1 and ATF sites in the human retinoblastoma gene. Nature 1991; 353: 83–86.

19   Draper GJ, Sanders BM, Brownbill PA, Hawkins MM. Patterns of risk of hereditary retinoblastoma and applications to genetic counselling. Br J Cancer 1992; 66: 211–219.

20   T'Ang A, Varley JM, Chakraborty S, Murphree AL, Fung Y-KT. Structural rearrangement of the retinoblastoma gene in human breast carcinoma. Science 1988; 242: 263–266.

21   Harbour JW, Lai S-L, Whang-Peng J, Gazdar AF, Minna JD, Kaye FJ. Abnormalities in structure and expression of the human retinoblastoma gene in SCLC. Science 1988; 241: 353–357.

22   Horowitz JM, Park S-H, Bogenmann E et al. Frequent inactivation of the retinoblastoma anti-oncogene is restricted to a subset of human tumour cells. Proc Natl Acad Sci USA 1990; 87: 2775–2779.

23   Onadim ZO, Mitchell CD, Rutland PC et al. Application of intragenic DNA probes in prenatal screening for retinoblastoma gene carriers in the United Kingdom. Arch Dis Child 1990; 65: 651–656.

24   Onadim Z, Hykin PG, Hungerford JL, Cowell JK. Genetic counselling in retinoblastoma: importance of ocular fundus examination of first degree relatives and linkage analysis. Br J Ophthalmol 1991; 75: 147–150.

25   Onadim Z, Hungerford J, Cowell JK. Follow-up of retinoblastoma patients having prenatal and perinatal predictions for mutant gene carrier status using intragenic polymorphic probes from the RB1 gene. Br J Cancer 1992; 65: 711–716.

26   Weinberg RA. Tumour suppressor genes. Science 1991; 254: 1138–1146.

27   Mihara K, Cao X-R, Yen A et al. Cell cycle-dependent regulation of phosphorylation of the human retinoblastoma gene product. Science 1989; 246: 1300–1303.

28   Horowitz JM. Regulation of transcription by the retinoblastoma protein. Genes, Chromosom Cancer 1993; 6: 124–131.

29   Nevins JR. Transcriptional activation by viral regulatory proteins. TIBS 1991; 1991: 435–439.

30   Lee EY-HP, Chang C-Y, Hu N et al. Mice deficient for Rb are nonviable and show defects in neurogenesis and haematopoiesis. Nature 1992; 359: 288–294.

31   Matsunaga E. Genetics of Wilms' tumour. Hum Genet 1981; 57: 231–246.

32   Knudson AG, Strong LC. Mutation and cancer: a model for Wilms' tumour of the kidney. J Natl Cancer Inst 1972; 48: 313–324.

33 Miller RW, Fraumeni JR, Manning MD. Association of Wilms' tumour with aniridia, hemihypertrophy, and other congenital malformations. N Engl J Med 1964; 270: 922–927.

34 Francke U, Holmes LB, Atkins L, Riccardi VM. Aniridia-Wilms' tumour association; evidence for specific deletion of 11p13. Cytogenet. Cell Genet 1979; 24: 185–192.

35 Riccardi VM, Sujansky E, Smith AC, Francke U. Chromosome imbalance in the aniridia-Wilms' tumour association: 11p interstitial deletion. Pediatrics 1978; 61: 604–610.

36 Narahara K, Kikkawa K, Kimira S et al. Regional mapping of catalase and Wilms' tumour, aniridia, genitourinary abnormalities, and mental retardation triad loci to the chromosome segment 11p1305-p1306. Hum Genet 1984; 66: 181–185.

37 Coppes MJ, Bonetta L, Huang A et al. Loss of heterozygosity mapping in Wilms tumour indicates the involvement of three distinct regions and a limited role for nondisjunction or mitotic recombination. Genes Chromosom Cancer 1992; 5: 326–334.

38 Mannens M, Slater RM, Heytig C et al. Molecular nature of genetic changes resulting in loss of heterozygosity of chromosome 11 in Wilms' tumours. Hum Genet 1988; 81: 41–48.

39 Wadey RB, Pal NP, Buckle B, Yeomans E, Pritchard J, Cowell JK. Loss of heterozygosity in Wilms' tumour involves two distinct regions of chromosome 11. Oncogene 1990; 5: 901–907.

40 Grundy P, Koufos A, Morgan K, Li FP, Meadows AT, Cavenee WK. Familial predisposition to Wilms' tumour does not map to the short arm of chromosome 11. Nature 1988; 336: 375–376.

41 Huff V, Compton DA, Chao L-Y, Strong LC, Geiser CF, Saunders GF. Lack of linkage of familial Wilms' tumour to chromosomal band 11p13. Nature 1988; 336: 377–378.

42 Schwartz CE, Haber DA, Stanton VP, Strong LC, Skolnick MH, Housman DE. Familial predisposition to Wilms' tumour does not segregate with the WT1 gene. Genomics 1991; 10: 927–930.

43 Maw MA, Grundy PE, Millow LJ et al. A third Wilms' tumour locus on chromosome 16q. Cancer Res 1992; 52: 3094–3098.

44 Huff V, Reeve AE, Leppert M et al. Nonlinkage of 16q markers to familial predisposition to Wilms' tumor. Cancer Res 1992; 52: 6117–6120.

45 Call KM, Glaser T, Ito CY et al. Isolation and characterization of a zinc finger polypeptide gene at the human chromosome 11 Wilms' tumour locus. Cell 1990; 60: 509–520.

46 Gessler M, Poustka A, Cavenee W, Neve RL, Orkin SH, Bruns GAP. Homozygous deletion in Wilms tumours of a zinc-finger gene identified by chromosome jumping. Nature 1990; 343: 774–778.

47 Bickmore WA, Oghene K, Little MH, Seawright A, van Heyningen V, Hastie ND. Modulation of DNA binding specificity by alternative splicing of the Wilms tumour WT1 gene transcript. Science 1992; 257: 235–237.

48 Beckwith JB, Kiviat NB, Bonadio JF. Nephrogenic rests, nephroblastomatosis, and the pathogenesis of Wilms' tumor. Pediatr Pathol 1990; 10: 1–36.

49 Pritchard-Jones K, Fleming S. Cell types expressing the Wilms' tumour gene (WT1) in Wilms' tumours: implications for tumour histogenesis. Oncogene 1991; 6: 2211–2220.

50 van Heyningen V, Hastie ND. Wilms' tumour: reconciling genetics and biology. Trends Genet 1992; 8: 16–21.

51 Breslow NE, Beckwith JB. Epidemiological features of Wilms tumour: results of the National Wilms' tumour study. J Natl Cancer Inst 1982; 68: 429.

52 Cowell JK, Wadey RB, Haber DA, Call KM, Housman DE, Pritchard J. Structural rearrangements of the WT1 gene in Wilms' tumour cells. Oncogene 1991; 6: 595–599.

53 Tadokoro K, Fujii H, Ohshima A et al. Intragenic homozygous deletion of the WT1 gene in Wilms' tumour. Oncogene 1992; 7: 1215–1221.

54   Huff V, Miwa H, Haber DA, Call KM, Housman D, Strong LC et al. Evidence for WT1 as a Wilms tumour (WT) gene: intragenic germinal deletion in bilateral WT. Am J Hum Genet 1991; 48: 997–1003.

55   Pelletier J, Bruening W, Li FP, Haber DA, Glaser T, Housman DE. WT1 mutations contribute to abnormal genital system development and hereditary Wilms' tumour. Nature 1991; 353: 431–434.

56   Coppes MJ, Liefers GJ, Paul P, Yeger H, Williams BRG. Homozygous somatic WT1 point mutations in sporadic unilateral Wilms tumor. Proc Natl Acad Sci USA 1993; 90: 1416–1419.

57   Little MH, Prosser J, Condie A, Smith PJ, van Heyningen V, Hastie ND. Zinc finger point mutations within the WT1 gene in Wilms tumor patients. Proc Natl Acad Sci USA 1992; 89: 4791–4795.

58   Haber DA, Buckler AJ, Glaser T, Call KM, Pelletier J, Sohn RL et al. An internal deletion within an 11p13 zinc finger gene contributes to the development of Wilms' tumour. Cell 1990; 61: 1257–1269.

59   Cowell JK, Groves N, Baird PN. Loss of heterozygosity at 11p13 in Wilms' tumour does not necessarily involve mutations in the WT1 gene. Br J Cancer 1993; 67: 1259–1261.

60   Santos A, Osorio-Almeida L, Baird PN, Silva JM, Boavida MG, Cowell JK. Insertional inactivation of the WT1 gene in tumour cells from a patient with WAGR syndrome. Hum Genet 1993; 92: 83–86.

61   Baird PN, Groves N, Haber DA, Housman DE, Cowell JK. Identification of mutations in the WT1 gene in tumours from patients with the WAGR syndrome. Oncogene 1992; 7: 2141–2149.

62   Brown KW, Watson JE, Poirier V, Mott MG, Berry PJ, Maitland NJ. Inactivation of the remaining allele of the WT1 gene in a Wilms' tumour from a WAGR patient. Oncogene 1992; 7: 763–768.

63   Rauscher FJ, Morris JF, Tournay OE, Cook DM, Curran T. Binding of the Wilms' tumour locus zinc finger protein to the EGR-1 consensus sequence. Science 1990; 250: 1259–1262.

64   Madden SL, Cook DM, Morris JF, Gashler A, Sukhatme VP, Rauscher FJ. Transcriptional repression mediated by the WT1 Wilms tumour gene product. Science 1991; 253: 1550–1553.

65   Drummond IA, Madden SL, Rohwer-Nutter P, Bell GI, Sukhatme VP, Rauscher FJ. Repression of the insulin-like growth factor II gene by the Wilms tumor suppressor WT1. Science 1992; 257: 674–678.

66   Gashler AL, Bonthron DT, Madden SL, Rauscher FJ, Collins T, Sukhamtme VP. Human platelet derived growth factor A chain is transcriptionally repressed by the Wilms tumour suppressor gene WT1. Proc Natl Acad Sci 1992; 89: 10984–10988.

67   Pelletier J, Bruening W, Kashtan CE, Mauer SM, Manivel JC, Striegel JE et al. Germline mutations in the Wilms' tumour suppressor gene are associated with abnormal urogenital development in Denys-Drash syndrome. Cell 1991; 67: 437–447.

68   Madden SL, Cook DM, Rauscher FJ. A structure-function analysis of transcriptional repression mediated by the WT1, Wilms' tumor suppressor protein. Oncogene 1993; 8: 1713–1720.

69   Morris JF, Madden SL, Tournay OE, Cook DM, Sukhatme VP, Rauscher FJ. Characterization of the zinc protein encoded by the WT1 Wilms' tumor locus. Oncogene 1991; 6: 2339–2348.

70   Denys P, Malvaux P, Van den Berghe H, Tanghe W, Proesmans W. Association d'un syndrome anatomo-pathologique de pseudohermaphrodisme masculin, d'une tumeur de Wilms, d'une nephropathie parenchymateuse et d'un mosaicism XX/XY. Arch Fr Pediatr 1967; 24: 729–739.

71   Drash A, Sherman F, Hartman WH, Blizzard RM. A syndrome of pseudohermaphroditism, Wilms' tumour, hypertension, and degenerative renal disease. J Pediatr 1970; 76: 585–593.

72 Jadresic L, Leake J, Gordon I, Dillon MJ, Grant DB, Pritchard J et al. Clinicopathologic review of twelve children with nephropathy, Wilms' tumor, and genital abnormalities (Drash syndrome). J Pediatr 1990; 117: 717–725.

73 Jadresic L, Wadey RB, Buckle B, Barratt TM, Mitchell CD, Cowell JK. Molecular analysis of chromosome region 11p13 in patients with Drash syndrome. Hum Genet 1991; 86: 497–501.

74 Baird PN, Santos A, Groves N, Jadresic L, Cowell JK. Constitutional mutations in the WT1 gene in patients with Denys-Drash syndrome. Hum Mol Genet 1992; 1: 301–305.

75 Ogawa O, Eccles MR, Yun K, Mueller RF, Holdaway MDD, Reeve AE. A novel insertional mutation at the third zinc finger coding region of the WT1 gene in Denys-Drash syndrome. Hum Mol Genet 1993; 2: 203–204.

76 Coppes MJ, Liefers GJ, Higuchi M, Zinn AB, Balfe JW, Williams BRG. Inherited WT1 mutation in Denys-Drash syndrome. Cancer Res 1992; 52: 6125–6128.

77 Beckwith JP. Extreme cytomegaly of the adrenal fetal cortex, omphalocele hyperplasia of kidneys and pancreas, and Leydig-cell hyperplasia: another syndrome? West Soc Pediatr Res 1963;

78 Wiedemann HR. Complexe malformatif familial avec hernie ombilicle et macro-glossie: un syndrome nouveau? J Genet Hum 1964; 13: 223–232.

79 Wiedemann HR. Tumours and hemihypertrophy associated with Wiedemann-Beckwith syndrome. Eur J Pediatr 1983; 141: 129.

80 Scrable HJ, Witte DP, Lampkin BC, Cavenee WK. Chromosomal localisation of the human rhabdomyosarcoma locus by mitotic recombination mapping. Nature 1987; 329: 645–647.

81 Best LG, Hoekstra RE. Wiedemann-Beckwith syndrome: Autosomal-dominant inheritance in a family. Am J Med Genet 1981; 9: 291–299.

82 Ping AJ, Reeve AE, Law DJ, Young MR, Boehnke M, Feinberg AP. Genetic linkage of Beckwith-Wiedemann syndrome to 11p15. Am J Hum Genet 1989; 44: 720–723.

83 Koufos A, Grundy P, Morgan K et al. Familial Wiedemann-Beckwith syndrome and a second Wilms' tumour locus both map to 11p15.5. Am J Hum Genet 1989; 44: 711–719.

84 Turleau C, De Grouchy J, Chavin-Colin F, Martelli H, Voyer M, Charlas R. Trisomy 11p15 and Beckwith-Wiedemann syndrome: A report of two cases. Hum Genet 1984; 67: 219–221.

85 Waziri M, Patil SR, Hanson JW, Bartley JA. Abnormalities of chromosome 11 in patients with features of Beckwith-Wiedemann syndrome. J Pediatr 1983; 102: 873–876.

86 Sapienza C. Genome imprinting and dominance modification. Ann N Y Acad Sci 1989; 564: 24–38.

87 Pal N, Wadey RB, Buckle B, Yeomans E, Pritchard J, Cowell JK. Preferential loss of maternal alleles in sporadic Wilms' tumour. Oncogene 1990; 5: 1665–1668.

88 De Chiara TM, Efstratiadis A, Robertson E. A growth-deficiency phenotype in heterozygous mice carrying an insulin-like growth factor II gene disrupted by targeting. Nature 1990; 345: 78–80.

89 De Chiara TM, Robertson EJ, Efstratiadis A. Parental imprinting of the mouse insulin-like growth factor II gene. Cell 1991; 64: 849–859.

90 Feinberg AP. Genomic imprinting and gene inactivation in cancer. Nature Genet 1993; 4: 110–113.

91 Scott J, Cowell JK, Robertson M et al. Insulin-like growth factor-II gene expression in Wilms' tumour and embryonic tissues. Nature 1985; 317: 260–262.

92 Werner H, Re GG, Drummon IA et al. Increased expression of the insulin-like growth factor I receptor gene, IGF1R in Wilms tumour is correlated with modulation of IGF1R promoter activity by the WT1 Wilms tumour gene product. Proc Natl Acad Sci USA 1993; 90: 5828–5832.

93 Ogawa O, Eccles MR, Szeto J et al. Relaxation of insulin-like growth factor II gene imprinting implicated in Wilms' tumour. Nature 1993; 362: 749–751.

94 Rainer S, Johnson LA, Dobry CJ, Ping AJ, Grundy PE, Feinberg AP. Relaxation of imprinted genes in human cancer. Nature 1993; 362: 747–749.

95 Koi M, Johnson LA, Kalikin LM, Little PFR, Nakamura Y, Feinberg AP. Tumor cell growth arrest caused by subchromosomal transferable DNA fragments from chromosome 11. Science 1993; 260: 361–364.

96 Maheswaran S, Park S, Bernard A, Morris JF, Rauscher FJ, Hill DE et al. Physical and functional interaction between WT1 and p53 proteins. Proc Natl Acad Sci USA 1993; 90: 5100–5104.

97 Lemoine NR, Hughes CM, Cowell JK. Abnormalities of the tumour suppressor gene p53 are very frequent in Wilms' tumours. J Pathol 1992; 168: 237–242.

98 Kreidberg JA, H. S, Loring JM, Maeda M et al. WT-1 is required for early kidney development. Cell 1993; 74: 679–691.

99 Knudson AG, Strong LC. Mutation and cancer: neuroblastoma and pheochromocytoma. Am J Hum Genet 1972; 24: 514–532.

100 Kushner BH, Gilbert F, Helson L. Familial neuroblastoma: Case reports, literature review and etiologic considerations. Cancer 1986; 57: 1887–1893.

101 Brodeur GM, Sekon GS, Goldstein MN. Chromosome aberrations in human neuroblastomas. Cancer 1977; 40: 2256–2263.

102 Fong C-T, Dracopoli NC, White PS et al. Loss of heterozygosity for the short arm of chromosome 1 in human neuroblastomas: correlation with N-myc amplification. Proc Natl Acad Sci 1989; 86: 3753–3757.

103 Weith A, Martinsson T, Cziepluch C, Bruderlein S, Amler LC, Berthold F et al. Neuroblastoma consensus deletion maps to 1p36:1-2. Genes Chromosom Cancer 1989; 1: 159–166.

104 Suzuki T, Yokata J, Mugishima H, Okabe I, Ookuni M, Sugimura T et al. Frequent loss of heterozygosity on chromosome 14 in neuroblastoma. Cancer Res 1989; 49: 401–407.

105 Laureys G, Speleman G, Opdenakker G, Benoit Y, Leroy J. Constitutional translocation t(1;17)(p36;q12-21) in a patient with neuroblastoma. Genes Chromosom Cancer 1990; 2: 252–254.

106 Biegel JA, White PS, Marshall HN et al. Constitutional 1p36 deletion in a child with neuroblastoma. Am J Hum Genet 1993; 52: 176–182.

107 Michalski AJ, Cotter FE, Cowell JK. Isolation of chromosome-specific DNA from an Alu polymerase chain reaction library to define the breakpoint in a patient with a constitutional translocation t(1;13)(q22;q12). Oncogene 1992; 7: 1595–1602.

108 Seeger RC, Brodeur GM, Sather H, Dalton A, Siegel SE, Wong KY et al. Association of multiple copies of the N-myc oncogene with rapid progression of neuroblastomas. N Engl J Med 1988; 311: 1111–1116.

109 Cowell JK. Double minutes and homogeneously staining regions: gene amplification in mammalian cells. Ann Rev Genet 1982; 16: 21–59.

110 Cohn SL, Salwen H, Quasney MW et al. Prolonged N-myc protein half-life in a neuroblastoma cell line lacking n-myc amplification. Oncogene 1990; 5: 1821–1827.

111 Douglass EC, Valentine M, Etcubanas E et al. A specific chromosomal abnormality in rhabdomyosarcoma. Cytogenet Cell Genet 1987; 45: 148–155.

112 Douglass EC, Rowe ST, Valentine M, Parham DM, Bekow R, Bowman WP et al. Variant translocations of chromosome 13 in alveolar rhabdomyosarcoma. Genes Chromosom Cancer 1991; 3: 480–482.

113 Barr FG, Galili N, Holick J, Biegel JA, Rovera G, Emanuel BS. Rearrangement of the PAX3 paired box gene in the paediatric solid tumour alveolar rhabdomyosarcoma. Nature Genet 1993; 3: 113–117.

114 Burri M, Tromvoukis Y, Bopp D, Frigerio G, Noll M. Conservation of the paired domain in metazoans and its structure in three isolated human genes. EMBO J 1989; 8: 1183–1190.

115 Turc-Carel C, Aurias A, Mugneret F et al. Chromosomes in Ewing's sarcoma. An evaluation of 85 cases and remarkable consistency of t(11;22)(q24;q12). Cancer Genet Cytogenet 1988; 32: 229–238.

116 Whang-Peng J, Triche TJ, Knutsen T, Hiser J, Douglass EC, Israel MA. Chromosome translocation in peripheral neuroepithelioma. N Engl J Med 1984;311: 584–585.
117 Zucman J, Delattre O, Desmaze C et al. Cloning and characterization of the Ewing's sarcoma and peripheral neuroepithelioma t(11;22) translocation breakpoints. Genes Chromosom Cancer 1992; 5: 271–277.
118 Delattre O, Zucman J, Plougastel B et al. Gene fusion with an ETS DNA-binding domain caused by chromosome translocation in human tumours. Nature 1992; 359: 162–165.

British Medical Bulletin (1994) Vol. 50, No. 3, pp. 624–639
© The British Council 1994

Familial cancer syndromes and clusters

J M Birch

University of Manchester, CRC Paediatric and Familial Cancer Research Group, Christie Hospital NHS Trust, Manchester, UK

The study of rare families in which a variety of cancers occur, usually at an early age and with patterns consistent with a common hereditary mechanism, has contributed much to our understanding of the process of carcinogenesis. So far, genes identified as having a role in cancer predisposition in these families have also been important in the histogenesis of sporadic cancers. In the two most clearly defined cancer family syndromes, the Li-Fraumeni syndrome and Lynch syndrome II, the genes involved predispose to diverse but specific constellations of cancers. Genes associated with site-specific familial cancer clusters may also give rise to increased susceptibility to other cancers, and site-specific clusters may represent one end of a spectrum.

A consistent feature of familial cancer syndromes is the variable expression within and between families. A challenge for the future will be to determine other factors which may interact with the principal genes involved, giving rise to this variability.

In recent years the study of rare families in which multiple members are affected with cancers in a pattern suggesting Mendelian inheritance of a trait conferring cancer susceptibility has yielded many important advances in our understanding of processes involved in carcinogenesis. A number of cancer susceptibility genes which, when altered in the germline, confer a high risk of malignancy, have now been characterized. Families in which such genes are transmitted in the germline are rare, but in all cases so far identified, the genes have been shown to be important in the development of corresponding sporadic cancers, and in many cases also in sporadic forms of other cancers which are not seen in association with germline mutations. All common cancers which have been studied have been shown to display a degree of familial clustering. Thus, systematic studies of the relatives of patients with specific cancers have consistently demonstrated an increased risk for that cancer in the relative. Among first degree relatives of cancer patients, relative risks of between 2 and 3 for the specific cancer have been found.[1] Site-specific genetic predisposition to common cancers is dealt with elsewhere in this volume.

The subject of the present chapter will encompass those families in whom a variety of cancers occur with patterns consistent with a common hereditary mechanism. In the majority of such families the genetic basis of cancer predisposition is either thought to be, or known to be, the result of constitutional mutations in tumour suppressor genes. These include syndromes with non-malignant phenotypic characteristics associated with an increased risk of specific malignancies and the cancer family syndromes in which an increased risk of a variety of rare and common cancers is the only phenotypic feature.

THE LI-FRAUMENI SYNDROME (LFS)

Li and Fraumeni in 1969 reported 4 families in which siblings or cousins were affected with rhabdomyosarcoma. The pairs of cases had been identified as part of a survey of nearly 650 children with rhabdomyosarcoma in the United States. They investigated the families of these 4 pairs of cases, and found an unusually high incidence of premenopausal breast cancer, soft tissue sarcomas diagnosed at young ages, and other unusually early onset cancers in close relatives of the index children. Li and Fraumeni proposed that the observed clustering of cancers within these families was due to inherited predisposition.[2] Following this publication, a number of case reports of other families consistent with Li and Fraumeni's findings appeared – eg Pearson et al, Lynch et al.[3,4] However, it was uncertain whether these observations were due to genetic susceptibility to these cancers, or simply represented chance clusters of cancers in these families. Subsequently, systematic studies of families and patient populations provided strong evidence in support of inherited susceptibility to a diverse but specific range of cancers. Li and Fraumeni conducted follow-up studies in their original 4 families, and after a 12-year period found that the number of cancers occurring in previously unaffected members of the families greatly exceeded chance expectation. Furthermore, the pattern of cancers was similar to that originally observed, that is, the cancers were predominantly sarcomas, premenopausal breast cancer, and other cancers diagnosed at young ages. A number of family members had also developed second primary cancers, and these second primaries were also of similar types, supporting the idea of genetic susceptibility.[5] Cancer incidence in the families of a population-based series of children with soft tissue sarcoma and a hospital-based series of survivors of childhood soft tissue sarcoma was reported by two groups. Both studies found that there was an increased risk of cancer in the first degree relatives of the childhood sarcoma patients, with the highest risk in relatives of patients in whom the cancers were diagnosed at younger ages and were of the types found in Li and Fraumeni's families, notably breast cancer in young women.[6,7] Segregation analysis in the families of children included in the hospital-based series found that the distribution of cancers was compatible with a rare autosomal gene. The gene frequency was estimated to be 0.00002 and penetrance was approximately 50% by age 30 years and 90% by age 60 years.[8]

Li et al collected details of 24 families in order to study the components of the syndrome. Each of the families conformed to standard criteria, as follows: a proband with bone or soft tissue sarcoma, diagnosed under the age of 45 years; one first-degree relative with cancer under 45 years; and one first or second-degree relative in the same lineage with cancer under 45, or sarcoma diagnosed at any age. These criteria subsequently became accepted as the standard clinical definition of the syndrome. In these 24 families, in addition to breast cancer and bone and soft tissue sarcoma, other tumours which were found to excess compared with US cancer incidence data were: brain tumours, adrenocortical carcinoma, and leukaemia. The study also confirmed the high frequency of individuals with multiple primary cancers in families with the syndrome.[9]

Studies of families of unselected series of children with sarcomas also indicate that brain tumours, adrenocortical carcinoma and leukaemia, in addition to bone and soft tissue sarcoma and breast cancer, form the principal components of the syndrome. These studies have suggested that melanoma, germ cell tumours and Wilms' tumour may also represent syndrome cancers.[6,7,10–12]

Epidemiologically, therefore, the syndrome has been well characterized in terms of cancer phenotype. However, with regard to identifying the responsible gene(s) giving rise to this diverse array of malignancies, there were difficulties in terms of classic genetic linkage analysis, due to the lethal nature of the component tumours. This made collection of sufficient biological samples from affected family members a problem; and furthermore, because the component cancers are frequent in the general population, the difficulty of phenocopies also arose. For these reasons, Malkin et al[13] chose to analyse candidate genes. The p53 gene on chromosome 17p was selected as the primary candidate, because mutations and/or deletions in p53 had frequently been observed in sporadic tumours characteristic of the syndrome. Germline mutations in the p53 gene in affected individuals from each of the 5 families included in this study were detected. Soon after this report a sixth LFS family with a germline p53 mutation was published.[14] These 6 mutations all occurred within a stretch of 14 codons in exon 7 of the p53 gene, and initially this resulted in some speculation about the possible significance of this positional clustering. However, following these initial reports, a number of other groups carried out analyses of the p53 gene in groups of patients and families, not all of whom conformed to the syndrome definition of Li et al.[9] Germline p53 mutations were detected in a small minority of breast cancer families, in families with a pattern of cancers resembling those in Li-Fraumeni syndrome, but where the syndrome criteria of Li et al were not fulfilled, eg families where the proband had an adrenocortical carcinoma or brain tumour, rather than a sarcoma; in patients with multiple primary cancers, regardless of family history; and in patients with sporadic sarcomas, as well as a number of additional examples in families with the classic form of the syndrome. These various reports are reviewed by Birch et al.[15]

In contrast to the initial reports, in these subsequent patients and families germline mutations were observed in exons 4, 5, 6, 8 and 9, as well as in exon 7. The majority of mutations were single-base changes, leading to aminoacid substitutions, predominantly transitions, but with some transversions. Nonsense mutations leading to truncated protein products have been observed, and in addition two intronic mutations have been reported. An example of a family with a germline mutation in codon 248 of the p53 gene is shown in Figure 1. This family conforms to the definition of Li et al and shows all the features of classic LFS, including bone and soft tissue sarcomas, very early onset breast cancer and the occurrence of multiple primary cancers in two members. The distribution of cancers in patients and families with germline p53 mutations is shown in Table 1.

The p53 gene acts as a tumour suppressor; but in contrast to the retinoblastoma gene, where loss of function by mutation or deletion of both copies of the gene leads to cellular transformation, in the case of p53, in addition to loss of normal function, certain mutant proteins show a gain of function[16] (see Lane, this issue). It is possible that the type of p53 mutation occurring constitutionally in Li-Fraumeni and Li-Fraumeni-like families may have an influence on the pattern of cancers occurring in particular families, with gain of function mutations possibly conferring a more highly penetrant cancer phenotype in terms of age at onset and occurrence of multiple primary tumours. Such variations may at least in part explain the wide variations seen between families. At present there are too few fully-documented families to enable studies of correlations between genotype and phenotype to be carried out. The

Table 1 Cancers in known carriers of germline p53 mutations and their first degree relatives

Cancers	Age at diagnosis*						Total
	0–9	10–19	20–29	30–39	40–49	50+	
Soft tissue sarcoma	18 (11.4)	3 (1.9)	3 (1.9)	3 (1.9)	1 (0.6)	1 (0.6)	29 (18.3)
Osteosarcoma and chondrosarcoma	4 (2.5)	22 (13.9)	5 (3.7)	1 (0.6)	–	–	32 (20.3)
Breast	–	–	12 (7.6)	14 (8.9)	11 (7.0)	1 (0.6)	38 (24.1)
Central nervous system	6 (3.8)	1 (0.6)	2 (1.3)	2 (1.3)	1 (0.6)	2 (1.3)	14 (8.9)
Leukaemia	2 (1.3)	3 (1.9)	–	1 (0.6)	–	–	6 (3.8)
Adrenocortical carcinoma	6 (3.8)	–	–	–	–	–	6 (3.8)
Other	2 (1.3)	6 (3.8)	5 (3.2)	8 (5.1)	6 (3.8)	6 (3.8)	33 (20.9)
Total	38 (24.1)	35 (22.2)	27 (17.1)	29 (18.3)	19 (12.0)	10 (6.3)	158

*number of cases (% total)

frequency of new germline mutations in the p53 gene, and the contribution of cancers arising as a result of germline p53 mutations to the
total population cancer burden, is unknown, but is likely to be small.

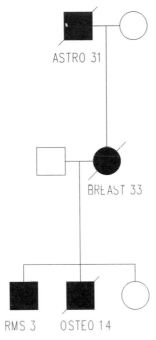

Fig. 1 Pedigree of a Li-Fraumeni family with germline mutation in codon 248 of
the p53 gene. Astro = astrocytoma; Breast = infiltrating carcinoma breast; RMS =
rhabdomyosarcoma; Osteo = osteosarcoma; Numbers indicate ages at diagnosis.

Two studies in which series of families with classic LFS or showing
features of LFS have been analysed for the presence of germline p53
mutations, have interestingly demonstrated that a substantial proportion
of these families do not carry such mutations. It appears that among
families fulfilling the classic definition of Li et al,[9] about 50% do not
have p53 coding mutations in the germline.[15,17] It is possible that some
of these families may have intronic mutations, but in at least one family
direct involvement of p53 has been excluded on the basis of lack of
shared p53 alleles in a pair of cancer-affected sibs.[18]

The genetic basis of cancer predisposition in LFS families without
germline mutations in the p53 gene is not known, but a clue was pro-

vided from the study of expression of p53 protein in one such family. Barnes et al[19] found increased expression of p53 protein in both tumour tissue and normal tissue by immunohistochemical analysis in two members of a family with a pattern of cancers consistent with LFS, although not fulfilling the classic criteria. After careful analyses, no germline mutation in p53 could be detected. The implication of this finding is that in this family there may be a constitutional abnormality in a gene other than p53, which is acting to stabilize p53 protein, and which results in a constitutional dysfunction in p53, which confers a Li-Fraumeni type phenotype by an indirect route. It is possible, therefore, that in other LFS families, negative for the presence of a germline p53 mutation, normal p53 function may be compromised. Germline mutations in possible candidate genes which are known to interact with p53 in this way, eg the MDM2 oncogene on chromosome 12q,[20] should be sought in LFS families negative for p53 germline mutations. Although families with LFS are rare, it is likely that any gene which when constitutionally mutated can produce the LFS phenotype, will also be important in the histogenesis of a number of common cancers, eg breast cancer.

OTHER CANCER FAMILY SYNDROMES

Lynch syndrome II

Genetic susceptibility to colon cancer occurs in association with familial adenomatous polyposis coli (FAP), but striking examples of familial colon cancer in the absence of FAP have also been described. Such families are said to exhibit hereditary non-polyposis colorectal cancer (HNPCC). Adenocarcinomas at sites other than the large bowel, and occurring at unusually early ages, have also been observed in some families with HNPCC. Lynch has proposed that there are two forms of HNPCC: Lynch syndrome I, characterized by autosomal dominant inheritance of susceptibility to early onset colorectal cancer in the absence of diffuse polyposis, and Lynch syndrome II, in which cancers other than colorectal carcinoma, notably endometrial carcinoma, also occur in affected family members. In families with Lynch syndrome II adenocarcinomas of ovary, stomach, ureter, renal pelvis and other sites have also been reported to occur to excess.[21]

In order to investigate whether there was sufficient evidence to support a distinction betweem Lynch syndromes I and II, Mecklin and Järvinen[22] analysed the tumour spectrum of 40 families with HNPCC included in a specialist register in Finland. The families were divided into two groups: those without endometrial cancer (group I, 17 families), and those with endometrial cancer (group II, 23 families). They found that group II families had more affected family members, particularly female affected members, than those without endometrial cancer.

Group I families were smaller and had more affected males than affected females. The proportions and distributions of other malignancies did not differ between group I and group II patients. The authors concluded that the subdivision of HNPCC families into two categories has no clinical significance, and the occurrence of endometrial and other cancers in families with HNPCC depends on the family size and proportions of males and females.

Recently, linkage analyses in two large families with HNPCC, both of which included endometrial carcinomas and carcinomas of other sites, have demonstrated the existence of a gene linked to the syndrome on chromosome 2p. Interestingly, it appears that, unlike other cancer susceptibility genes which act as tumour suppressors, eg Rb1, p53, the chromosome 2p gene when mutated may act to create a generalized genetic instability, manifest as multiple replication errors. Although tight linkage to the locus on chromosome 2p in these two families with multiple cases of colorectal, endometrial and other cancers was demonstrated, it was possible to exclude linkage in 3 other families. There appears therefore to be genetic heterogeneity in HNPCC.[23,24]

Other familial cancer clusters

Site specific familial breast cancer has been the subject of intense study for many years, but the extent to which other types of cancer may also cluster in breast cancer families had not been formally assessed until recently. Results of 3 studies in which the occurrence of cancer in close relatives of large unselected series of breast cancer patients have now been reported.[25–27] Tulinius et al found that among the first degree relatives of 947 breast cancer patients from Iceland, there was an excess of prostate cancer and ovarian cancer, and among all relatives, excesses of prostate, ovarian and endometrial cancer were found. Thus the study provided evidence of co-aggregation between breast cancer and cancers of prostate, ovary and endometrium.[25]Anderson et al analysed the cancer mortality among mothers and sisters of 740 breast cancer patients diagnosed under age 36. Excess mortality below age 60 was found in these relatives for cancers of cervix, ovary and endometrium.[26] Teare et al[27] found an excess of cancers overall in all first degree relatives of an unselected series of 402 breast cancer patients. A significant excess of cancers was seen in both male and female relatives. When individual types of cancers were considered, a marked excess of bone and soft tissue sarcoma in males and females was seen, and males also had a statistically significant excess of carcinomas of lip, oral cavity and pharynx. No excess of prostate or ovarian cancer was found.

These studies demonstrate that in addition to the previously documented excess risk of breast cancer among relatives of patients with breast cancer, close relatives of such patients may also be at increased risk of a variety of other cancers. To what extent this is due to common genetic factors, which predispose to more than one cancer type, is unknown. However, both of the genes associated with genetic predisposition to breast cancer which have already been identified (BRCA1 and p53), confer a high risk of a number of cancers other than of breast. Germline mutations in the p53 gene predispose to bone and soft tissue sarcoma, brain tumours, leukaemia, and other cancers as well as breast cancer, in the Li-Fraumeni syndrome, as described above; and the BRCA1 gene is also associated with predisposition to ovarian, prostate and possibly other cancers.[28,29]

Familial breast cancer is known to be heterogeneous, and when other genes associated with predisposition to breast cancer are identified, it is likely that these genes also will confer an increased risk of cancers at other sites. All genes associated with heritable predisposition to cancer which have so far been identified as being associated with a specific cancer, can also confer increased risk to other cancers, eg Rb1.[30] As with site-specific HNPCC and site-specific familial breast cancer, other apparently site-specific familial cancer clusters may simply represent one end of a spectrum arising as a result of ascertainment bias. As genes conferring predisposition to cancer are cloned, population-based studies can be carried out to determine penetrance and full range of expression.

SYNDROMES ASSOCIATED WITH INCREASED RISK OF CANCER

This heading includes those inherited syndromes characterized by congenital anomalies and other benign phenotypic features, and where increased risk of specific cancers is also a characteristic. Examples of these syndromes include neurofibromatosis type I (NF1), Gorlin syndrome and von Hippel-Lindau syndrome. These 3 examples serve to illustrate a number of points, and in each the responsible gene has recently been located and/or cloned. A number of other cancer-prone syndromes exist and are dealt with elsewhere in this volume.

Neurofibromatosis type 1 (NF1)

NF1 (von Recklinghausen neurofibromatosis) is a relatively common condition, which is transmitted in a pattern consistent with autosomal dominant inheritance. The main characteristics of the disorder include presence of café-au-lait patches on the skin, lisch nodules (hamartomas) of the iris, and multiple benign neurofibromata with axillary and inguinal freckling and various skeletal anomalies. The incidence of NF1 is between 1 in 5000 and 1 in 3000 live births, and it is thus one of the most common monogenic conditions in man.[31] Penetrance appears to be close to 100% but is variable with some patients manifesting only minor phenotypic characteristics.[32]

Individuals with NF1 are at high risk of developing a variety of tumours, the majority of which arise in tissues derived from the neural crest. They include central nervous system tumours (characteristically optic gliomas and astrocytomas and glioblastomas); malignant peripheral nerve sheath tumours (MPNST) are also common. The latter frequently arise as a result of malignant transformation in benign 'plexiform' neurofibromata (these are not to be confused with the usually much more numerous neurofibromata of the skin). Sarcomatous change may occur in as many as 10% of patients, although estimates vary.

Other malignancies which have been said to be associated with NF1 include rhabdomyosarcoma and leukaemias, and it is probable that these are a manifestation of the syndrome. Wilms' tumour and neuroblastoma have also been reported in patients with NF1. However, it is not certain whether these latter malignancies are part of the syndrome or chance occurrences.[33]

In 1987 the NF1 gene was assigned to chromosome 17 by genetic linkage analysis, and subsequent linkage studies localized the gene to band 17q112.[34–36] The gene was isolated and characterized in 1990.[37,38] The NF1 gene encodes a GTPase-activating product with tumour suppressor function.[39] Given the considerable variation in phenotypic expression in patients with NF1, it will be interesting to see whether particular mutations are associated with specific phenotypes, and in particular whether certain mutations confer a higher risk of malignancy than others. In this context possible interaction with other cancer-associated genes is relevant, and this is considered further below.

Von Hippel-Lindau syndrome

Von Hippel-Lindau syndrome (VHLS), in common with NF1, is an inherited syndrome conferring predisposition to a number of benign and malignant neoplasms, including retinal angiomas, haemangioblastoma of the central nervous system, phaeochromocytoma, and renal cell carcinoma. Pancreatic, renal and epididymal cysts are also features of the syndrome. The pattern of disease in affected families suggested autosomal dominant inheritance.

Maher et al conducted complex segregation analysis based on 38 kindreds with at least two affected members, which supported dominant inheritance with virtually complete penetrance by age 70, and with no evidence of heterogeneity. In the same study the birth incidence was estimated to be 1 in 36 000.[40] The disease has a very variable expression, with some individuals manifesting only one symptomatic lesion while others may have a number of lesions with considerable associated morbidity. The most common cause of death in affected individuals is renal cell carcinoma. Neumann and Wiestler[41] studied the clustering of the various features characteristic of VHLS in 29 kindreds with the disease, and found evidence of a marked tendency for familial clustering of specific features in the affected kindreds. Thus retinal angioma and hemangioblastomas in the central nervous system were found in most families, but rcnal cell carcinoma, renal cysts and/or pancreatic cysts were not found in families with phaeochromocytoma, and vice versa. On the basis of these observations, the authors concluded that VHLS occurs as the result of different mutations within a complex genetic locus, with a linear sequence giving rise to the various features.

The VHLS gene appears to act as a tumour suppressor. It was assigned to chromosome 3p25 by genetic linkage,[42] and has recently been cloned.[43] The structure of the gene suggests that it may be involved in signal transduction or cell adhesion. It will now be interesting to see whether specific mutations are correlated with the pattern of associated lesions in affected families.

Gorlin syndrome (The naevoid basal cell carcinoma syndrome)

The first clear description of the syndrome was published by Gorlin and Goltz in 1960.[44] It is characterized by multiple basal cell carcinomas, odontogenic cysts, skeletal deformities, skin pits on palms and soles, soft tissue calcification, and other neoplasms, including medulloblastoma and ovarian fibromas. Mental retardation can also be a feature. The pattern of inheritance is consistent with autosomal dominant predisposition, with high penetrance, but very variable expression. The syndrome is rare, with a minimum prevalence of 1 per 57 000. Affected individuals may spontaneously develop numerous basal cell carcinomas during their lifetime, but onset of these lesions may rapidly follow radiotherapy. This effect is characteristically seen in children with medulloblastoma associated with Gorlin syndrome, following treatment with cranio-spinal irradiation (Fig. 2). In such patients, large numbers of basal cell carcinomas may develop within months of the radiotherapy and occur throughout the radiation field, but they tend to cluster particularly at the edges of the field. This effect can result in severe morbidity.[45] It is therefore particularly important that the possibility of Gorlin syndrome is considered in treatment planning for very young children with medulloblastoma. At the time of diagnosis in the child there may be no obvious clinical manifestations of the syndrome in an affected parent.[46]

The gene for Gorlin syndrome has not yet been cloned, but has been located to chromosome 9q31 by genetic linkage analysis, and appears to behave as a tumour suppressor gene.[47,48] The rapid develop-

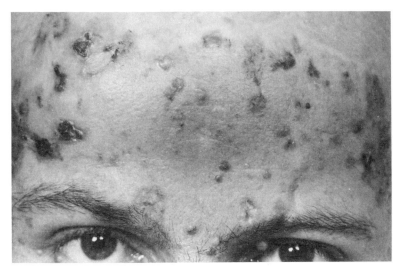

Fig. 2 Patient with Gorlin syndrome showing multiple basal cell carcinoma following radiotherapy for medulloblastoma.

ment of basal carcinomas following radiotherapy in patients with Gorlin syndrome provides a dramatic example of the interaction between genetic (intrinsic) and extrinsic factors in carcinogenesis. The main characteristics of NF1, VHLS and Gorlin syndrome are summarized in Table 2.

CONCLUSIONS

Both in the cancer predisposition syndromes, which include benign phenotypic characteristics as well as malignancies, and in the cancer family syndromes, a striking feature is the very variable expression between families and within families. Thus in families with NF1 some individuals may exhibit only mild symptoms while others are severely affected.[32] Also, the tendency to develop malignancies associated with NF1 appears to be present in some families.[49] Some of this variation may be due to shared environmental exposures giving rise to specific patterns of cancer in certain families; alternatively, specific exposures in individual family members may account for severity of affection where other family members are less severely affected. As a series of families with known cancer-predisposing mutant genes are built up, genetic epidemiological studies can address these issues.

Table 2 Characteristics of cancer predisposition syndromes

Syndrome	Benign characteristics	Associated cancers	Location of gene
von Recklinghausen neurofibromatosis NF1	*Café-au-lait* patches Multiple benign neurofibromata Lisch nodules of the iris Axillary and inguinal freckling Skeletal abnormalities (scoliosis, pseudoarthrosis)	Central nervous system tumours (especially optic nerve gliomas) Malignant peripheral nerve sheath tumours Rhabdomyosarcoma Leukaemia	17q11.2
von Hippel Lindau	Renal, pancreatic and epididymal cysts Phaeochromocytoma	Haemangioblastomas of central nervous system Retinal angioma Renal cell carcinoma Phaeochromocytoma	3p25
Gorlin syndrome (naevoid-basal-cell-carcinoma syndrome)	Skin pits on palms and soles Keratocysts of jaw Other dental malformations Bifid ribs Other skeletal anomalies Mesenteric cysts Ectopic calcification Ovarian fibromas	Multiple basal cell carcinomas Medulloblastoma Other brain tumours	9q31

In some instances, penetrance and expression may be influenced by the genetic background within families or individuals. In this context the extent to which constitutional mutations or variation in more than one cancer predisposition gene in an individual or family, may contribute to cancer development, is unknown. Of interest is a report of a patient with NF1 who also had a germline mutation in the p53 gene. The patient was diagnosed with multiple colon carcinomas, following apparent cure of a non-Hodgkin's lymphoma.[50] This example raises the possibility that the wide range of penetrance and expression observed in families with germline p53 mutations may in part be due to the presence of constitutional lesions in other cancer-associated genes. Contributions from more than one gene should be considered in the analysis of familial cancer clusters. Similarly, the presence of familial polyposis coli and NF1 in the same patient has been reported.[51] Given the relative frequency of NF1 in the population, examples such as the two given are to be expected. As more cancer-susceptibility genes are characterized, including those with lower penetrance than the genes so far identified, further such examples will come to light.

The ways in which genes conferring an increased risk of cancer interact with environmental hormonal and dietary factors etc., and with each other, are of profound importance in genetic counselling and screening in cancer families. The elucidation of such interactions represents a major research challenge for the future.

ACKNOWLEDGEMENTS

Jillian M. Birch is a Cancer Research Campaign Reader in Oncology.

REFERENCES

1 Easton D, Peto J. The contribution of inherited predisposition to cancer incidence. Cancer Surv 1990; 9: 395–416

2 Li FP, Fraumeni Jr JF. Soft-tissue sarcomas, breast cancer, and other neoplasms. A familial syndrome? Ann Intern Med 1969; 71: 747–752.

3 Pearson ADJ, Craft AW, Ratcliffe JM, Birch JM, Morris-Jones PH, Roberts DF. Two families with the Li-Fraumeni cancer family syndrome. J Med Genet 1982; 19: 362–365.

4 Lynch HT, Mulcahy GM, Harris RE, Guirgis HA, Lynch JF. Genetic and pathologic findings in a kindred with hereditary sarcoma, breast cancer, brain tumors, leukemia, lung, laryngeal, and adrenal cortical carcinoma. Cancer 1978; 41: 2055–2064.

5 Li FP, Fraumeni JF Jr. Prospective study of a family cancer syndrome. JAMA 1982; 247: 2692–2694.

6 Birch JM, Hartley AL, Blair V et al. Cancer in the families of children with soft tissue sarcoma. Cancer 1990; 66: 2239–2248.

7 Strong LC, Stine M, Norsted TL. Cancer in survivors of childhood soft tissue sarcoma and their relatives. J Natl Cancer Inst 1987; 79: 1213–1220.

8 Lustbader ED, Williams WR, Bondy ML, Strom S, Strong LC. Segregation analysis of cancer in families of childhood soft-tissue–sarcoma patients. Am J Hum Genet 1992; 51: 344–356.

9 Li FP, Fraumeni Jr JF, Mulvihill JJ et al. A cancer family syndrome in twenty-four kindreds. Cancer Res 1988; 48: 5358–5362.

10 Hartley AL, Birch JM, Kelsey AM, Marsden HB, Harris M, Teare MD. Are germ cell tumors part of the Li-Fraumeni Cancer Family Syndrome? Cancer Genet Cytogenet 1989; 42: 221–226.

11 Hartley AL, Birch JM, Marsden HB, Harris M. Malignant melanoma in families of children with osteosarcoma, chondrosarcoma and adrenal cortical carcinoma. J Med Genet 1987; 24: 664–668.

12 Hartley AL, Birch JM, Tricker K et al. Wilms' tumour in the Li-Fraumeni cancer family syndrome. Cancer Genet Cytogenet 1993; 67: 133–135.

13 Malkin D, Li FP, Strong LC et al. Germ line p53 mutations in a familial syndrome of breast cancer, sarcomas, and other neoplasms. Science 1990; 250: 1233–1238.

14 Srivastava S, Zou Z, Pirollo K, Blattner W, Chang EH. Germ-line transmission of a mutated p53 gene in a cancer-prone family with Li-Fraumeni syndrome. Nature 1990; 348: 747–749.

15 Birch JM, Hartley AL, Tricker KJ et al. Prevalence and diversity of constitutional mutations in the p53 gene among 21 Li-Fraumeni families. Cancer Res 1994; 54: 1298–1304.

16 Dittmer D, Pati S, Zambetti G et al. Gain of function mutations in p53. Nature Genet 1993; 4: 42–45.

17 Brugiéres L, Gardes M, Moutou C et al. Screening for germ line p53 mutations in children with malignant tumors and a family history of cancer. Cancer Res 1993; 53: 452–455.

18 Santibáñez-Koref MF, Birch JM, Hartley AL et al. p53 germline mutations in Li-Fraumeni syndrome. Lancet 1991; 338: 1490–1491.

19 Barnes DM, Hanby AM, Gillett CE et al. Abnormal expression of wild type p53 protein in normal cells of a cancer family patient. Lancet 1992; 340: 259–263.

20 Momand J, Zambetti GP, Olson DC, George D, Levine AJ. The mdm-2 oncogene product forms a complex with the p53 protein and inhibits p53-mediated transactivation. Cell 1992; 69: 1237–1245.

21 Lynch HT, Lanspa S, Smyrk T, Boman B, Watson P, Lynch J. Hereditary nonpolyposis colorectal cancer (Lynch syndromes I and II). Genetics, pathology, natural history, and cancer control, Part I. Cancer Genet Cytogenet 1991; 53: 143–160.

22 Mecklin J-P, Järvinen HJ. Tumor spectrum in cancer family syndrome (hereditary nonpolyposis colorectal cancer). Cancer 1991; 68: 1109–1112.

23 Peltomäki P, Aaltonen LA, Sistonen P et al. Genetic mapping of a locus predisposing to human colorectal cancer. Science 1993; 260: 810–812.

24 Aaltonen LA, Peltomäki P, Leach FS et al. Clues to the pathogenesis of familial colorectal cancer. Science 1993; 260: 812–816.

25 Tulinius H, Egilsson V, Olafsdóttir GH, Sigvaldason H. Risk of prostate, ovarian and endometrial cancer among relatives of women with breast cancer. BMJ 1992; 305: 855–857.

26 Anderson KE, Easton DF, Matthews FE, Peto J. Cancer mortality in the first degree relatives of young breast cancer patients. Br J Cancer 1992; 66: 599–602.

27 Teare MD, Wallace SA, Harris M, Howell A, Birch JM. Cancer experience in the relatives of an unselected series of breast cancer patients. Br J Cancer 1994 ;70: July.

28 Easton DF, Bishop DT, Ford D, Crockford GP, Breast Cancer Linkage Consortium. Genetic linkage analysis in familial breast and ovarian cancer: results from 214 families. Am J Hum Genet 1993; 52: 678–701.

29 Arason A, Barkardóttir RB, Egilsson V. Linkage analysis of chromosome 17q markers and breast-ovarian cancer in Icelandic families, and possible relationship to prostatic cancer. Am J Hum Genet 1993; 52: 711–717.

30 Cowell JK. The genetics of retinoblastoma. Br J Cancer 1991; 63: 333–336.

31 Riccardi VM. von Recklinghausen neurofibromatosis. N Engl J Med 1981; 305: 1617–1627.
32 Riccardi VM, Lewis RA. Penetrance of von Recklinghausen neurofibromatosis: a distinction between predecessors and descendants. Am J Hum Genet 1988; 42: 284–289.
33 Hope DG, Mulvihill JJ. Malignancy in neurofibromatosis. In: Riccardi VM, Mulvihill JJ, eds. Neurofibromatosis (von Recklinghausen Disease) New York: Raven Press, 1981: 33–56.
34 Barker D, Wright E, Nguyen K et al. Gene for von Recklinghausen neurofibromatosis is in the pericentromeric region of chromosome 17. Science 1987; 236: 1100–1102.
35 Seizinger BR, Houleau GA, Ozelius LJ et al. Genetic linkage of von Recklinghausen neurofibromatosis to the nerve growth factor receptor gene. Cell 1987; 49: 589–594.
36 Goldgar DE, Green P, Parry DM, Mulvihill JJ. Multipoint linkage analysis in neurofibromatosis type 1: an international collaboration. Am J Hum Genet 1989; 44: 6–12.
37 Wallace MR, Marchuk DA, Andersen LB et al. Type 1 neurofibromatosis gene: identification of a large transcript disrupted in three NF1 patients. Science 1990; 249: 181–186.
38 Viskochil D, Buchberg AM, Xu G et al. Deletions and a translocation interrupt a cloned gene at the neurofibromatosis type 1 locus. Cell 1990, 62. 187–192.
39 Gutmann DH, Wood DL, Collins FS. Identification of the neurofibromatosis type 1 gene product. Proc Natl Acad Sci USA 1991; 88: 9658–9662.
40 Maher ER, Iselius L, Yates JRW et al. Von Hippel-Lindau disease: a genetic study. J Med Genet 1991; 28: 443–447.
41 Neumann HPH, Wiestler OD. Clustering of features of von Hippel-Lindau syndrome: evidence for a complex genetic locus. Lancet 1991; 337: 1052–1054.
42 Seizinger BR, Rouleau GA, Ozelius LJ, Lane AH, Farmer GE, Lamiell JM et al. Von Hippel-Lindau disease maps to the region of chromosome 3 associated with renal cell carcinoma. Nature 1988; 332: 268–269.
43 Latif F, Tory K, Gnarra J et al. Identification of the von Hippel-Lindau disease tumor suppressor gene. Science 1993; 260: 1317–1320.
44 Gorlin RJ, Goltz RW. Multiple naevoid basal cell epithelioma, jaw cysts and bifid ribs: a syndrome. N Engl J Med 1960; 262: 908–912.
45 Evans DGR, Birch JM, Orton CI. Brain tumours and the occurrence of severe invasive basal cell carcinoma in first degree relatives with Gorlin syndrome. Br J Neurosurg 1991; 5: 643–646.
46 Evans DGR, Farndon PA, Burnell LD, Gattamaneni R, Birch J. The incidence of Gorlin syndrome in 173 consecutive cases of medulloblastoma. Br J Cancer 1991; 64: 959–961.
47 Farndon PA, Del Mastro RG, Evans DGR, Kilpatrick MW. Location of gene for Gorlin syndrome. Lancet 1992; 339: 581–582.
48 Gailani MR, Bale SJ, Leffell DJ, DiGiovanna JJ, Peck GL, Pollak S et al. Developmental defects in Gorlin syndrome related to a putative tumor suppressor gene on chromosome 9. Cell 1992; 69: 111–117.
49 Hartley AL, Birch JM, Kelsey AM, Harris M, Morris Jones PH. Sarcomas in three generations of a family with neurofibromatosis. Cancer Genet Cytogenet 1990; 45: 245–248.
50 Shearer P, Parham D, Kovnar E et al. Neurofibromatosis Type 1 and malignancy: review of 32 pediatric cases treated at a single institution. Med Pediatr Oncol 1994; 22: 78–83.
51 Lynch HT, Fitzgibbons Jr RJ, Lanspa SJ, Marcus JN, Lynch JF, Kopelovich L. Familial polyposis coli and neurofibromatosis in the same patient: a family study. Cancer Genet Cytogenet 1987; 28: 245–251.

British Medical Bulletin (1994) Vol. 50, No. 3, pp. 640–655

Genetics of colorectal cancer

C Cunningham
M G Dunlop

MRC Human Genetics Unit, Western General Hospital, Edinburgh, UK

Recent advances in understanding the genetic basis of malignant disease have been dominated by research in colorectal cancer. In familial adenomatous polyposis, characterisation of the causative gene had immediate clinical relevance allowing confident prediction of disease inheritance. Somatic mutations in this gene have been demonstrated to have a fundamental role in the development of sporadic colorectal cancer. More recently, efforts have focused on the genetic abnormalities responsible for hereditary non-polyposis colorectal cancer which may possibly account for up to 15% of all colorectal malignancies. In the foreseeable future, it is possible that significant population-based genetic screening for this condition will be available. As the molecular basis of colorectal cancer is elucidated, it will inevitably lead to radical changes in clinical management, particularly with the possible introduction of gene therapy and chemoprevention. This review discusses the current developments in colorectal cancer genetics which will be central to such changes.

Colorectal cancer is a common malignancy responsible for around 20 000 deaths in the UK each year and consuming considerable health care resources. Traditional diagnostic and therapeutic approaches have made little impact on survival over the last 30 years. Advances in molecular biology with regard to both fundamental knowledge and practical application hold great promise for the future early detection, prevention and treatment of colorectal cancer.

In recent years the cloning and identification of a number of genes involved in colorectal cancer development and susceptibility has resulted in an unprecedented expansion in the knowledge of fundamental genetic aspects of cancer biology. This review discusses the background and recent advances made in understanding the role of a number of important colorectal cancer genes, including *APC, hMSH2, p53, DCC* and *ras* genes.

FAMILIAL ADENOMATOUS POLYPOSIS

Role of *APC* gene in familial adenomatous polyposis

Constitutional mutations in the *APC* gene are responsible for familial adenomatous polyposis (FAP) and data suggest that somatic mutations in *APC* are ubiquitous in colorectal adenomas and carcinomas.[1,2] FAP is an autosomal dominant disorder with an annual incidence of around 1/7000 births. It is characterised by the development of hundreds to thousands of adenomatous polyps in the colon and rectum with the inevitable development of malignancy unless prophylactic colectomy is undertaken. The syndrome is also associated with a number of extracolonic features. Some of these are innocuous, such as epidermoid cysts and retinal pigmentation; but others are more sinister, including multiple osteomata, desmoid tumours and gastroduodenal polyposis and malignancy (which includes ampullary carcinoma, cholangiocarcinoma and hepatoblastomas).[3]

   Initial localisation of the *APC* gene was suggested by cytogenetic studies and further mapping by genetic linkage analysis, localised the gene to a region on the long arm of chromosome 5. DNA was eventually cloned from chromosome 5q21 and several candidate genes identified for further analysis. DNA sequencing identified mutations in one of these candidate genes which showed germline transmission to affected offspring in FAP families, indicating that it was the causative gene. The gene was named *APC* and had features of a tumour suppressor gene.[4,5] *APC* is a fairly large gene consisting of 15 exons encoding a 2843 amino acid polypeptide. Exons 1–14 are small and exon 15 is large, accounting for 77% of the coding region. There are alternatively spliced forms of *APC*, and it is likely that more than 15 exons will eventually be identified. In FAP, 97% of mutations occur in the 5′ half of the gene, 60% in a region of 600 codons within exon 15. Within this region 10% of mutations occur at two specific sites at codons 1061 and 1309.[6] The mutations detected so far are mainly deletions or insertions of short sequences which suggests errors of replication rather than the action of mutagens.[7] Only about 40% of germline mutations are single nucleotide substitutions (most commonly C to T transitions). However, the analyses employed to detect mutations may have introduced bias, preferentially detecting insertions or deletions rather than substitutions. It is almost certain that all mutations causing the FAP syndrome result in a premature STOP codon, either directly or by frame shift, resulting in premature termination of transcription and truncation of the protein.[6] In some FAP patients, mutations in *APC* have not yet been identified. It is likely that such mutations will ultimately be shown to affect transcription, occurring within promoter regions, splice sites or introns. Although mutations at codons 1061 and 1309 are relatively frequent, the majority of mutations show no evidence of clustering and, therefore, attempts at mutation identification are time consuming and laborious.

The adenomas of FAP acquire somatic mutations in the remaining wild type (normal) copy of the *APC* gene with increasing frequency as the adenomas increase in size and dysplasia.[8] Approximately half of these somatic events are large genetic rearrangements or deletions detected by loss of heterozygosity, and the remainder are mutations with a similar profile to those occurring in the germline, resulting in truncation of the protein. There are 2 possibilities with regard to the generation of somatic *APC* mutations occurring in the colon. First, mutagens in the faecal stream directly cause mutations and the subsequent expansion occurs due to an acquired growth advantage. The second possibility is that cells carrying an impairment in DNA repair mechanisms, such as occurs in *hMSH2* mutation (see below) may have a specific difficulty in repairing *APC* frameshift mutations. The net result is selective growth advantage caused by the *APC* mutation and clonal expansion of cells carrying such a defect. Overall, it is possible that both mechanisms may operate to varying extents between individuals, thereby accounting for the variety of somatic genetic lesions in adenomas of FAP. The colorectal cancers arising in FAP patients are very similar to sporadic colorectal cancers in terms of distribution, histology and indeed in molecular alterations.[6]

Presymptomatic screening and diagnosis

Genetic linkage analysis has been of considerable value in presymptomatic diagnosis enabling the identification of affected individuals who had previously been discharged from clinical follow-up.[9] With new polymorphic intragenic markers based on highly informative microsatellite polymorphisms, the predictive power of linkage analysis increases such that it can identify those inheriting the disease with a reliability of more than 99%. However, this depends on the availability of DNA from (usually) at least 2 affected individuals in the family. Problems such as early death of gene carriers, uncertain paternity within families and the fact that 25% of FAP patients carry a new mutation with no family history, substantially reduces the value of linkage studies in many clinical situations. In addition, linkage-based prediction always carries a residual uncertainty, which should be absent when diagnosis is offered by analysis of mutations.

Mutation analysis relies on identifying the specific mutation causing FAP in an affected individual. Since the mutation is inherited by all affected members in the family, its subsequent detection in at-risk relatives confirms the presence of the disease susceptibility. The presence of a mutation is initially determined by screening analyses which exploit the ability to detect single base pair changes in a sequence of a few hundred nucleotides. Such techniques, including single stranded conformation polymorphism (SSCP) analysis, denaturing gel electrophoresis, heteroduplex analysis and chemical mismatch analysis, only allow the identification of a region likely to contain a mutation.[10] Sequence analysis is then used to determine the details of the mutation in terms of the exact location and nature of the defect – ie whether deletion, insertion or substitution. Once a mutation is detected, more user-friendly techniques can be designed to identify the same mutation in other family members. These may utilise PCR primers which will specifically amplify mutant alleles or exploit changes in restriction endonuclease cutting sites which can be detected by PCR and enzyme digest. In the near future it is likely that preliminary screening analyses will concentrate on the identification of mutant protein as opposed to DNA by means of in vitro synthesis of mutant protein or by functional assays. In vitro transcription/translation systems can be applied to wildtype and mutant *APC* gene and the peptides produced separated by gel electrophoresis. The products can be visualised by monoclonal antibodies or the incorporation of radiolabelled amino acids. This technique allows exploitation of the truncation of APC protein generated by mutations resulting in STOP codons. Hence, a single screening analysis may detect a wide array of mutations, all of which result in the generation of a STOP codon. In one recent example of a functional assay, a PCR-amplified *APC* fragment was cloned into a plasmid vector with the *Lac Z* gene.[11] When the plasmid is transfected into bacteria, those bacteria which produce a 'normal' fusion *APC* fragment-Lac Z protein product have an active galactosidase gene and produce deep blue colonies on appropriate medium. However, those with mutant *APC* gene containing a premature STOP codon cannot efficiently transcribe the *Lac Z* gene and produce light blue colonies. This is an elegant example of how knowledge of the mutation spectrum in a specific disease can be used to practical effect. These strategies will be applicable to other genes where mutations alter the protein structure through premature truncation or alternative splicing.

Individuals in FAP families who are shown not to carry the mutant gene need not be subjected to clinical screening. Indeed, in the near future, those family members known to carry an *APC* mutation will be the only at-risk individuals requiring follow up and this will be performed as a management exercise to assess the optimum timing for surgery. Mutation analysis will soon be the most frequently used technique in routine presymtomatic testing in FAP. Linkage analyses will be reserved for confirmation of carrier status predictions in those where no *APC* mutation is detected and the underlying genetic lesion is presumed to have subtle effects on splicing or transcription. Although a laborious activity, identification of every mutation responsible for FAP is desirable in elucidating possible genotype-phenotype correlations and providing ultimate diagnostic reliability.

APC gene function and genotype-phenotype correlation in FAP

The function of the *APC* gene product is under intense study. An association with α- and β-catenins has been recently demonstrated. These proteins bind to the cell surface molecule E-cadherin, and are essential for its role in cellular adhesion. It is proposed that APC protein may affect the interaction between catenins and E-cadherin, thus influencing cellular adhesion and possibly intercellular communication.[12,13]Antibodies to the APC protein have identified a 300 kD cytoplasmic protein expressed in epithelial cells in the upper portions of the colonic crypts, suggesting it is functional in the mature colonocyte.[14] Short repeat sequences within APC protein have been identified which are predicted to form coiled coil structures. This may allow the molecule to form dimers with other proteins including itself, thereby modifying protein function. Mutant APC protein is known to interact with normal *APC* resulting in a heterodimer with reduced function. Thus the mutant *APC* is acting in a dominant-negative manner.[15] The extent to which normal *APC* function is impaired may be related to the structure and residual ability of the mutant protein to form dimers. Short 5' truncations may fail to form mutant/wild type dimers whereas more 3' mutations may form dimers with wild type protein, reducing overall function and creating a more aggressive phenotype. Recently, a more definite correlation between the specific type of germline *APC* mutation and disease phenotype has been proposed. Analysis of 7 families displaying an attenuated phenotype with few colorectal polyps identified 4 separate mutations in exons 3 and 4, all of which resulted in a very short mutant protein.[16] The position of these mutations appeared to define a functional boundary between codons 157 and 168. Markedly truncated proteins from mutations 5' to this boundary resulted in an attenuated phenotype and those more 3' produced a larger protein causing classical FAP with multiple polyposis. Such findings support the existence of dominant-negative behaviour in larger truncations. However, the presence of classical FAP phenotype when one entire copy of the *APC* gene is lost in a constitutional chromosomal deletion indicates that the dominant-negative effect of mutant protein is not the only phenotypic determinant. A similar relationship between the site of the mutation and phenotype with congenital hypertrophy of the retinal pigment epithelium (CHRPE) is noted.[17] However, in this instance the critical boundary lies in exon 9. Mutations 3′ to this region are associated with CHRPE lesions, whereas those more 5′ mutations which produce a shorter protein product, are not. These recent reports provide the most convincing evidence that an independent relationship exists between type of mutation and phenotype. However, the number of reported mutations and quality of clinical data produced to date have not permitted the complete elucidation of the clinical effects of different APC mutations. Indeed, identical APC mutations have been associated with diverse FAP phenotypes.[17]

Overall, there is considerable evidence to support the existence of factors other than simply the type of mutation which can influence expression of the APC gene defect. There may be environmental components. Evidence from the Min (multiple intestinal neoplasia) mouse, which is a model for FAP, indicates that phenotypic expression can also be modulated by an unlinked genetic locus.[19] Identification of the murine and homologous human modifier genes will be of great importance with regard to understanding and treating the human condition. The variation in phenotype apparent in individuals carrying identical APC mutation[17] may be explained by such modifier effects.

The role of APC in sporadic colorectal tumorigenesis

Study of the APC gene in FAP, and in the neoplasms which develop in patients with FAP and non-FAP colorectal cancer, has provided insight into the mechanisms of sporadic colorectal carcinogenesis. Somatic mutations in the APC gene have been shown in over 80% of sporadic colorectal cancers and adenomas and, indeed, are likely to be ubiquitous in colorectal neoplasia.[6] Furthermore, inactivation of APC appears to be one of the earliest events in sporadic colorectal tumourigenesis.[2] The data suggest that a double knock-out of APC is a frequent, if not essential, event in sporadic colorectal cancer. One copy of APC is inactivated by point mutation and the other most frequently by loss or rearrangement of a larger sequence of DNA, although inactivating point mutations of both alleles are well documented.

Novel therapeutic approaches in FAP

Gene therapy

Single gene disorders, such as FAP, are potentially attractive candidates for gene therapy where the delivery of a normal APC gene under the control of a suitable promoter by means of a viral vector may correct the phenotypic changes. However, in FAP, colectomy is associated with such low operative mortality and provides such a drastic reduction in the risk of cancer, that there would have to be considerable evidence of potential benefit before surgical prophylaxis could be abandoned. Even so, gene therapy may still be useful. There will undoubtedly be a place for local gene therapy to the retained rectum after colectomy and ileorectal anastomosis. The delivery of replacement genes may allow control of upper GI polyposis and malignancy (which is a major cause of mortality) and provide some control of desmoid disease, another of the capricious problems associated with FAP. The development of methods of administration of novel gene therapies is an area of intense interest. For local delivery of gene therapy to the rectum in FAP patients following ileorectal anastomosis, the normal gene and its vector (delivered to the cells by a either viral or liposome system) would be administered by enema and the effects on rectal polyposis could be readily assessed. The intraluminal delivery of *APC* gene is unlikely to provide an efficient means of reaching every stem cell in all parts of the colon. However, treatment of the rectum after ileorectal anastomosis may allow retention of the rectum even for patients with rectal carpeting. In view of this, the authors believe that it may be wise to avoid restorative proctocolectomy for FAP patients at the present time, unless rectal polyposis is uncontrollable.

Chemoprevention in FAP

Recent reports have suggested that the administration of aspirin or sulindac may have a role in controlling both rectal and upper GI polyposis in FAP.[20] Chemical carcinogenesis studies in animals suggest that aspirin and other non-steroidal anti-inflammatory drugs (NSAIDs) have a strong protective effect in colorectal cancer.[21] In addition there are several series suggesting that aspirin prophylaxis reduces death from colorectal cancer in humans.[22] These effects are believed to be mediated by inhibition of prostaglandin H synthetase and offer a potential mode of therapeutic intervention in FAP and in prevention of non-FAP colorectal cancer. Unfortunately, recent reports suggest that the observed reduction in the number of colorectal polyps in FAP patients may be only transient.[23] However, second generation NSAIDs could be designed specifically for their anti-neoplastic effect.

Advances in our understanding of cancer genetics have revolutionised approaches in the screening and diagnosis of FAP and there is encouraging evidence that gene therapy will transform management. There is every reason to believe that the methodology and principles underlying these advances will be applicable to non-FAP colorectal cancer.

THE HNPCC LOCUS IN SUSCEPTIBILITY TO COLORECTAL CANCER

The identification of the *APC* gene was aided by the dominant, fully penetrant nature of FAP. However, more common heritable forms of colorectal cancer are described, which lack any phenotype other than the development of cancer at an early age. Of this group, hereditary non-polyposis colorectal cancer (HNPCC) is the most well defined. HNPCC is an autosomal dominant disorder with high penetrance which may account for up to 5–15% of cases of colorectal cancer. Adenomatous polyps are found in HNPCC patients, but the numbers are much smaller than FAP (usually <10); which is comparable to the frequency of ademonas in the general population. There is a propensity for both adenomas and carcinomas to develop in the proximal part of the colon and the age of onset is earlier than in the general population. HNPCC can be inherited as a site-specific colorectal cancer susceptibility trait (Lynch Type 1) or associated with breast, ovarian, uterine and other malignancies (Lynch Type 2 or cancer family syndrome).

Recently, 2 reports have identified a gene on chromosome 2p which appears to be responsible for colorectal cancer susceptibility in many HNPCC families.[24,25] The importance of the discovery of such a gene cannot be overestimated as its involvement in both familial and sporadic forms of the disease may dramatically alter the traditional clinical approach to colorectal cancer. The initial localisation of this gene was achieved by linkage studies in 2 large unrelated HNPCC pedigrees.[26] DNA from each family member was used in a systematic genetic linkage analysis employing 345 polymorphic markers spread throughout the human genome. The aim was to identify any marker which co-segregated with the disease phenotype. The majority of markers employed were highly polymorphic short repeat microsatellite polymorphisms, known as $(CA)_n$ repeats.

The disease phenotype was found to co-segregate with an anonymous marker, D2S123, mapping to the short arm of chromosome 2 in both large families studied. This indicated the presence of a causative gene near the location of D2S123. The gene has subsequently been named *hMSH2*. The frequency of involvement of *hMSH2* in colorectal cancer susceptibility was determined by analysis of 14 smaller HNPCC kindreds. Most were either definitely or likely to be linked to this locus, however, one-third showed no evidence of linkage to D2S123, clearly establishing genetic heterogeneity in HNPCC.[26] The genetic heterogeneity of HNPCC has also been indicated by further independent studies which have excluded linkage to the chromosome 2 locus in some families. In one report the HNPCC families had late onset colorectal cancer, suggesting heterogenecity based on age at onset,[27] while others have found co-segregation between HNPCC families and a locus on chromosome 3.[28] It would therefore appear that, although most HNPCC families appear phenotypically homogenous, more than one locus is involved.

Colorectal cancers from patients in families linked to chromosome 2p and, indeed, those linked to chromosome 3p displayed a form of genomic instability in tumour DNA.[28,29] This was noted by a change in the electrophoretic mobility of the microsatellite $(CA)_n$ alleles in tumour as compared to normal DNA. This instability was found throughout the genome at random sites unrelated to any described colorectal cancer genes. A similar form of instability in microsatellite DNA markers was demonstrated in yeast and was shown to be caused by mutations in mismatch repair genes.[30] This putative association between mismatch repair genes and genomic instability in human colorectal cancers was exploited by one of the 2 groups responsible for the cloning and identification of the susceptibility gene. Fishel et al[24] determined the chromosomal location of the human homologs of yeast and bacterial mismatch repair genes (*MSH2* and *MutS*, respectively) which was possible because genes with such fundamental function tend to show considerable inter-species homology. One such homolog, *hMSH2*, was localised to human chromosome 2p in the region already shown by linkage studies to be likely to contain the HNPCC susceptibility locus. The group proposed that this mismatch repair gene was a strong candidate for the susceptibility gene. Fishel et al also determined the location of the mouse homolog of the mismatch repair gene, on mouse chromosome 17, which will allow the development of important mouse models of HNPCC.

Leach et al[25] employed a combination of positional cloning and a candidate gene strategy, generating multiple markers within the region of 25 cM which linkage studies suggested contained the susceptibility gene.[26] These were applied to 6 HNPCC families shown to be linked to the chromosome 2p gene. Recombination events were identified which designated a 0.8 Mb region containing the locus of interest. Candidate genes in this 0.8 Mb region were identified and sequenced for the presence of germline mutations in HNPCC kindreds. These genes included a homolog of the bacterial mismatch repair gene *MutS*. cDNA was generated from the human homolog, which was named *hMSH2*. The sequence was similar between species and contained a highly conserved region between codons 615–788. Several mutations were identified in the highly conserved region of *hMSH2*, which co-segregated with the disease in HNPCC families, implying that this is the causative gene.

These mutations comprise both missense and nonsense mutations, and a single splice defect.

Many of the genes involved in colorectal carcinogenesis are tumour suppressor genes, recognisable by loss of heterozygosity (LOH) in tumours. There was no evidence of significant LOH at the hMSH2 or chromosome 3p locus in any of the colorectal cancers examined, suggesting that hMSH2 mutation causes cancer by a different mechanism. Mutation in hMSH2 results in a defect in the fidelity of DNA replication. This is manifest in cancer DNA as shifts in electrophoretic mobility of the $(CA)_n$ repeat microsatellite markers, described earlier. Such replication errors could be responsible for the mutation of other important genes involved in the various stages of development of colorectal neoplasia such as APC, or could cause variation which may have a role in the control of transcription.[31]

Evidence of genomic instability has also been identified in apparently sporadic tumours, although at a lower frequency.[29,31-33] The majority of sporadic cancers displaying microsatellite instability have features similar to HNPCC tumours: that is, location primarily in the proximal colon, younger age at onset and a tendency to have a diploid karyotype. Hence, these apparently 'sporadic' cancers may also be generated by a constitutional hMSH2 mutation, or a similar mutation in another 'mutator' gene.

Mutation analysis of the hMSH2 gene in colorectal cancer families linked to chromosome 2p will provide invaluable information for predictive testing. Population-based mutation studies will be required to determine the penetrance of the hMSH2 mutations and the population prevalence of mutation in the gene. This must be known before population screening can be considered. For the present, efforts could be targeted on individuals developing colorectal cancer before 45 years of age. The identification of this gene is likely to radically change the selection of individuals for screening, and possibly the treatment of patients with bowel cancer. Eventually, it may lead to new prophylactic drug treatments to counter the tendency to develop replication errors in individuals who carry the hMSH2 mutation.

p53 GENE IN COLORECTAL CARCINOGENESIS

Abnormalities of p53 are the commonest genetic events associated with human cancers.[34] There has been considerable impetus to understand the normal cellular functions of p53 and how these may be altered in carcinogenesis (see Lane, this issue). p53 is a phosphoprotein which enters the nucleus during DNA synthesis, exerting control over the transcription of other genes and regulating the onset of DNA replication at the G1-S boundary.[35] Elevated levels of stabilised p53 protein are detected on exposure of cells to DNA-damaging agents, such as ionising radiation. In these conditions p53 appears to block cell growth, thereby allowing DNA repair prior to cell division. Alternatively p53 may induce apoptosis. Recent work has indicated that apoptosis in response to ionising radiation and etoposide is p53 dependent.[36,37] This may have important clinical implications, as apoptotic tumour cell death in response to radiation and chemotherapy is likely to be reduced in the absence of *p53* function. Cancers lacking *p53* might therefore be more resistant to treatment.[38] It is possible that restoration of *p53* function would increase response to conventional therapies. Loss of function of wild type *p53* also appears to result in chromosome instability and aneuploidy.[39] This is demonstrated in fibroblast cell lines from Li-Fraumeni patients, which have constitutional *p53* mutations. These cell lines readily become aneuploid and acquire immortality in vitro.[40] The exact significance of this instability is uncertain, but it may favour the appearance of neoplastic clones.

The *p53* mutational spectrum exhibits tissue specificity. Most mutations in colorectal cancer are found in codons 175, 248, 278 and 282. These are most commonly single base transitions in CpG nucleotides causing mis-sense mutations.[41] Such mutations result in a full length protein with altered conformation and abnormal function. The exact relationship between the type of *p53* mutation and the effects on cellular function is undetermined. Under normal conditions *p53* functions as a tumour suppressor gene. However, it appears that certain types of mutation may result in *p53* acting as a dominant oncogene with gain of function rather than simply loss of tumour suppressor function[42] (*see also* Lane, this issue).

p53 mutation is rare in colorectal adenomas, indicating that it occurs late in the process of tumourgenesis.[39] Constitutional *p53* mutations have been shown to be responsible for the rare, autosomal dominant Li-Fraumeni syndrome[43] which is characterised by predisposition to a variety of cancers including brain tumours, breast carcinomas, soft tissue sarcomas, leukaemia, osteosarcomas and adrenocortical carcinomas. However, colorectal cancer is very rare in Li-Fraumeni gene carriers and despite an extensive search, we have shown that constitutional *p53* mutations are not involved in the development of colorectal cancer in patients who succumb to the disease at an early age.[44]

SOMATIC EVENTS IN OTHER COLORECTAL CANCER GENES

Deleted in colon cancer (*DCC*) gene

Cytogenetic studies in colorectal cancer demonstrated frequent deletions involving the long arm of chromosome 18, and molecular genetic studies detected frequent allele loss on 18q21-ter in tumour DNA.[45]

A large gene was identified by positional cloning, in a region defined by a chromosome 18q rearrangement in a single cancer. This gene was named *DCC*. It encodes a 12.5kb transcript which is expressed at a low level in many tissues including normal colonic mucosa, but expression is reduced or absent in colorectal cancer tissue.[46] This strongly suggests that the *DCC* gene is indeed a tumour suppressor gene, consistent with the finding that in colorectal cancer both copies of the gene are apparently inactivated by mutation, deletion or rearrangement as detected by LOH.[47] LOH involving the *DCC* gene is found in large adenomas as well as carcinomas indicating that inactivation of this gene is important in the intermediate stages of colorectal tumorigenesis.[45]

Preliminary data suggested that *DCC* may also be involved in colorectal cancer susceptibility. This was based on the description of a family which exhibited genetic linkage of the Kidd blood group to a dominant non-polyposis trait developing colorectal cancer at an early age.[48] The Kidd blood group has been shown to map to a region very close to *DCC* on chromosme 18q. However, published data and our own unpublished findings have not detected any evidence for linkage of intragenic *DCC* markers in a number of HNPCC kindreds.[49] As genetic heterogeneity in HNPCC is well documented, it remains possible that *DCC* is a colorectal cancer susceptibility locus in a minority of families. It will be of great interest to carry out further analysis of *DCC* in HNPCC families who are shown not to be linked to the *hMSH2* gene on chromosome 2 or the putative chromosome 3p locus.

The *ras* genes

Activated proto-oncogenes have been shown to play a major role in many human cancers. The *ras* gene family are cytoplasmic proto-oncogenes with signal transduction functions. Activating mutations in codons 12 and 13 of Kirsten *ras* occur in 50% of colorectal cancers and adenomas greater than 1 cm in diameter.[45] The frequency of Kirsten *ras* mutations is much lower in adenomas <1cm and it appears that this oncogene is involved in the progression of adenoma to carcinoma.[50] Kirsten *ras* expression, although high in primary carcinomas, tends to be lower in clinically advanced cases, indicating that when the tumour progresses to a certain stage, *ras* activation is no longer required.

There is some evidence to suggest that the *ras* genes may also be involved in colorectal cancer susceptibility. Recently, a meta-analysis of all published studies identified a clear association between rare alleles of a microsatellite sequence adjacent to Harvey *ras* and risk of cancer at several sites. The authors propose from their findings that 1 in 11 colorectal cancers might be attributable to the occurence of predisposing Harvey *ras* alleles in the population.[51] It is possible that inheritance of a rare Harvey *ras* allele may indicate an increased risk of colorectal cancer and that this predisposition may interact with predisposition due to inheritance of a *hMSH2* or other DNA repair gene mutation.

Chromosome 8p tumour suppressor locus

A number of chromosome loci exhibit frequent non-random LOH, indicating the presence of a putative tumour suppressor gene. LOH at loci on chromosome 8p is seen in 50% of colorectal cancers,[52] but in less than 10% of adenomas, suggesting a role for this locus late in tumourigenesis.[53] No candidate gene has yet been described but this locus also appears to be important in bladder, prostate and hepatocellular cancer,[54-56] providing further evidence that its overall contribution to carcinogenesis is substantial. Recent work suggests there may be 2 tumour suppressor genes in this region.[57] With improved localisation the exact contribution of these genes will be ascertained, including any role in cancer predisposition.

PERSPECTIVE

Over the last 5 years increased understanding of the molecular mechanisms of carcinogenesis has resulted in an unprecedented change in approaches to screening for colorectal cancer associated with FAP. In the future it seems likely that manipulation of the disease process will be possible by means of gene therapy and chemoprevention. Improvements in predictive testing will continue, particularly through the use of in vitro transcription/translation systems and functional assays. With the discovery of the *hMSH2* gene and characterisation of its function, every aspect of current detection, diagnosis and treatment of colorectal cancer will require re-evaluation. Constitutional *hMSH2* mutations and other human mutator gene defects (eg the 3p locus) could account for a substantial proportion of all colorectal cancer. Within HNPCC families, predictive testing will force important management dilemmas, particularly the use of prophylactic colectomy. However, as understanding of the function of the *hMSH2* gene and DNA repair mechanisms progresses, through the use of mouse models with the defective gene, it is possible that novel gene therapy approaches will be developed with the potential to radically alter current management.

In the light of the recent discoveries outlined above and the rapid advances in the technological aspects of molecular genetics, a significant reduction in the death rate from colorectal cancer now seems a realistic possibility in the foreseeable future.

ACKNOWLEDGEMENTS

Christopher Cunningham is supported by a University of Edinburgh Medical Faculty Fellowship.

REFERENCES

1 Miyoshi Y, Nagase H, Ando H et al. Somatic mutations in the *APC* gene in colorectal tumours: mutation cluster region in the *APC* gene. Hum Mol Genet 1992; 1: 229–233.

2 Powell SM, Zilz N, Beazer-Barclay Y et al. *APC* mutations occur early during colorectal tumorigenesis. Nature 1992; 359: 235–237.

3 Parks TG. Extracolonic manifestations associated with familial adenomatous polyposis. Ann R Coll Surg Engl 1990; 72: 181–184.

4 Groden J, Thliveris A, Samowitz W et al. Identification and characterisation of the familial adenomatous polyposis coli gene. Cell 1991; 66: 589–600.

5 Kinzler, KW, Nilbert MC, Su L-K et al. Identification of FAP locus genes from chromosome 5q21. Science 1991; 253: 661–665.

6 Nagase H, Nakamura Y. Mutations of the *APC* (adenomatous polyposis coli) gene. Hum Mutat 1993; 2: 425–434.

7 Nagase H, Miyoshi Y, Horii A et al. Screening for germ-line mutations in familial adenomatous polyposis patients: 61 new patients and a summary of 150 unrelated patients. Hum Mutat 1992; 1: 467–473.

8 Miyaki M, Seki M, Okamoto M et al. Genetic changes and histopathological types in colorectal tumours from patients with familial adenomatous polyposis. Cancer Res 1990; 50: 7166–7173.

9 Dunlop MG, Wyllie AH, Steel CM, Piris J, Evans HJ. Linked DNA markers for presymptomatic diagnosis of familial adenomatous polyposis. Lancet 1991; 337: 313–316.

10 Grompe M. The rapid detection of unknown mutations in nucleic acids. Nature Genet 1993; 5: 111–117.

11 Varesco L, Groden J, Spirio L et al. A rapid screening method to detect nonsense and frameshift mutations: identification of disease-causing alleles. Cancer Res 1993; 53: 5581–5584.

12 Rubinfeld B, Souza B, Albert I et al. Association of the *APC* gene product with β-catenin. Science 1993; 262: 1731–1734.

13 Su L-K, Vogelstein B, Kinzler K. Association of the *APC* tumour suppressor protein with catenins. Science 1993; 262: 1734–1737.

14 Smith KJ, Johnson KA, Bryan T et al. The *APC* gene product in normal and tumour cells. Proc Natl Acad Sci USA 1993; 90: 2846–2850.

15 Su L-K, Johnson KA, Smith KJ, Hill DE, Vogelstein B, Kinzler KW. Association between wild type and mutant *APC* gene products. Cancer Res 1993; 53: 2728–2731.

16 Spirio L, Olshwang S, Groden J et al. Alleles of the *APC* gene: an attenuated form of familial polyposis. Cell 1993; 75: 951–957.

17 Olshwang S, Tiret A, Laurent-Puig P, Muleris M, Parc R, Thomas G. Restriction of ocular fundus lesions to a specific subgroup of *APC* mutations in adenomatous polyposis coli patients. Cell 1993; 75: 959–968.

18 Paul P, Letteboer T, Gelbert L, Groden J, White R, Coppes MJ. Identical *APC* exon 15 mutations result in a variable phenotype in familial adenomatous polyposis. Hum Mol Genet 1993; 2: 925–931.

19 Moser AR, Pitot HC, Dove WF. A dominant mutation that predisposes to multiple intestinal neoplasia in the mouse. Science 1990; 247: 322–324.

20 Giardiello FM, Hamilton SR, Krush AJ et al. Treatment of colonic and rectal adenomas with sulindac in familial adenomatous polyposis. N Engl J Med 1993; 328: 1313–1316.

21 Pollard M, Lockert PH. Effect of indomethacin on intestinal tumours in rats by the acetate derivative of dimethylnitrosamine. Science 1981; 214: 558–559.

22 Thun MJ, Namboodiri MM, Heath CW. Aspirin use and reduced risk of fatal colon cancer. N Engl J Med 1991; 325: 1593–1596.

23 Tonelli F, Valanzano R. Sulindac in familial adenomatous polyposis. Lancet 1993; 342: 1120.

24 Fishel R, Lescoe MK, Rao MRS et al. The human mutator gene homolog *MSH2* and its association with hereditary nonpolyposis colon cancer. Cell 1993; 75: 1027–1038.

25 Leach FS, Nicolaides NC, Papadopolous N et al. Mutations of a MutS homolog in hereditary non-polyposis colorectal cancer. Cell 1993; 75: 1215–1225.

26 Peltomaki P, Aaltonen LA, Sistonen P et al. Genetic mapping of a locus predisposing to human colorectal cancer. Science 1993; 260: 810–812.

27 Lewis CM, Cannon-Albright RW, Burt JD et al. Linkage analysis of colorectal cancer to chromosome 2 in Utah kindreds. Am J Hum Genet 1993; 53 (3): A23.

28 Lindblom A, Tannergard P, Werelius B, Nordenskjold M. Genetic mapping of a second locus predisposing to hereditary non-polyposis colon cancer. Nature Genet 1993; 5: 279–282.

29 Aaltonen LA, Peltomaki P, Leach FS et al. Clues to the pathogenesis of familial colon cancer. Science 1993; 260: 812–816.

30 Strand M, Prolla TA, Liskay RM, Petes TD. Destabilization of tracts of simple repetitive DNA in yeasts by mutations affecting DNA mismatch repair. Nature 1993; 365: 274–276.

31 Ionov Y, Peinado MA, Malkhosyan S, Shibata D, Perucho M. Ubiquitous somatic mutations in simple repeated sequences reveal a new mechanism for colonic carcinogenesis. Nature 1993; 363: 558–561.

32 Young J, Leggett B, Gustafson C et al. Genomic instability occurs in colorectal carcinomas but not in adenomas. Hum Mutat 1993; 2: 351–354.

33 Thibodeau SN, Bren G, Schaid D. Microsatellite instability in cancer of the proximal colon. Science 1993; 260: 816–819.

34 Hollstein M, Sidransky D, Vogelstein B, Harris CC. *p53* mutations in human cancers. Science 1991: 253: 49–53.

35 Vogelstein B, Kinzler KW. *p53* function and dysfunction. Cell 1992; 70: 523–526.

36 Clarke AR, Purdie CA, Harrison DJ et al. Thymocyte apoptosis induced by *p53*-dependent and independent pathways. Nature 1993; 362: 849–851.

37 Lowe SW, Schmitt EM, Smith SW, Osborne BA, Jacks T. *p53* is required for radiation-induced apoptosis in mouse thymocytes. Nature 1993; 362: 847–849.

38 Lowe SW, Ruley HE, Jacks T, Housman DE. *p53*-dependent apoptosis modulates the cytotoxicity of anticancer agents. Cell 1993; 74: 957–967.

39 Carder P, Wyllie AH, Purdie CA et al. Stabilised *p53* facilitates aneuploid clonal divergence in colorectal cancer. Oncogene 1993; 8: 1397–1401.

40 Bischoff JR, Friedman PN, Marshak DR, Prives C, Beach D. Human *p53* is phosphorylated by p60-cdc2 and cyclin B-cdc2. Proc Natl Acad Sci USA 1990; 87: 4766–4770.

41 Prives C, Manfredi JJ. The *p53* tumour suppressor protein: meeting review. Genes Dev 1993; 7: 529–534.

42 Halvey O, Michalovitz D, Oren M. Different tumour derived *p53* mutants exhibit distinct biological activities. Science 1990; 250: 113–116.

43 Malkin D, Li FP, Strong LC et al. Germ line *p53* mutations in a familial syndrome of breast cancer, sarcomas, and other neoplasms. Science 1990; 250: 1233–1238.

44 Bhagirath T, Condie A, Dunlop MG, Wyllie AH, Prosser J. Exclusion of constitutional *p53* mutations as a cause of genetic susceptibility to colorectal cancer. Br J Cancer 1993; 68: 712–714.

45 Vogelstein B, Fearon ER, Hamilton SR et al. Genetic alterations during colorectal tumour development. N Engl J Med 1988; 319: 525–532.

46 Fearon ER, Cho KR, Nigro JM et al. Identification of a chromosome 18q gene that is altered in colorectal cancers. Science 1990; 247: 49–56.

47 Tanaka K, Oshimura M, Kikuchi R et al. Suppression of tumorigenicity in human colon carcinoma cells by introduction of normal chromosome 5 or 18. Nature 1991; 349: 340–342.

48 Lynch HT, Schuelke GS, Kimberling WJ et al. Hereditary non-polyposis colorectal cancer (Lynch Syndromes 1 and 2): Biomarker studies. Cancer 1985; 56: 939–951.

49 Peltomaki P, Sistonen P, Mecklin J-P et al. Evidence supporting exclusion of the DCC gene and a portion of chromosome 18q as the locus for susceptibility to hereditary nonpolyposis colorectal carcinomas in five kindreds. Cancer Res 1991; 51: 4135–4140.

50 Shibata L, Schaeffer J, Li Z-H et al. Genetic heterogeneity of c-K-ras locus in colorectal adenomas but not adenocarcinomas. J Natl Cancer Inst 1993; 85: 1058–1063.
51 Krontiris TG, Devlin B, Karp DD et al. An association between the risk of cancer and mutations in the HRAS1 minisatellite locus. N Engl J Med 1989; 329: 517–523.
52 Cunningham C, Dunlop MG, Wyllie AH, Bird CC. Deletion mapping in colorectal cancer of a putative tumour suppressor gene in 8p22–p21.3. Oncogene 1993; 8: 1391–1396.
53 Cunningham C, Dunlop MG, Bird CC, Wyllie AH. Deletion analysis of chromosome 8p in sporadic colorectal adenomas. Br J Cancer 1994 (In press).
54 Knowles MA, Shaw ME, Proctor AJ. Deletion mapping of chromosome 8 in cancers of the urinary bladder using restriction fragment length polymorphisms and microsatellite polymorphisms. Oncogene 1993; 8: 1357–1364.
55 Bergerheim US, Kunimi K, Collins P, Ekman P. Deletion mapping of chromosomes 8, 10, and 16 in human prostatic cancer. Genes Chromosom Cancer 1991; 3: 215–220.
56 Emi M, Fujiwara Y, Nakajima T et al. Frequent loss of heterozygosity for loci on chromosome 8p in hepatocellular carcinoma, colorectal cancer and lung cancer. Cancer Res 1992; 52: 5368–5372.
57 Fujiwara Y, Emi M, Ohata H et al. Evidence for the presence of two tumour suppressor genes on chromosome 8p for colorectal cancer. Cancer Res 1993; 53. 1172–1174.

British Medical Bulletin (1994) Vol. 50, No. 3, pp. 656–676

Genetics of breast and ovarian cancer

S A Narod

Department of Medicine, Division of Medical Genetics, McGill University, Montreal, Canada

Studies of familial breast and ovarian cancer have traditionally been directed towards a single type of cancer, but recent evidence leads us to consider these two types of cancer together. The original evidence for a common hereditary basis for breast and ovarian cancer comes from the observation of large families with several cases of both types.[1] The number of cancers in these families was too great to be explained by chance and none of the known environmental risk factors are sufficient to account for the clustering. Statistical analysis performed on a number of breast-ovary cancer families identified by Dr Henry Lynch and his colleagues led them to conclude that the clustering could be explained by the effect of a single dominant gene.[2] Women with breast cancer are at increased risk of developing a second primary cancer of the ovary;[3] and relatives of women with breast or ovarian cancer are at roughly double the risk for either tumour.[4] The most convincing evidence, however, for a common predisposition for breast and ovarian cancer comes from genetic linkage studies. In a linkage study cancer susceptibility in a family is shown to be transmitted with a particular allele of genetic marker of known chromosomal location. A gene from chromosome region 17q12–q21, designated BRCA1, identified in 1990 by Dr Mary-Claire King and colleagues, predisposes to both cancer of the breast and the ovary.[5–7]

It is important to distinguish between the terms hereditary and familial cancer. Hereditary cancer is used to refer to a cancer which occurs in a woman who is believed to carry a mutation of a gene which predisposes to breast or ovarian cancer (eg p53 or BRCA1). The presence of a constitutional mutation is inferred either from the observation of extensive familial clustering, by direct DNA sequencing (in the case of p53 mutations) or by linkage analysis (eg BRCA1). In the case of a new mutation, or if a woman's family is small, or if the history is incomplete, a woman with hereditary cancer may have no documented family history of the disease. The term familial cancer is mostly used by epidemiologists to define a subgroup of cancer patients with a positive family history of breast or ovarian cancer (eg one or more cases in first or second degree relatives). Familial breast cancer may be hereditary or may simply be a chance occurrence, given the high frequency of the breast cancer in Western populations. There is likely to be considerable mis-classification when a single relative with breast cancer is used to define a predisposed subgroup.

Families with a small number of cancer cases may also be due to mutations, or to polymorphic variants, of common genes which confer a small increased risk of cancer. For example, a frequent genetic variant which doubles the risk of breast cancer may contribute to a considerable proportion of cancers in the population, but is unlikely to be the cause of large families with many affected women. Some possible candidate genes of this type will also be discussed.

CLINICAL FEATURES OF HEREDITARY BREAST AND OVARIAN CANCER

The clinical cancer geneticist is often asked to estimate the probability that a particular case of breast or ovarian cancer is hereditary. This probability is used in turn to estimate the risk of cancer occurrence in family members, or of recurrence in the patient herself. Several lines of evidence must be considered, including the number and sites of cancer in the woman's family, her past history of cancer, and the age-of-onset, laterality and histology of her tumour.

Hereditary cancer syndromes

The familial breast and ovarian cancer syndromes are usually divided into 5 groups: site-specific breast cancer; site-specific ovarian cancer; the breast-ovarian cancer syndrome; the Li-Fraumeni syndrome and hereditary non-polyposis colon cancer. The most important criterion used in making a diagnosis of hereditary breast or ovarian cancer is the total number of family members affected with cancer. The Breast Cancer Linkage Consortium currently considers 4 early-onset breast cancer cases in a family to be sufficient to qualify for hereditary site-specific breast cancer.[7] Because it is considerably less frequent, 3 cases of ovarian cancer in first-degree relatives is considered to be hereditary. A family with a total number of 5 cases of breast or ovarian cancers, including 2 cancers of each type, qualifies as the breast-ovarian cancer syndrome.

An excess of soft tissue sarcomas and early-onset breast cancer was found in the relatives of children with soft tissue sarcomas.[8] This familial cancer association, now designated the Li-Fraumeni syndrome, has been extended to include osteosarcomas, adrenocortical cancers, leukaemia, lung cancer and brain tumours, and should be considered when a woman with early-onset breast cancer is found to have a relative with childhood cancer. The most frequent manifestation of the Li-Fraumeni syndrome is breast cancer; in a follow-up study of 24 families, breast cancer accounted for 15 of 52 new cases of cancer.[9] The relative risk for breast cancer among relatives under the age of 45 years was 17.9, much greater than the relative risk of 1.8 observed for women over age 45. It is estimated that 50% of susceptibles in Li-Fraumeni families will develop cancer by the age of 30 years. Surprisingly, there appears to be no excess cancer risk after the age of 60. The role of the p53 gene in Li-Fraumeni syndrome is discussed later.

Hereditary non-polyposis colon cancer (HNPCC) is a dominant predisposition to cancer of the colon, in the absence of familial adenomatous polyposis. Cancers at other sites, most notably the endometrium, may be seen in colon cancer families.[10] Cancer of the ovary appears in excess in some HNPCC families, but probably accounts for less than 5% of the total burden of cancers.[10] HNPCC is genetically heterogeneous; at least two colon cancer families[11] have been shown to be linked to a locus on the short arm of chromosome 2 and several others are unlinked. Cancer of the ovary was present in both of the HNPCC families which were linked to chromosome 2 in the original report. A family history in a woman with ovarian cancer should include the documentation of additional cases of cancer of the breast, ovary, colon and endometrium.

The association of birth defects and childhood cancer may be a clue to an underlying genetic etiology, but adult cancer syndromes are rarely associated with developmental abnormalities or other physical signs. One exception is Cowden syndrome, which is the infrequent association of breast cancer and hamartomatous polyps of the skin, mucous membranes and the thyroid.[12] Children with XY gonadal dysgenesis are at increased risk for gonadal germ cell tumours[13] and males with androgen insufficiency due to androgen receptor defects are at increased risk of breast cancer.[14] Ovarian tumours, benign and malignant, may complicate the Peutz-Jegher syndrome[15] and the basal cell nevus syndrome. These rare conditions will not be considered further.

Past history of cancer

Multiple primary cancers diagnosed in a single individual may result from the treatment of the first malignancy, may be due to environmental carcinogens or to hereditary predisposition, or to chance. The proportion of women with both cancer of the breast and ovary who are affected because of inherent cancer susceptibility has not yet been determined. A past history of breast cancer was reported in 6 of 130 (4.6%) sporadic ovarian cancers, versus 5 of 19 (26.3%) patients with familial ovarian cancer in Italy.[16] In a study of Schildkraut et al,[4] 10 of 493 (2.0%) women with ovarian cancer had a past history of breast cancer, but only women diagnosed with cancer before age 55 were included in this study.[4] A past history of breast cancer was documented in 23 of 450 unselected ovarian cancer cases in Southern Ontario.[17] The majority of the women with multiple primary cancers in this study were from families with additional cases of breast or ovarian cancer. It is important to extend these studies to estimate better the cancer risk for female relatives of women with double primaries.

Histology

All histologic types of breast cancer may be familial, and several different types may be found in a single family. Medullary cancer of the breast is probably over-represented in cancer families (H. Lynch, personal communication).

The predominant histologic type of hereditary ovarian cancer is serous papillary cystadenocarcinoma.[18] It is important to know all of the types of ovarian cancer which are over-represented in cancer families in order to estimate accurately risks for relatives. In the Gilda Radner Familial Ovarian Cancer Registry cases of mucinous adenocarcinoma and cystadenocarcinoma were significantly under-represented.[19] Only 6 of 439 familial ovarian cancers were described as mucinous (1.4%), compared to 12.7% of unselected ovarian cancers in the SEER database. Mucinous carcinoma of the ovary is believed to arise from the surface epithelium of the ovary and shares histologic features with the uterine endocervix. There were no mucinous carcinomas among the 37 hereditary ovarian cancers reported by Bewtra et al[18] or among the 11 familial ovarian cancers of Greggi et al.[16] In a recent study, only 1 of 31 familial ovarian cancers was mucinous.[17] Schildkraut et al[20] found an excess risk of ovarian cancer in first-degree relatives of all 3 types of epithelial ovarian tumours, however the relative risk associated with mucinous tumours (2.4) was slightly lower than that associated with serous or endometroid forms (3.4). Among the 16 BRCA1-linked breast-ovary cancer families in the Creighton University Registry, there were a total of 49 ovarian cancers. Of these cancers, 5 were described as mucinous and 1 was 'pseudomucinous'. By haplotype analysis, using chromosome 17q markers, it was possible to determine the BRCA1 carrier status of 40 of the cases. 36 of the ovarian carcinomas occurred in BRCA1 mutation carriers and 4 were sporadic (ie occurred in non-carriers). Of the 36 ovarian cancers in BRCA1-carriers 2 were described as mucinous, versus 3 of the 4 carcinomas observed in BRCA1-non-carriers (p = 0.008).

Schildkraut et al[20] did not see an excess risk of ovarian cancers in the family members of women with borderline ovarian tumours. Borderline carcinomas comprised 5 of 439 familial ovarian cancers in the Gilda Radner Registry;[19] 2 of 37 hereditary ovarian cancers at Creighton [18] and 1 of 31 familial ovarian cancers in Ontario.[17] In the Creighton Registry a single case of borderline ovarian carcinoma appeared in 16 BRCA1-linked families.

These data cast doubt on whether ovarian cancer susceptibility genes, including BRCA1, predispose to mucinous epithelial cancer or to ovarian cancers of borderline differentiation.

Age-of-onset

The risk of breast cancer among relatives increases with early age-of-onset in the index case;[21] the relative risk for a sister was estimated to be 4.3 for breast cancer cases diagnosed at age 30, 2.7 for cases diagnosed at age 40 and 1.7 for cases diagnosed at age 50. Similar results have been observed by others.

Early age-of-onset is not as predictive of hereditary ovarian cancer as it is for hereditary breast cancer. Amos et al[22] found that the age-of-onset of hereditary ovarian cancer (two or more relatives affected with ovarian cancer), but not of familial ovarian cancer (one affected relative) was younger than expected. The median age of diagnosis of hereditary ovarian cancer was 47 years, 14 years earlier than the US median. Women with a single relative affected with ovarian cancer were at higher risk, but the age distribution of familial ovarian cancers was not shifted. Bewtra et al[18] also found the average age of diagnosis of hereditary cases (50.2 years) to be younger than controls (59 years). No significant differences in age of onset between sporadic, familial and hereditary cases were found by Narod et al.[17] The median age of onset of ovarian tumours associated with hereditary non-polyposis colon cancer is 40 years,[10] considerably younger than the general population. Houlston et al[23] found a strong correlation between ages of death from ovarian cancer between sisters, but not between mothers and daughters. Because germ cell and mucinous ovarian cancers occur on average at an earlier age than serous and endometrioid tumours[24] but are not characteristic of hereditary ovarian cancer syndromes, age comparisons may be slightly biased, unless adjusted for histology.

Bilaterality

The risk of breast cancer is greater for relatives of bilateral cases than for unilateral cases.[25,26] This cannot be said for ovarian cancer; borderline tumours of the ovary are frequently bilateral,[27] but are rarely familial.[17,20] The lack of association is not surprising because bilateral ovarian tumours are often metastatic,[28] but bilateral breast cancers are usually separate primaries.

Pre-neoplastic lesions

Several dominant cancer syndromes are characterized by a precancerous hyperplastic state in tissues at risk for malignancy, including familial adenomatous polyposis and multiple endocrine neoplasia type 2. There is no convincing evidence for the existence of a characteristic preneoplastic state in the hereditary breast or ovarian cancer syndromes. Among women undergoing breast biopsy, atypical hyperplasia is associated with a 4-fold risk of developing breast cancer.[29] There appears to be a positive association between atypical hyperplasia and a family history of breast cancer. Carter et al[30] documented a first-degree relative with breast cancer for 20.0% of women with atypical hyperplasia, but for only 11.9% of controls ($P < 0.01$). In a similar study Skolinck et al[31] reported ductal or atypical hyperplasia in 35% of women from high risk families, compared to 13% of controls. Dupont and Page found the risk of breast cancer to be increased 11 times if a woman had both atypical hyperplasia and a family history of disease.[32] To date there is no evidence that atypical hyperplasia or carcinoma-in-situ are frequent features of breast cancers associated with BRCA1 mutations.

POPULATION GENETICS

Approximately 4% of cases of breast cancer are from families with multiple affected women.[33] The risk for a woman with an affected mother and sister may reach 50%, the same as for an autosomal dominant gene.[34] Using the population-based CASH registry, which contained data on families of 4 370 cases of breast cancer, Claus et al[35] hypothesized the existence of a rare (q = .0033) dominant breast cancer gene with a lifetime penetrance of 92%. Other segregation analyses give similar results[36–38] with the exception of that of Goldstein and Amos (who also studied the CASH data) who found the data best fit a recessive model.[39]

In a recent Swedish study, Lindblom et al[40] approached 2 694 patients with breast cancer for family histories. Among the 1 976 patients who responded to a mailed questionnaire 29 families, with from 2–6 cases of breast cancer, were identified. Of these, 5 families contained 4 or more cases, and 2 contained 5 or more cases. There were no hereditary breast-ovary cancer families identified in this series.

A family history of ovarian cancer is a consistent risk factor for ovarian cancer.[41] Schildkraut et al[20] found a relative risk of 3.6 for first-degree relatives and 2.9 for second-degree relatives with ovarian cancer in the CASH data base. Amos et al[22] obtained an odds ratio of 3.6 for a history of ovarian cancer in a first-degree relative, in a meta-analysis of data combined from 4 American studies. Koch et al[42] estimated a slightly lower relative risk for first-degree relatives using mortality data reported to the Alberta Cancer Registry. Some of the difference in risk between studies may be due to information bias; women with cancer may be more aware of the same diagnosis in a relative, or may be more likely to confuse benign conditions with malignancy, than are healthy controls.

Based on the records of the Office of Population Censuses and Surveys (UK) it was found that the lifetime risk of death from ovarian cancer was 1 in 40 when one relative was affected.[43] This incidence is 3 times greater than the general population. If a woman had an affected mother and sister, or 2 affected sisters, the risk reached 30–40%. These figures imply that a large proportion of sister pairs, or mother-daughter pairs, with ovarian cancer are due to the effect of a major gene, with a lifetime penetrance of 50% or greater.

Eight ovarian cancer families (2 or more total cases) were identified from 138 consecutive ovarian cancer cases by Greggi et al.[16] In a study by Cramer et al,[29] 34 of 493 women with ovarian cancer reported a relative with the disease (6.9%), but only 3 reported 2 or more affected relatives (0.6%). This group also found an excess of consanguinity among parents of ovarian cancer cases compared with controls, further evidence in favor of a recessive component for ovarian cancer. By segregation analysis using the mixed model Houlston et al[49] predicted the existence of a dominant ovarian cancer gene with a mutant frequency of 0.0015–0.0026, and which is responsible for 13% of the total burden of ovarian cancer. This proportion seems to be high in comparison to other studies, given that tumours at other sites were not included in the phenotype, however the pedigrees were ascertained through women who were self-referred to an ovarian screening clinic.

Subtypes of hereditary ovarian cancer are site-specific ovarian cancer, the breast-ovarian cancer syndrome and hereditary nonpolyposis colon cancer (HNPCC). HNPCC is a distinct entity, but it is not yet proven that site-specific familial ovarian cancer and the breast-ovarian cancer syndrome are due to different genes. Hereditary site-specific ovarian cancer is rare. Only 0.6% of ovarian cancer patients in the CASH study reported 2 or more affected relatives with ovarian cancer. Families with site-specific ovarian cancer, when followed, have been found to contain cases of breast cancer[45] and vice-versa.[46]

In order to estimate adequately the frequency of hereditary breast or ovarian cancer it is necessary to document relatives with both types of cancer. In an Ontario study only 1 family with hereditary site-specific (3 or more cases) ovarian cancer was identified from 450 unselected cases of ovarian cancer.[17] The breast-ovarian cancer syndrome was much more common. 25 families with a total of 4 or more cases of breast or ovarian cancer were identified. The breast-ovarian cancer syndrome accounted for 12 of 17 ovarian cancer families in the Creighton University Registry[18] and 3 of 6 ovarian cancer families identified by Fraumeni et al.[47]

LINKAGE ANALYSIS

In 1990, Mary-Claire King and her colleagues[5] identified linkage of breast cancer susceptibility to the D17S74 locus (probe CMM86) on chromosome 17q21. Not all of the families in the original report showed linkage; the positive LOD scores occurred in the subset of families with a mean age of onset of breast cancer below age 45 (LOD = 5.98). Little evidence for linkage was observed in families of later onset. Overall, it was estimated that 40% of the 23 families were linked to D17S74. Shortly after, linkage to D17S74 was confirmed in 3 of 5 families with hereditary breast-ovarian cancer.[6] An international consortium studying linkage to hereditary breast ovarian cancer, consisting of 13 study groups from 8 countries, has reported BRCA1 mapping results using a total of 214 families.[7] These data place BRCA1 approximately 20 cM centromeric to the position of the original linked marker, D17S74. The current region of assignment for BRCA1 from the Consortium Group data, and more recent data, is between the markers THRA1 and D17S579, a region of approximately 6 cM. Multiple crossovers, derived from several families, support this assignment.[46,48–50]

Because of genetic heterogeneity and because it is possible that sporadic cases (ie non-hereditary) of breast or ovarian cancer may also occur in linked families, no single recombinant is definitive. In at least 2 instances[51,52] it has been erroneously inferred that BRCA1 was distal to D17S579. Since the Consortium report, new recombinant events have been identified which narrow the region of assignment of BRCA1. Simard et al[49] place BRCA1 distal to RARA based on 2 cases of breast cancer in a sibship occurring at ages 35 and 32 (LOD = 3.62 for this family). Kelsell et al[53] and Tonin et al[54] each have identified crossovers in families which place BRCA1 distal to D17S800. Goldgar et al[50] map

BRCA1 distal to D17S776 (MFD191); this appears to be the closest proximal flanking marker reported to date. An affected woman in this large breast-ovarian family developed ovarian cancer at the age of 45 years (her mother developed ovarian cancer at 58 years old). The family provided a maximum LOD score of 8.52 at the locus ED2. The closest reported[49] marker to be telomeric to BRCA1 is D17S78, based on the appearance of breast-cancer in a 34-year-old woman in a small linked breast-ovary family (LOD = 0.52).

Several candidate genes which map to chromosome 17q12–q21 have been excluded by linkage analysis,[7,49,55] including retinoic acid receptor alpha (RARA), thyroid hormone receptor A1, the HER2 (or ERBB2) proto-oncogene, growth hormone and insulin-like-growth factor binding protein type 4 (IGFBP4) (D. Black, personal communication). The gene for estradiol 17β dehydrogenase, EDH17B2, has not yet been excluded by linkage analysis. This enzyme converts the hormone estrone to the more metabolically active estradiol. Sequence analysis of 5 affected BRCA1 carriers has failed to reveal any sequence variation in EDH17B2,[49,53] but it remains possible that a BRCA1 mutation could alter the tissue regulation of this enzyme.

BRCA1 EPIDEMIOLOGY

Gene frequency

Claus et al[35] estimate the frequency of a dominant breast cancer susceptibility gene in the population to be 0.0033, or roughly 1 in 150 women is predisposed. This estimate is based on the CASH data set and is theoretically the sum of the frequencies of all of the dominant genes associated with breast cancer. This figure was used initially as the estimated frequency of mutant BRCA1 alleles by the Breast Cancer Linkage Consortium.[7] However, because it is now estimated that only 60% of hereditary breast cancer families are linked to BRCA1, the frequency for carriers of mutant BRCA1 alleles is likely to be less than 1 in 150. Easton et al[56] estimate the frequency of BRCA1 mutant alleles to be 0.0007, based on 44 breast cancer deaths occurring among the relatives of 1203 cases of ovarian cancer (31.8 expected). It is therefore likely that the frequency of carriers of BRCA1 mutations in the population is closer to 1 in 500.

Penetrance

The relative risk for breast cancer among BRCA1 carriers[56] varies from 100 for cancer below at the age of 30 years to 1.6 at 75 years. Based on a gene frequency of 0.002 for mutant BRCA1 alleles, this implies that the proportion of breast cancers due to BRCA1 in the population varies from 28% below the age of 30 years to less than 1% over 70 years.

By studying 33 linked families submitted to the Breast Cancer Linkage Consortium, Ford et al[57] estimate a cumulative risk of 48% to age 70 for ovarian cancer and 85% for breast cancer. However, the data best fit a model with a mix of two susceptibility genes;[56] one with a risk of breast cancer of 71% and ovarian cancer of 87% to age 70, and a second gene with a risk of breast cancer of 86% to age 70 and a risk of ovarian cancer of only 18%. By studying a single large BRCA1 linked pedigree Goldgar et al[50] estimate the penetrance of breast or ovarian cancer to be 40% by 50 years old and 90% by 70 years old.

Genetic heterogeneity

It was estimated by the Breast Cancer Linkage Consortium[7] that 45% of 157 site-specific breast cancer families (confidence limits 25–66%) were linked to chromosome 17. Linkage was more likely if the average age of breast cancer onset was young. It is interesting that in several countries there has been little or no evidence to date for linkage for site specific breast cancer to the BRCA1 locus, including France, Sweden, and Canada.[40,54,58] Most of the evidence for BRCA1-linked site-specific breast cancer families comes from the the USA.

In contrast to site-specific breast cancer it was estimated that 100% of the 57 breast-ovary families were linked to BRCA1 (confidence limits 79–100%). A more recent investigation of newly identified Consortium families indicates that a small proportion of breast-ovarian cancer families are probably unlinked (unpublished data). It is important to know if the breast-ovarian syndrome is genetically heterogeneous, both for purposes of genetic counselling and to expedite positional cloning.

Little linkage data are available for site-specific ovarian cancer, but a few rare families have been linked to BRCA1, including one with 6 cases of ovarian cancer and no breast cancer with a LOD of 1.13 to BRCA1 (Y. J. Bignon, personal communication). No unlinked site-specific ovarian cancer families have been reported.

Other cancers

Breast cancer has been associated in families with other tumour types as well. A family history of prostate cancer was found to be a risk factor for breast cancer.[59,60] 13 cases of prostate cancer were found among 5 breast cancer kindreds studied for chromosome 17q linkage to BRCA1 in Iceland;[61] 9 of the 13 cases were in men believed to carry predisposing cancer genes, including at least 2 who carried BRCA1 mutations. 2 further cases of prostate cancer (ages 58 and 68) were diagnosed in BRCA1 carriers in a large 17q-linked pedigree reported by Goldgar et al.[50] In the Breast Cancer Linkage Consortium study 76 cancers other than breast or ovary were observed among 33 BRCA1-linked families (62 expected).[57] Prostate cancer accounted for a portion of the excess (relative risk 2.0).

The other site found to be significantly over-represented in the BRCA1-linked families was cancer of the colon (RR = 2.8). There is a modest increased risk of colorectal cancer in women diagnosed with breast cancer and vice-versa.[62] One unusual family with a striking susceptibility to both early-onset breast and early-onset colon cancer has been described.[63] This family does not show linkage to BRCA1 or to markers on chromosome 2p associated with HNPCC (S. Narod, unpublished data).

Breast cancer and malignant melanoma share several risk factors related to reproductive history. Males with breast cancer were found to have a past history of melanoma more frequently than expected.[59] Skolnick et al[64] reported 7 cases of maignant melanoma among cases and relatives of BRCA1-linked families in Utah. 9 families with breast cancer, ovarian cancer and malignant melanoma were identified in the Creighton University Cancer Family Registry (CFR). All of these families show evidence of linkage to chromosome 17 markers (total LOD = 11.22). However, haplotype analysis revealed that only 4 of the 10 cases of melanoma appearing in these families were among carriers of BRCA1 mutations.[65]

2 cases of Wilms' tumour have also been seen among the BRCA1-linked breast-ovary families in Creighton University (unpublished data). 1 of these children has been typed with chromosome 17q markers and has been found to be a BRCA1 carrier.

OTHER GENES

HRAS

It is possible that polymorphic variants of several genes exist which are associated with a small or moderate inbcreased risk of breast cancer. A gene associated with risk ratio of 2–5 would rarely lead to large family clusters of cancer, but could be responsible for a significant proportion of breast cancer in the population. One candidate gene is HRAS1. The presence of one of the 'rare alleles' of a minisatellite polymorphism located near to the HRAS1 proto-oncogene was found in a meta-analysis to be associated with a 1.93 times increased risk of breast cancer.[66] The 24 or so rare alleles of HRAS1 make up only 6% of the total alleles seen at this locus. Whether variation within the HRAS1 gene itself, or a closely linked gene is responsible for this association is yet to be determined.

Ataxia-telangiectasia

Another gene that has attracted interest as a candidate breast cancer gene is the gene for ataxia-telangiectasia (AT). The homozygote frequency of this recessive disease[67] is 1 in 100 000. This prevalence is equivalent to a gene frequency of 0.006 (ie 1.2% of the population are heterozygote carriers) assuming AT is a single gene condition. Swift et al[68] found 23 cases of breast cancer in relatives of cases of ataxia-telangiectasia. This rate was 5.1 times higher than that expected, based on the observation of 3 cases of breast cancer in a spouse control group. However, based on North American tumour registry data there were 4.0 cases expected in this control group, so the true relative risk is likely to be smaller (eg 3.8). On the other hand, because of complementation in AT, the gene frequency of carriers is likely to be higher than 0.006. For example, assuming 2 equally frequent complementation groups, the carrier frequency for AT increases from 1.2–1.8% and the population attributable risk would increase from 3.3–5.3%. Approximately 80% of AT patients fall into complementation groups A and C.[69,70] When a diagnostic test for the AT heterozygotes is identified the confirmation of the Swift hypothesis will be straightforward. Easton et al[56] estimate the proportion of breast cancer due to AT heterozygotes to be 7%. Swift et al[68]also reported a greater use of diagnostic and therapeutic X-rays in the cases of breast cancer than among healthy controls. Markers from the AT locus have been now typed on 16 breast cancer families, including 10 which appear to be unlinked to BRCA1, but there was no evidence that the AT gene accounted for the cancer susceptibility observed in these families.[70]

p53

In 1990, Dr David Malkin and colleagues reported that germ line mutations of the p53 gene were present in 5 of 5 families studied with the Li-Fraumeni syndrome.[71] Sporadic p53 mutations have been implicated in a wide range of human tumours,[72] including those characteristic of the Li-Fraumeni syndrome. 3 of the 5 original families contained cases of early onset breast cancer (ages 27–34 years). Breast cancers associated with germ line p53 mutations tend to be very young. The effect of p53 gene is restricted to pre-menopausal cancer and germ line mutations in the gene probably account for less than 1% of all cases of breast cancer. 3 p53 mutations were found in a total of 463 women with breast cancer in 2 studies (at ages 24, 33, and 41 years).[73,74] 2 of these 3 women were from families with features of the Li-Fraumeni syndrome.

MALE BREAST CANCER

Female relatives of male breast cancer patients have a 2-fold increased risk for breast cancer, similar to the risk of breast cancer in the relatives of female patients.[59] Breast cancer in men comprises less than 1% of all breast cancers, but is found more commonly in males with Klinefelter syndrome (XXY karyotype).[75] Klinefelter males typically have features of androgen insufficiency and may have decreased expression of the androgen receptor.[76] In 3 males, including 2 brothers, with breast cancer, mutations in the DNA-binding domain of the androgen receptor have been found.[14,77] All 3 had developmental features of androgen insufficiency, including hypospadias, undescended testes, bifid scrotum and gynecomastia.

Male breast cancer is seen in a minority of families with hereditary breast cancer.[7] Early data suggest that families with male breast cancer cases are not likely to be linked to the BRCA1 locus (D. Easton, personal communication).

COFACTORS

Early age at first birth and multiple parity are associated with a reduced risk of breast cancer in the general population,[78] but the effects of these reproductive factors on familial or hereditary breast cancer are not yet clear. Dupont and Page reported an 8-fold risk of breast cancer associated with first birth over the age of 30 (versus below age 20) among women with a positive family history of the disease.[29] Sellers and colleagues studied a cohort of 37 105 women, of whom 493 developed breast cancer.[79] They found that the risks associated with low parity and early menarche were greater among women with a family history of breast cancer (1 or more affected first-degree relatives). First pregnancy after age 30 years was associated with a 5.8-fold risk of breast cancer in the familial subgroup. No positive interaction between family history and early menarche was found by Brinton et al.[80] It should again be emphasized that the potential for significant mis-classification is present when family history is used to infer genetic susceptibility; a large proportion of sister pairs, or mother-daughter pairs, will be affected with breast cancer by chance.

Parity has been found to be protective for ovarian cancer, and is one reason used to justify the 'incessant ovulation' hypothesis of ovarian cancer etiology. Greggi et al[16] found a smaller proportion of nulliparous women among familial (5.6%) than among sporadic ovarian cancer cases (26%)[16] and inferred that low parity was not a risk factor for familial ovarian cancer. Neither parity nor early birth appear to protect against ovarian cancer in carriers of BRCA1 mutation[50] (and S. Narod, unpublished data).

An interesting family was reported in the UK in which 7 consecutive cases of ovarian cancer were followed by 2 cases of early-onset breast cancer.[45] The possibility that hereditary breast cancer may be more frequent in recent generations is also supported by the observation of a large, multi-generation BRCA1-linked family.[81] It is possible that non-genetic factors modify the risk of cancer among BRCA1 carriers. The nature of these factors is unknown.

MANAGEMENT ISSUES

Oophorectomy

Because of the uncertain benefits of screening for ovarian cancer, many high-risk women opt for prophylactic oophorectomy. The prophylactic removal of ovaries from high risk women at the completion of child-bearing to prevent ovarian cancer is increasingly common in North America. The logic of this approach is appealing, but it is not yet been proven that this procedure decreases mortality and the optimum age for the operation has not yet been determined. Early surgery is expected to maximize the chances of preventing ovarian cancer (or removing cancers at an early stage), but increases the risk of complications of surgical menopause, including osteoporosis and cardiovascular disease.[82–84] A further concern is post-surgical peritoneal cancer. Among a group of 28 women who underwent prophylactic oophorectomy because of high risk of ovarian cancer, 3 subsequently developed disseminated intra-abdominal carcinomatosis, indistiguishable histologically from ovarian carcinoma.[85] In none of the 3 was an ovarian or uterine abnormality identified. This report led to increased caution about the prophylactic removal of ovaries in high risk women, although it has not been determined if peritoneal carcinoma is a complication of surgery or is part of the natural history of the disease (either as latent ovarian metastases or primary cancer). Piver et al[86] estimate the rate of this complication to be low (2.8%) – 9 cases of primary peritoneal carcinoma developed among 324 women who underwent prophylactic oophorectomy. The omentum was involved in 6 of the cases. It is possible that the peritoneum is at risk for malignant transformation in ovarian cancer families. It has not yet been established if women with primary peritoneal neoplasms, identified through the general population, are genetically predisposed.

Early menopause, whether natural or surgically induced, offers some protection against breast cancer.[78] It has not yet been determined to what extent oophorectomy diminishes the risk of hereditary breast cancer, if at all.

Prophylactic mastectomy

Current strategies for breast cancer prevention in high risk women are inadequate. Because of the limitations of screening mammography, and because the benefit of Tamoxifen or other chemopreventive agents in preventing breast cancer is unproven, some women at very high risk opt for prophylactic surgical removal of breasts. In the Consortium study 23 contralateral breast cancers were observed more than 3 years after the initial diagnosis of breast cancer.[57] The cumulative risk for contralateral cancer among affected carriers was 85% to the age of 70. Because of the high risk of recurrent cancer in BRCA1 carriers, some authors recommend that contralateral mastectomy be considered at the time of the initial surgery.[87]

Mammography

Mammographic screening is routinely recommended for high risk women in most family cancer clinics. Mammography has not been proven to reduce mortality from breast cancer in young women,[88] but the subgroup of women with a strong family history has not been extensively studied. Evans et al[45] reported a 40-year-old woman in a hereditary site-specific ovarian cancer family who detected breast cancer by self-examination shortly after a negative mammogram. In a large BRCA1-linked family, followed at Creighton University, 14 of 14 breast cancers were diagnosed in the presence of a palpable mass, despite extensive counselling and routine mammography. Post-menopausal screening may be more effective. Lalle et al[89] reported a case of hereditary post-menopausal breast cancer in a BRCA1 carrier that was detected by mammography at an early stage.

Screening for ovarian cancer

Screening for ovarian cancer may include physical examination, CA-125, abdominal or trans-vaginal ultrasound. Because of the poor specificity of trans-abdominal ultrasound for detecting early ovarian cancer the predictive value of a positive test is low.[90] The performance of screening tests improves when individuals at high risk are screened (ie the prevalence is effectively increased). The use of trans-vaginal probes in combination with colour Doppler flow imaging may increase the ability to discriminate between benign and malignant ovarian lesions. So far none of these techniques has been proven to be of benefit for reducing mortality. In a study of trans-vaginal ultrasound the positive predictive value for cancer was 7.7%. Of 776 screened women, 3 had ovarian cancer detected, but 39 women underwent surgery.[91] Other evaluative trials are underway.

Hormone replacement therapy

The potential for modification of cancer risk in BRCA1 carriers by levels of exogenous and endogenous hormones deserves study. The safety of post-menopausal estrogen replacement in women who are at high risk for cancer is under debate. Women for whom the question is most relevant are those who have undergone surgical menopause to prevent ovarian cancer and who then become at increased risk for osteoporosis and cardiovascular disease. There is probably a modest increase in breast cancer risk for women taking prolonged hormone replacement,[92,93] but this is offset by a reduction in cardiovascular disease incidence and mortality.[94] In a meta-analysis of hormone replacement therapy and breast cancer risk, it was concluded that women with a positive family history of breast cancer had a 3.4-fold increase in breast cancer risk if they had ever used hormone replacement therapy ($P < 0.05$).[92] The size of the effect was smaller for those women without a family history of breast cancer. Colditz et al[93] did not find family history to modify the risk of estrogen use, which they estimate as 1.23 for greater than 10 years of estrogen use. It may be that Tamoxifen will become a useful drug in this setting; it is hoped that Tamoxifen will prevent breast cancer and offer protection to the bone and cardiovascular system as well. A large trial evaluating the use of Tamoxifen in preventing breast cancer in high risk women is now underway.

There is little evidence of an association between hormone replacement therapy and ovarian cancer, in keeping with the hypothesis that ovulation *per se* is the major determinant of risk. For this reason, it is suspected that fertility-promoting drugs which stimulate the ovary may be a risk factor for ovarian cancer.[95]

Oral contraceptives

Most risk factors for ovarian cancer relate to the number of ovulatory cycles experienced by the woman – factors that are associated with diminished ovulation tend to reduce the risk of ovarian cancer, including oral contraceptives. The protection afforded by oral contraceptives against ovarian cancer is one of the best established associations in epidemiology. In a recent review, 19 of 21 studies found relative risks below unity.[41] Long-term use of oral contraceptives is associated with risk reductions of 60% or more. It has not yet been established if the risk reduction is equal in women with familial, or hereditary ovarian cancer. Oral contraceptive use has been associated with a modest increase in risk of early-onset breast cancer in some studies (eg[96]), but there have been negative studies as well.[97] In the UK data there is a suggestion that the risk may be greater for familial breast cancer. It is an important question to establish the relative risks and benefits of oral contraceptives in women from breast-ovarian cancer families. Currently, few clinicians consider a family history of breast cancer to be a contraindication for oral contraceptive use.

Genetic counselling

The risk of breast and ovarian cancer to relatives of women diagnosed with these forms of cancer has been established and there are several papers published which present empiric risks which can be used in most counselling situations.[34,98,99]

Although BRCA1 is not yet cloned, it is now possible, using linkage analysis, to identify with a high degree of probability, women in predisposed families (of sufficient size) who carry BRCA1 mutations before the onset of clinical cancer.[87] The use of genetic linkage in counselling women from high-risk breast cancer families is now established in several centers.[87,89,100-102] Genetic risk assessment was provided to 28 women and 4 men in the first family counselled with DNA markers.[87] 8 women were told they were at high risk of being carriers (above 90%) and others were given risk estimates that fell below 10%. Genetic counselling using BRCA1 markers may be considered if it can be established that a family segregates a BRCA1 mutation. Genetic heterogeneity must be taken into account (ie first establish the probability that a given family is linked to BRCA1). It is hoped that specific mutation analysis will be available shortly and risks will be more precise. With the cloning of BRCA1 it should be possible to identify gene carriers within the general population, although the risks associated with different mutant alleles will require further study. The potential demand for such testing is not yet known, but the implications deserve our attention.

REFERENCES

1   Lynch HT, Krush AJ, Lemon HM, Kaplan AR, Condit PT, Bottomley RH. Tumour variations in families with breast cancer. JAMA 1972; 220: 1631–1635.
2   Go RCP, King MC, Bailey-Wilson J, Elston RC, Lynch HT. Genetic epidemiology of breast cancer and associated cancers in high-risk families. I Segregation analysis. J Natl Cancer Inst 1983; 71: 455–461.
3   Prior P, Waterhouse JAH. Multiple primary cancers of the breast and ovary. Brit. J. Cancer 1981; 44: 628–636.
4   Schildkraut JM, Risch N, Thompson WD. Evaluating genetic association among ovarian, breast, and endometrial cancer: evidence for a breast/ovarian cancer relationship. Am J Hum Genet 1989; 45: 521–529.
5   Hall JM, Lee MK, Newman B et al. Linkage of early-onset familial breast cancer to chromosome 17q21. Science 1990; 250: 1684–1689.
6   Narod SA, Feunteun J, Lynch H et al. A familial breast-ovarian cancer locus on chromosome 17q12-23. Lancet 1991; 338: 82–83.
7   Easton DF, Bishop DT, Ford D, Crockford GP and the Breast Cancer Linkage Consortium. Genetic linkage analysis in familial breast and ovarian cancer – results from 214 families. Am J Hum Genet 1993; 52: 678–701.
8   Li FP, Fraumeni J. Soft tissue sarcomas, breast cancers and other neoplasms: A familial syndrome? Ann Intern Med 1969;71: 747–752.

9   Garber JE, Goldstein AM, Kantor AF, Dreyfus MG, Fraumeni JF, Li FP. Follow-up study of twenty-four families with the Li-Fraumeni syndrome. Cancer Res 1991; 51: 6094–6097.

10   Watson P, Lynch HT. Extracolonic cancer in hereditary nonpolyposis colorectal cancer. Cancer 1993; 71: 677–685.

11   Peltomaki P, Aaltonen LA, Sistonen P et al. Genetic mapping of a locus predisposing to human colorectal cancer. Science 1993; 260: 810–812.

12   Lloyd KM, Dennis M. Cowden's disease: a possible new symptom complex with multiple system involvement. Ann Intern Med 58: 136–142.

13   Verp MS, Simpson JL. Abnormal sexual development and neoplasia. Cancer Genet Cytogenet 1987; 25: 191–218.

14   Wooster R, Mangion, Eeles R et al. A germline mutation in the androgen receptor gene in two brothers with breast cancer and Reifenstein syndrome. Nature Genet 1992; 132–134.

15   Christian CD. Ovarian tumours: an extension of the Peutz-Jegher syndrome. Am J Obstet Gynecol 1971; 111: 529–534.

16   Greggi S, Genuardi M, Benedetti-Panici P et al. Analysis of 138 consecutive ovarian cancer patients: Incidence and characteristics of familial cases. Gynecolog Oncol 1990; 39: 300–304.

17   Narod SA, Madlensky L, Bradley L, Cole D, Tonin P, Rosen B, Risch H. Hereditary and familial ovarian cancer in Southern Ontario. 1993 (Submitted)

18   Bewtra C, Watson P, Conway T, Read-Hippee C, Lynch HT. Hereditary ovarian cancer: a clinicopathological study. Int J Gynecol Path 1992; 11: 180–187.

19   Piver MS, Baker TR, Jishi MF et al. Familial ovarian cancer. A report of 658 families from the Gilda Radner Familial Ovarian Cancer Registry 1981–1991. Cancer 1993; 71: 582–588.

20   Schildkraut JM, Thompson WD. Familial ovarian cancer: a population-based case-control study. Am J Epidemiol 1988; 128: 456–466.

21   Claus EB, Risch N, Thompson WD. Age of onset as an indicator of familial risk of breast cancer. Am J Epidemiol 1990; 131: 961–972.

22   Amos CI, Shaw GL, Tucker MA, Hartge P. Age at onset for familial epithelial ovarian cancer. J AM Heart Assoc 1992; 268: 1896–1899.

23   Houlston RS, Path MRC, Hampson J et al. Correlation in ages at death from familial ovarian cancer among sisters. Gynecol Oncol 1992; 47: 253–254.

24   Cramer DW, Hutchison GB, Welch WR et al. Determinants of ovarian cancer risk. I. Reproductive experiences and family history. J Natl Cancer Inst 1983; 71: 711–716.

25   Bernstein JL, Thompson WD, Risch N, Holford TR. The genetic epidemiology of second primary breast cancer. Am J Epidemiol 1992; 136: 937–948.

26   Anderson DE, Badzioch MD. Bilaterality in familial breast cancer patients. Cancer 1985; 56: 2092–2098.

27   Merino MJ, Jaffe G. Age contrast in ovarian pathology. Cancer 1993; 71: 537–544.

28   Tsao S W, Mok C-H, Knapp RC et al. Molecular genetic evidence of a unifocal origin for human serous ovarian carcinomas. Gynecol Oncol 1993; 48: 5–10.

29   Dupont WD, Page DL. Breast cancer risk associated with proliferative disease, age at first birth and a family history of breast cancer. Am J Epidemiol 1987; 125: 769–779.

30   Carter CL, Corle DK, Micozzi MS, Schatzkin A, Taylor PR. A prospective study of the development of breast cancer in 16,692 women with benign breast disease. Am J Epidemiol 1988; 128: 467–477.

31   Skolnick MH, Cannon-Albright, Goldgar DA et al. Inheritance of proliferative breast disease in breast cancer kindreds. Science 1990; 250: 1715–1720.

32   Dupont WD, Page DL. Risk factors for breast cancer in women with proliferative disease. N Engl J Med 1985; 312: 146–151.

33   Lynch HT, Lynch JF. Breast cancer genetics in an oncology clinic: 328 consecutive patients. Cancer Genet Cytogenet 1986; Vol: 369–371.

34   Schwartz AG, King MC, Belle SH, Satariano WA. Risk of breast cancer to relatives of young breast cancer patients. J Natl Cancer Inst 1985; 75: 665–668.

35 Claus EB, Risch N, Thompson WD. Genetic analysis of breast cancer in the Cancer and Steroid Hormone Study. Am J Hum Genet 1991; 48: 232–242.

36 Bishop DT, Cannon-Albright L, Mclellan T, Gardner EJ, Skolnick MH. Segregation and linkage analysis of nine Utah breast cancer pedigrees. Genetic Epidemiol 1988; 5: 151–169.

37 Newman B, Austin MA, Lee M, King MC. Inheritance of human breast cancer: evidence for autosomal dominant transmission in high-risk families. Proc Natl Acad Sci USA 1988; 85: 3044–3048.

38 Iselius L, Slack J, Littler M, Morton NE. Genetic epidemiology of breast cancer in Britain. Ann Hum Genet 1991; 55: 151–159.

39 Goldstein AM, Amos CI. Segregation analysis of breast cancer from the Cancer and Steroid Hormone Study: Histologic subtypes. J Natl Cancer Inst 1990; 82: 1911–1917.

40 Lindblom A, Rotstein S, Nordensjkold M, Larsson M. Linkage analysis with markers on 17q in 29 Swedish breast cancer families. Am J Hum Genet 1993; 52: 749–754.

41 Parazzinni F, Franchesi S, La Vecchia C, Fasoli M. The epidemiology of ovarian cancer. Gynecol Oncol 1991; 43: 9–23.

42 Koch M, Gaedke J, Jenkins H. Family history of ovarian cancer patients: A case-control study. Am J Epidemiol 1988; 128: 456–466.

43 Ponder BAJ, Easton DF, Peto J. Risk of ovarian cancer associated with a family history: preliminary report of the OPCS study. In: Sharp F, Mason WP, Leake RE, eds. Ovarian cancer: biological and therapeutic challenges. New York: WW Norton 1991: 3–6.

44 Houlston RS, Collins A, Slack J, Campbell S, Collins WP, Whitehead MI, Morton NE. Genetic epidemiology of ovarian cancer: segregation analysis. Ann Hum Genet 1991; 55: 291–299.

45 Evans DGR, Ribiero G, Warrell D, Donnai D. Ovarian cancer family and prophylactic choices. J Med Genet 1992; 29: 416–418.

46 Bowcock AM, Anderson LA, Friedman LS et al. THRA1 and D17S183 flank and interval of < 4 cM for the breast-ovarian cancer gene. Am J Hum Genet 1993; 52: 718–722.

47 Fraumeni JF, Grundy GW, Creagan ET, Everson RB. Six families prone to ovarian cancer. Cancer 1975; 36: 364–369.

48 Chamberlain JS, Boehnke M, Frank TS et al. BRCA1 maps proximal to D17S579 on chromosome 17q21 by genetic linkage analysis. Am J Hum Genet 1993; 52: 792–798.

49 Simard J, Feunteun J, Lenoir GM et al. Genetic mapping of the breast-ovarian cancer syndrome to a small interval on chromosome 17q12-21: exclusion of candidate genes EDH17B2 and RARA. Hum Mol Genet 1993; 2: 1193–1199.

50 Goldgar DE, Fields P, Lewis CM et al. A large kindred with 17q-linked breast and ovarian cancer: genetic, phenotypic and genealogic analysis. J Natl Cancer Inst 1994; 86: 200–209.

51 Feunteun J, Narod SA, Lynch HT et al. A breast-ovarian cancer susceptibility gene maps to chromosome 17q21. Am J Hum Genet 1993; 52: 736–742.

52 Porter DE, Cohen BB, Wallace MR, Carothers A, Steel CM. Int J Cancer 1993; 53:188–198.

53 Kelsell DP, Black DM, Bishop DT, Spurr NK. Genetic analysis of the BRCA1 region in a breast/ovarian family: refinement of the minimal region containing BRCA1. Hum Mol Genet 1993; 2: 1823–1828.

54 Tonin P, Moslehi R, Normand R et al. Linkage analysis of 13 Canadian breast and breast-ovarian cancer families. 1993 (submitted).

55 Tonin P, Ehrenborg E, Lenoir GM et al. Human insulin-like growth factor-binding protein maps to chromosome 17q12-q21.1 and is close to the gene for hereditary breast-ovarian cancer. Genomics 1993; 18: 414–417.

56 Easton D, Ford D, Peto J. Inherited susceptibility to breast cancer. Cancer Surv 1993; 18: 1–17.

57 Ford D, Easton DF, Bishop DT, Narod SA and the Breast Cancer Linkage Consortium. The risks of cancer in BRCA1 mutation carriers. Am J Hum Genet 1993; 53: A298.

58   Mazoyer S, Lalle P, Narod SA et al. Linkage analysis of 19 breast cancer families, with five chromosome 17q markers. Am J Hum Genet 1993; 52: 754–760.
59   Anderson DE, Badzioch MD. Breast cancer risks in relatives of male breast cancer patients. J Natl Cancer Inst 1992; 84: 1114–1117.
60   Tulinius H, Egilsson V, Olafsdottir GH, Sigvaldson H. Risk of prostate, ovarian, and endometrial cancer among relatives of women with breast cancer. BMJ 1992; 305: 855–857.
61   Arason A, Barkardottir RB, Egilsson V. Linkage analysis of chromosome 17q markers and breast-ovarian cancer in Icelandic families, and possible relationship to prostatic cancer. Am J Hum Genet 1993; 52: 711–717.
62   Neugut AI, Murray TI, Lee WC, Robinson E. The association of breast cancer and colorectal cancer in men. Cancer 1991; 68: 2069–2073.
63   Miller S, Jothy S, Shibata H, Parboosingh J, Narod SA. Early onset breast and ovarian cancer in a large sibship. Am J Hum Genet 1992; 51: A66.
64   Skolnick MH, Goldgar D, Albright LA et al. Phenotypic effects of the BRCA1 locus in 8 linked kindreds. Am J Hum Genet 1992; 51: A38.
65   Tonin P, Cutler C, Conway T et al. Linkage analysis of 10 families with breast cancer and malignant melanoma. 1993 (Submitted).
66   Krontiris TG, Devlin B, Karp DD, Robert NJ, Risch N. An association between the risk of cancer and mutations in the HRAS1 minisatellite locus. N Engl J Med 1993; 329: 517–523.
67   Pippard EC, Hall AJ, Barker DJP, Bridges BA. Cancer in homozygotes and heterozygotes of ataxia-telangiectasia and xeroderma pigmentosum in Britain. Cancer Res 1988; 48: 2929–2932.
68   Swift M, Morrell D, Massey RB, Chase CL. Incidence of cancer in 161 families affected by ataxia-telangiectasia. N Engl J Med 1991; 325: 1831–1836.
69   Lehman AR, Jaspers NGJ, Gatti RA. Meeting report: Fourth International workshop on ataxia-telangiectasia. Cancer Res 1989; 49: 6162–6163.
70   Wooster R, Ford D, Mangion J et al. Absence of linkage to the ataxia-telangiectasia locus in familial breast cancer. Hum Genet 1993; 92: 91–94.
71   Malkin D, Li FP, Strong LC et al. Germ line p53 mutations in a familial syndrome of breast cancer, sarcomas and other neoplasms. Science 1990; 250: 1233–1238.
72   Hollstein M, Sidransky D, Vogelstein B, Harris CC. p53 mutations in human cancers. Science 1991; 253: 49–53.
73   Borresen AL, Anderson TI, Garber J et al. Screening for germline TP53 mutations in breast cancer patients. Cancer Res 1992; 52: 3234–3236.
74   Sidransksy D, Tokino T, Helzsouer K et al. Inherited p53 gene mutations in breast cancer. Cancer Res 1992; 52: 2984–2986.
75   Everson RB, Fraumeni JF, Wilson RE et al. Familial male breast cancer. Lancet 1976; i: 9–12.
76   Meurer M et al. Androgen receptor in Klinefelter syndrome. Lancet 1993; 341: 1351.
77   Lobaccarro J M, Lumbroso S, Belon C et al. Male breast cancer and the androgen receptor gene. Nature Genet 1993; 5: 109–110.
78   Kelsey JL. A review of the epidemiology of human breast cancer. Epidemiol Rev 1979; 1: 74–109.
79   Sellers TA, Kushi LH, Potter JD et al. Effect of family history, body-fat distribution and reproductive factors on the risk of pre-menopausal breast cancer. N Engl J Med 1992; 326: 1323–1329.
80   Brinton LA, Hoover R, Fraumeni JF. Interaction of familial and hormonal risk factors for breast cancer. J Natl Cancer Inst 1982; 69: 817–822.
81   Narod SA, Lynch HT, Conway T, Feunteun J, Lenoir GM. The incidence of cancer is increasing in a large family with hereditary breast-ovarian cancer. Lancet 1993; 341: 1101–1102.
82   Cann CE, Genant HK, Ettinger B, Gordon GS. Spinal mineral loss in oophorectomized women. JAMA 1980; 244: 2056–2059.
83   Colditz GA, Willett WC, Stampfer J et al. Menopause and the risk of coronary heart disease in women. N Engl J Med 1987; 316: 1103–1108.

84   Wuest JH, Dry TJ, Edwards JE. The degree of coronary atherosclerosis in bilaterally oophorectomized women. J Am Heart Assoc 1953; 7: 801–809.

85   Tobacman JK, Tucker MA, Kase R, Greene MH, Costa J, Fraumeni JF. Intra-abdominal carcinomatosis after prophylactic oophorectomy in ovarian cancer prone families. Lancet 1982; 2: 795–797.

86   Piver MS, Jishi MF, Tsukada Y, Nava G. Primary peritoneal carcinoma after prophylactic oophorectomy in women with a family history of ovarian cancer. Cancer 1993; 71: 2751–2755.

87   Lynch HT, Watson P, Conway TA et al. Pilot study of DNA screening for breast/ovarian cancer susceptibility based on linked markers. Arch Int Med 1993; 153: 1979–1987.

88   Miller AB, Baines CJ, To T, Wall C. Canadian National Breast Screening Study: 1. Breast cancer detection and death rates among women aged 40–49 years. Can Med Assoc J 1992; 147: 1459–1476.

89   Lalle P, Bignon YV, Stoppa-Lyonnet D et al. Screening of inherited breast cancer with DNA markers. Lancet 1993; 341: 1422.

90   Campbell S, Bhan V, Royston P, Whitehead MI, Collins WP. Transabdominal ultrasound screening for early ovarian cancer. BMJ 1989; 299: 1363–1367.

91   Bourne TH, Whitehead MI, Campbell S, Royston P, Bhan V, Collins WP. Ultrasound screening for familial ovarian cancer. Gynecol Oncol 1991; 43: 92–97.

92   Steinberg K, Thacker S, Smith S et al. A meta-analysis of the effect of estrogen replacement therapy on the risk of breast cancer. JAMA 1991; 265; 1985–1990.

93   Colditz GA, Egan KM, Stampfer MJ. Hormone replacement therapy and risk of breast cancer; results from epidemiologic studies. Am J Obstet Gynecol 1993; 168: 1473–1480.

94   Stampfer MJ, Colditz GA, Willet WC et al. Post-menopausal estrogen therapy and cardiovascular disease. Ten-year follow-up from the Nurses' Health Study. N Engl J Med 1989; 321: 293–297.

95   Whittemore AS, Harris R, Intyre J and the Collaborative Ovarian Cancer Group. Characteristics relating to ovarian cancer risk: collaborative analysis of 12 US case-control studies. Am J Epidemiol 1992; 136: 1212–1220.

96   UK National Case-Control Study Group: Oral contraceptive use and breast cancer risk in young women: subgroup analyses. Lancet 1990; 335; 1507–1509.

97   The Cancer and Steroid Hormone Study of the Centers for Disease Control and the National Institute of Child Health and Human Development: Oral contraceptive use and the risk of breast cancer. N Engl J Med 1986; 315: 405–411.

98   Ottman R, Pike MC, King MC, Casagrande JT, Henderson BE. Familial breast cancer in a population-based series. Am J Epidemiol 1986; 123: 15–21.

99   Gail MH, Brinton LA, Byar DP et al. Projecting individualized probabilities of developing breast cancer for white females who are being examined annually. J Natl Cancer Inst 1989; 81: 1879–1886.

100   King M-C, Rowell S, Love S. Inherited breast and ovarian cancer. What are the risks? What are the choices? JAMA 1993; 269: 1975–1980.

101   Narod SA. Hereditary breast-ovarian cancer: How can we use the new DNA markers to improve patient management. Clin Invest Med 1993; 16: 314–317.

102   Biesecker BB, Boehnke M, Calzone K et al. Genetic counselling for families with inherited susceptibility to breast and ovarian cancer. JAMA 1993; 269: 1970–1974.

103   Narod SA. Counselling under genetic heterogeneity. A practical approach. Clin Genet 1991; 39: 125–131.

British Medical Bulletin (1994) Vol. 50, No. 3, pp. 677–687
© The British Council 1994

Genetics of melanoma

J A Newton

ICRF Skin Tumour Laboratory, Royal London Hospital, Whitechapel, London, UK

Melanoma may cluster in families with 'family cancer syndromes' in which there is a predisposition to a variety of different tumours. Other families seem vulnerable to melanoma alone. In the majority of these families, the propensity to melanoma is associated with the presence of abnormal melanocytic naevi, the so-called atypical mole syndrome (AMS) phenotype. However, in a smaller number of families, individuals are susceptible to melanoma but have normal naevi. There appears, therefore, to be clinical (and probably genetic) heterogeneity.

Segregation analysis does not support a predisposition by single dominant gene as an explanation for the AMS/melanoma syndrome. To date, a single gene which is clearly important for susceptibility to melanoma has not been identified.

Karyotypic studies of melanoma tumours have pointed to chromosomes 1,6,7,9 and 10 as possible sites for melanoma related genes. Loss of heterozygosity studies have suggested that chromosome 9 may carry a tumour suppressor gene important in familial disease, and linkage studies appear to confirm this. It is not yet clear, however, what percentage of familial melanoma is attributable to this gene. A more longstanding suggestion that a gene on chromosome 1 may be important has not been confirmed, but a chromosome/gene may be responsible for susceptibility in a small subset of melanoma families.

Even within AMS families, there is a lack of concordance between the AMS phenotype and susceptibility to melanoma. This might be explained either by the effects of modifying genes, or the environment.

EVIDENCE FOR CLUSTERING OF MELANOMA IN FAMILIES

5–10% of melanoma patients have been reported to give a family history of the same disease.[1,2] In a case control study of melanoma nearing completion in the UK, 2% of cases reported familial disease. Familial aggregation of melanoma has also been demonstrated in a large study from Utah, using the Utah genealogy data base.[3] The aggregation of melanoma was marked among the common cancers in the Mormon population. Melanoma showed the fourth highest level of family aggregation (after ovary, prostate and lip cancer).

Clustering of melanoma in families may conceivably occur because of shared environmental factors (exposure to ultraviolet light) and a common susceptible skin type, that is, fair skin and a tendency to sunburn. Excessive UV exposure and fair skin are well established risk factors for melanoma. This may be especially true, for example, in Australia where a susceptible population live an outdoor lifestyle in conditions of intense UV exposure.

There also appears however, to be genetic susceptibility to melanoma in several family cancer syndromes. For example, melanoma accounts for approximately 7% of second malignancies in familial retinoblastoma patients.[4] It is of note that in 2 of 6 melanoma patients from such families there were multiple primary melanomas, a finding characteristic of genetic predisposition.[4]

There is also an increased number of cases of melanoma in Li-Fraumeni families[5] and (although less well established) in families with the Lynch type II family cancer syndrome.[6] A small number of families have also been described in which there appears to be susceptibility to melanoma and breast cancer[7] which may or may not represent a distinct entity.

In the majority of families in which there is clustering of melanoma, however, the individuals seem predisposed to melanoma alone. In most such families described in the literature susceptibility to melanoma was associated with the presence of abnormal melanocytic naevi, or moles. This condition was first well delineated by Clark[8] and has been known by several names. Initially it was called the BK mole syndrome for the surnames of the two affected families, then the dysplastic naevus syndrome, also the familial atypical mole and malignant melanoma (FAMMM) syndrome.[9] Latterly the atypical mole syndrome (AMS) has found favour.

In Clark's original two families, abnormal naevi, and melanoma appeared to be inherited in an autosomal dominant pattern, and the similarities to adenomatous polyposis coli (the polyps being analogous to the atypical naevi) seemed obvious. In both types of family the increased risk of cancer seemed to occur only in individuals with precursor lesions.

CLINICAL STUDIES OF FAMILIES PRONE TO MELANOMA (AMS FAMILIES)

Families at risk of cutaneous melanoma were studied clinically by Bale et al[10] at the National Cancer Institute in Washington as a result of the initial report by Clark of the BK mole family, and these families later formed the basis of linkage studies. Utah families have been studied by Skolnick's group.[11] A very large family studied by Anderson in Texas[12] in which there were 28 cases of melanoma also subsequently formed part of the linkage study by the Utah group.[13] In all of these studies, the families were reported to have abnormal melanocytic naevi and were described as AMS families. In Australian studies,[14] however, the association between susceptibility to melanoma and atypical naevi was much less clear. In UK families the majority of susceptible families have the AMS phenotype, but not all.[15] The possibility exists therefore that familial susceptibility to melanoma may occur either in association with the AMS phenotype, or without such an association: in other words, that there may be heterogeneity.

An atypical or dysplastic naevus is usually defined as a naevus bigger in diameter than 5 mm, with variable pigmentation and an irregular edge (Fig. 1). Clark described typical corresponding histological features, with atypical melanocytic hyperplasia[16] and cellular atypia. There are, however, considerable difficulties in the definition of the AMS phenotype even within families found to have atypical melanocytic naevi. Clark believed that 'dysplastic' naevi were diagnostic of familial melanoma[16] so that in early linkage studies[17] family members without melanoma were considered to be gene carriers if they had 2 histologically 'proven' dysplastic naevi. Subsequently, however, poor correlation between histological and clinical features of these dysplastic or atypical naevi[18] was demonstrated. In addition, although atypical naevi are powerful indicators of risk of melanoma within and outside families,[19,20] the naevi were shown not to be restricted to AMS families, being present in 2–19%[20,21] of the normal population in Europe. Furthermore the AMS phenotype and melanoma frequently do not co-segregate in melanoma families.[9,15]

The difficulties of definition of phenotype have led several groups to pursue linkage analysis of these families based on melanoma alone as the criterion for an affected individual.[13,14] New definitions of the AMS phenotype of varying degrees of complexity have been developed[20,22] to try and overcome these difficulties. Most take into account several aspects of the AMS phenotype, in particular the presence of numerous

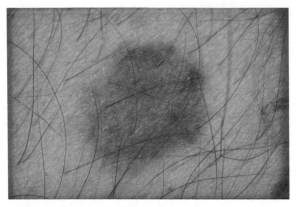

Fig. 1 A clinically atypical or dysplastic naevus, 1 cm in diameter, showing the usual characteristics of irregular shape and colour.

naevi as well as atypical ones. One such system, the Royal London Hospital system, also considers an abnormal distribution of naevi. Patients with AMS have such a marked tendency to melanocytic naevi that they develop them in sites such as the iris, dorsum of the foot, and on the buttocks. Table 1 is the AMS scoring system used.[20] Figure 2 shows typical features of the AMS phenotype.

These scoring systems certainly identify some gene carriers with a degree of confidence, but melanoma undoubtedly occurs even within AMS families in people with entirely normal moles. In the FAMMM families and in our UK families there was a lack of concordance between melanoma and the AMS phenotype. In only 54% and 57% of cases respectively did individuals with melanoma also have abnormal naevi: that is, the AMS phenotype. The absence of the AMS phenotype in an individual from an AMS family cannot therefore be confidently used in family counselling as a basis for reassurance. Furthermore in linkage studies the use of the AMS phenotype as a definition of an 'affected' individual remains problematic.

Melanoma families exhibit clinical characteristics common to most family cancer syndromes. The age of first melanoma tends to be earlier than in sporadic tumours. In our study of 13 AMS families the mean age of first melanoma was 42.3 years compared with 51.7 years in unselected melanoma cases in NE Thames, UK. Multiple tumours are also more likely. In these same 13 UK families, 9 of the 37 melanoma cases had multiple primary tumours (range 2 to 7). There is some evidence

Table 1 The Royal London Hospital's AMS scoring system. Individuals having 3 or more of the 5 features are considered to have the AMS phenotype

The atypical mole syndrome scoring system	
Clinical observation	**Score**
100 or more naevi 2 mm+ in diameter (50 or more if younger than 20 or older than 50 years)	1
2 or more clinically atypical naevi	1
2+ naevi dorsum of the foot or 1+ buttock	1
Naevus in the anterior scalp	1
Pigmented lesion iris	1
Total	Max of 5

that AMS families may also have an increased susceptibility to other tumours. In the FAMMM families in Leiden there appears to be an increased risk of gastrointestinal cancer (particularly pancreatic cancer) and ocular melanoma.[23] In the UK there also appears to be evidence of an association between choroidal or conjunctival melanoma and cutaneous melanoma.[24,25] Other authors, however, have been unable to confirm this association.[26]

The AMS phenotype in the general population and risk of melanoma

The presence of abnormal melanocytic naevi has been established as the most potent risk factor for melanoma[20] in case control studies of melanoma in the general population. Although the presence of clinically atypical naevi implies an increased risk of melanoma, large numbers even of banal naevi also implies increased risk.

A recent detailed study of melanoma patients in the UK quantified the risk associated with the various clinical features of melanocytic naevi which constitute the AMS phenotype.[20] Table 2 shows the increasing risk of melanoma associated with an increasing AMS score. The identification of individuals with the AMS phenotype in screening programmes would therefore identify people with a significantly raised risk of cutaneous melanoma. The approximate lifetime risk of cutaneous melanoma in the UK is 1 in 200; patients with AMS have a risk of 1 in 20.

It is of note that a similar study of melanoma patients with melanoma of the eye showed that the AMS phenotype was also a risk factor for

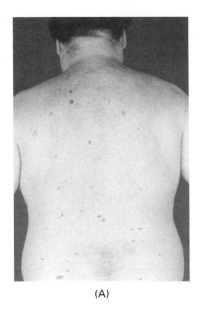

(A)

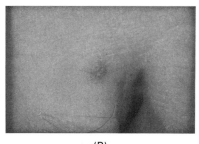

(B)

Fig. 2 (A) The typical appearance of an individual with the AMS phenotype. There are multiple banal naevi as well as atypical naevi and naevi in unusual sites such as on the dorsum of the foot **(B)**. The naevus in Figure 1 is from the same patient.

ocular melanoma.[27] The incidence of ocular melanoma in the UK is approximately 10 times lower than of cutaneous melanoma so that the absolute risk of ocular melanoma in an individual with AMS is low: approximately 1 in 200 lifetime risk. The explanation for the association between cutaneous melanocytic naevi and ocular melanoma is unclear but in the absence of strong evidence for common environmental factors, may be genetic.

Table 2 An increasing odds ratio for melanoma with an increasing AMS score. Results from a case control study[20]

	Increasing odds ratio for melanoma with increasing AMS score				
AMS score	Number cases	Controls	Odds ratio	P value	95% CI
0	102	179	1.00		
1	82	90	1.60	0.02	(1.09, 2.35)
2	42	29	2.54	0.0001	(1.49, 4.33)
3	29	6	8.48	<0.0001	(3.41, 21.12)
4	11	1	19.30	0.005	(2.46, 151.76)
Total	266	305			

WHAT IS THE MODE OF INHERITANCE OF MELANOMA IN AMS FAMILIES?

In many AMS families the pedigrees are suggestive of an autosomal dominant pattern of inheritance.[9,15,28] However, there has been controversy and several authors have suggested that a polygenic pattern of inheritance is more plausible.[29]

Linkage studies published subsequently have shown that, in some families at least, the tendency to melanoma is inherited, at least in part, in an autosomal dominant pattern. It is the relationship of melanoma risk to atypical naevi which remains difficult to elucidate.

Half of the Genetic Analysis Workshop, Number 7, in 1990, was devoted to the genetic epidemiology of melanoma. Data sets were available for twin studies from the UK and family studies from Utah, the NCI, Leiden and Australia.[30] The data were analysed in very different ways by a series of investigators variably experienced in the melanoma field. The twin data provided strong evidence of genetic determinants and a significant effect of sun exposure. Overall, the genetic model suggested by the analyses was of multiple genes possibly acting additively.

The Utah data (which was of clinical and linkage studies) provided the clearest information for the inheritance of abnormal naevi. The best fitting genetic model varied widely according to the type of analysis performed and the only consistent finding was that the dominant Mendelian model was rejected. The relationship between the AMS phenotype and risk of melanoma was also addressed. The theory that the naevi were precursors of melanoma and therefore that the association between naevi and melanoma was simply 'the more naevi, the more likely is melanoma' was rejected.

There is no doubt that the AMS phenotype is commonly associated with risk of melanoma in families. However, the association is not constant and even within AMS families two groups have shown that only 60% of melanoma patients express the AMS phenotype. It seems very plausible that there are at least two genes playing a role in these families and that the interaction of these mutliple genes leads to susceptibility to melanoma and the presence of abnormal naevi.

CYTOGENETICS OF MELANOCYTIC LESIONS AS A CLUE TO THE SITE OF PUTATIVE GENES FOR MELANOMA

Although there remain considerable difficulties in interpretation of the AMS phenotype and it is not known how many genes are important in determining genetic predisposition to melanoma, nevertheless it is clear that there are genes which predispose to melanoma in a small number of families. Cytogenetic abnormalities in melanoma tissue were performed in the hope that they may give a clue as to the site of such genes.

Non-random abnormalities of chromosomes 1,6,7,9 and 10 have been demonstrated most frequently.[31,32] Most of the karyotypic abnormalities were found to occur predominantly in metastatic melanoma, while family studies are most likely to identify tumour suppressor genes which act early in carcinogenesis. Particular attention was therefore paid to the demonstration of abnormalities in chromosome 9, which have been found in melanocytic naevi:[33] that is, early in the cascade of tumourigenesis. An identical pattern of loss of heterozygosity of 9p24 in 6 metastases from a single patient provided further evidence for a gene on chromosome 9 with effects before the stage of metastasis.[34]

Loss of alleles on the long arm of chromosome 6 is common in melanomas. This led Trent et al[35] to assess the control of tumourigenicity in melanoma lines by transfer of a normal chromosome 6 into melanoma cells. The resultant cell hybrids were no longer tumourigenic in nude mice, which provides some evidence that there may be a gene on chromosome 6, which is involved in the development of melanoma.

LINKAGE STUDIES TO LOCALISE A MELANOMA GENE

The observation that chromosomal abnormalities are commonest on chromosome 1 led the NCI group to perform genetic linkage studies with markers on chromosome 1, in their melanoma families. Initial weak evidence of linkage to the rhesus (Rh) gene was followed by a report claiming very significant LOD scores for linkage of the AMS/melanoma gene at 1p 36[17] using either melanoma or the AMS phenotype to define 'affected' individuals. Subsequently the same group revised their LOD score to lower but still significant levels. The LOD score was not significant if melanoma alone was considered. Other groups have failed to confirm this linkage.[11,36,37] The explanation may be genetic heterogeneity with only a subset of families exhibiting linkage to 1p.[38]

Despite the chromosome transfer experiments of Trent[35] there has been no evidence of linkage to chromosome 6 in families.

In 1992 several groups started to look for linkage to chromosome 9 because of Dracopoli's report of deletions in melanoma metastases,[34] but also because of a report by Petty in 1991 of melanoma and the AMS in a patient with a 5p/9p chromosomal rearrangement.[39] Karyotypic abnormalities in rare patients have provided the essential clues which led to the discovery of other cancer family syndrome genes, such as the gene for polyposis coli. In 1992 the Utah group published convincing evidence for linkage to chromosome 9[40] in their large melanoma pedigrees. This has now been confirmed by the groups in the Netherlands[41] and in Australia.[42] Although the Utah families have abnormal naevi, difficulties in interpretation of the AMS phenotype led the group to use melanoma alone as the criterion of being an 'affected' individual. The subsequent report from the Dutch group, however, demonstrated linkage for melanoma and the AMS phenotype.[41]

It is therefore clear that there is a gene on chromosome 9 which is responsible for familial susceptibility to melanoma around the world. It is not yet clear whether there are families not linked to this gene: that is, how much genetic heterogeneity exists. This is currently being established. The next phase will be to locate the gene itself using tumour deletion studies and positional cloning techniques. Once the gene is identified, it will be possible to determine how important it is in the aetiology of melanoma in the general population.

The possibility that multiple genes are involved in the pathogenesis of the AMS/melanoma syndrome has been discussed. It may be that further linkage studies will be necessary to explore this. Once the genotype of predisposition can be identified, the interacting effects of the environment on the final phenotype can also be studied.

REFERENCES

1 Cawley EP. Genetic aspects of malignant melanoma. Arch Dermatol 1952; 65: 440–450.
2 Greene MH, Fraumeni JF. The hereditary variant of malignant melanoma. In: Clark WH, Goldman LI, Mastrangelo MJ eds. Human malignant melanoma. New York: Grune and Stratton, 1979; pp 139–166.
3 Bishop DT and Skolnick MH. Genetic epidemiology of cancer in Utah geneologies: a prelude to the molecular genetics of common cancer. In: TW Mack, I Tannock, eds. Cellular and molecular biology of neoplasia. J Cell Physiol 1984 (Suppl 3); 63–77.
4 Traboulsi EI, Zimmerman LE , Manz HJ. Cutaneous malignant melanoma in survivors of heritable retinoblastoma. Arch Ophthalmol 1988; 109: 1059–1066.

5 Little JB, Nove J, Dahlberg WK et al. Normal cytotoxic response of skin firoblasts from patients from patients with Li-Fraumeni familial cancer syndrome to DNA-damaging agents in vitro. Cancer Res 1987; 47: 4229–4234.

6 Lynch HT, Watson P, Kriegler M et al. Differential diagnosis of hereditary nonpolyposis colorectal cancer (Lynch syndrome I and Lynch syndrome II). Dis Colon Rectum 1988; 31: 372–377.

7 Lynch HT, Frichot BC, Lynch P, Lynch J, Guirgis HA. Family studies of malignant melanoma and associated cancer. Surg Gynccol Obstet 1975; 141: 517–522.

8 Clark WH, Reimer RR, Greene MH et al. origin of familial malignant melanomas from hereditable melanocytic lesions: 'the B.K. mole syndrome'. Arch Dermatol 1978; 114: 732–773

9 Bergman W, Palan A, Went LN. Clinical and genetic studies in 6 Dutch kindreds with the DNS. Ann Hum Genet 1986; 50: 249–258.

10 Bale SJ, Goldstein AM, Tucker MA. Description of the National Cancer Institute melanoma families. Cytogenet Cell Genet 1992; 59: 159–160.

11 Cannon-Albright LA, Goldgar DG, Wright EC et al. Evidence against the reported linkage of the cutaneous melanoma dysplastic nevus syndrome locus to chromosome 1p 36. Am J Hum Genet 1990; 46: 912–918.

12 Anderson DE, Badzioch MD. Hereditary cutaneous melanoma: a 20 year family update. Anticancer Res 1991; 11: 433–438.

13 Cannon-Albright LA, Goldgar DE, Meyer LJ et al. Assignment of a locus for familial melanoma MLM to chromosome 9p13–p22. Science 1992; 258: 1148–1152.

14 Kefford RF, Salmon J, Shaw HM, Donald JA, McCarthy WH. Hereditary melanoma in Australia: variable association with dysplastic naevi and absence of genetic linkage to chromosome 1p. Cancer Genet Cytogenet 1991; 51: 45–55 1991.

15 Newton JA, Bataille V, Pinney E, Bishop DT. Family studies in melanoma: identification of the atypical mole syndrome (AMS) phenotype. Melanoma Res 1994 (In press).

16 Clark WH, Ackerman AB. An exchange of views regarding the dysplastic nevus controversy. Seminars in Dermatol 1989; 8: 229–250.

17 Bale SJ, Dracopoli NC, Tucker MA et al. Mapping the gene for hereditary cutaneous malignant melanoma-dysplastic nevus to chromosome 1p. N Engl J Med 1989; 329: 1367–1372.

18 Ahmed I, Piepkorn MW, Rabin MS et al. Histopathologic characteristics of dysplastic nevi. Limited association of conventional histologic criteria with melanoma risk group. J Am Acad Dermatol 1990; 22: 727–733.

19 Halpern AC, Gerry D, Elder DE, Trook B, Synnestvedt M. A cohort study of melanoma in patients with dysplastic nevi. J Invest Dermatol 1993; 100: 346S–349S.

20 Newton JA, Bataille V, Griffiths K et al. How common is the atypical mole syndrome in apparently sporadic melanoma? J Am Acad Dermatol 1994 (In press).

21 Stierner U, Augustsson A, Rosdahl I, Suurkula M. Regional distribution of common and dysplastic naevi in relation to melanoma site and sun exposure. A case control study. Melanoma Res 1990; 1: 367–375.

22 Meyer LJ, Goldgar DE, Cannon-Albright LA et al. Number, size, and histopathology of nevi in Utah kindreds. Cytogenet Cell Genet 1992; 59: 167–169.

23 Bergman W, de Jong J, Lynch HT, Fusaro RM. Systemic cancer and the FAMMM syndrome. Br J Cancer 1990; 61: 932–936.

24 Bataille V, Boyle J, Hungerford JL, Newton JA. Three cases of primary acquired melanosis of the conjunctiva as a manifestation of the atypical mole syndrome. Br J Dermatol 1993; 128: 86–90.

25 Bataille V, Pinney E, Hungerford JL, Cuzick J, Bishop DT, Newton JA. Five cases of primary ocular and cutaneous melanoma in the same individual. Arch Dermatol 1993; 129: 198–201.

26 Tucker MA, Fraser MC, Goldstein AM et al. Risk of melanoma and other cancers in melanoma-prone families. J Invest Dermatol 1993; 100: 350S–355S.

27 Bataille V, Sasieni P, Cuzick J, Hungerford JL, Swerdlow A, Newton JA. Risk factors of ocular melanoma in relation to cutaneous and iris naevi 1994 (In press).

28 Lynch HT, Fusaro RM, Kimberling WJ, Lynch JF, Danes BS. Familial atypical multiple mole-melanoma (FAMMM) syndrome: segregation analysis. J Med Genet 1983; 20: 342–344.

29 Happle R, Traupe H, Vakilzadeh F, Macher E. Arguments in favour of a polygeneic inheritance of precursor nevi. J Am Acad Dermatol 1982; 6: 540–543.

30 Risch N, Sherman S. Genetic analysis workshop 7: summary of the melanoma workshop. Cytogenet Cell Genet 1992; 59: 148–158.

31 Parmiter AH, Nowell PC. Cytogenetics of melanocytic tumors. J Invest Dermatol 1993; 100: 254S–258S.

32 Trent JM. Cytogenetics of human malignant melanoma. Cancer Metast Rev 1991; 10: 103–113.

33 Cowan JM, Halaban R, Francke U. Cytogenetic analysis of melanocytes from premalignant nevi and melanomas. J Natl Cancer Inst 1988; 80: 1159–1164.

34 Dracopoli NC, Alhadeff B, Houghton AN, Old LJ. Loss of heterozygosity at autosomal and X-linked loci during tumor progression in a patient with melanoma. Cancer Res 1987; 47: 3995–4000.

35 Trent JM, Stanbridge EJ, McBride HL et al. Tumorigenicity in human melanoma cell lines controlled by introduction of human chromosome 6. Science 1990; 247: 568–571.

36 Gruis NA, Bergman W, Frants RR. Locus for susceptibility to melanoma on chromosome 1p. N Engl J Med 1990; 322: 853–854.

37 Nancarrow DJ, Palmer JM, Walters MK. Exclusion of the familial melanoma locus (MLM) from the PND/D1S47 regions of chromosome arm 1p in 7 Australian families. Genomics 1992; 12: 18–25.

38 Goldstein AM, Dracopoli NC, Ho EC, et al Further evidence for a locus for cutaneous malignant melanoma-dysplastic nevus (CMM/DN) on chromosome 1p, and evidence for genetic heterogeneity. Am J Hum Genet 1993; 52: 537–550.

39 Petty EM, Bale AE, Bolognia JL et al. A constitutional cytogenetic abnormality associated with cutaneous malignant melanoma/dysplastic naevus syndrome (CMM/DNS). Am J Hum Genet 1991: 49(Suppl): Abstract 1353.

40 Cannon-Albright LA, Golgar DE, Meyer LJ et al. Assignment of a locus for familial melanoma MLM, to chromosome 9p13-p22. Science 1992; 258: 1148–1152.

41 Nancarrow DJ, Mann GJ, Holland EA, Walker GJ, Beaton SC, Walter. Confirmation of chromoosme 9p linkage in familial melanoma. Am J Hum Genet 1993; 53: 936–942.

42 Gruis NA, Sandkuijl JL, Weber A et al. Linkage analysis in Dutch familial atypical mutiple mole-melanoma (FAMMM) syndrome families. Effect of naevus count. Melanoma Res 1993: 3: 271–277.

British Medical Bulletin (1994) Vol. 50, No. 3, pp. 688–697

Genetic changes in the development of lung cancer

P H Rabbitts

MRC Clinical Oncology and Radiotherapeutics Unit, MRC Centre, Cambridge, UK

Both inherited predisposition and acquired somatic genetic changes contribute to lung tumour development but the former is likely to be the minor component. The relative ease with which lung tumours can be established as cell lines has resulted in extensive cytogenetic analysis, and, this together with molecular techniques which assess loss of genetic material has revealed consistent patterns of genetic damage. Some of these characteristic somatic genetic changes have been traced back to the pre-invasive stage of tumour development and this information may contribute to the future management of this currently intractable disease.

The majority of lung cancer patients have a history of smoking, yet the majority of smokers do not get lung cancer. While incidence is dose-related, many heavy smokers remain free of this disease and other smoking-related cancers. For those who do contract the disease, inherited genetic predisposition may be a contributing factor. For some adult tumours (breast cancer, for example) it is clear that a susceptibility gene can be inherited and patients carrying such a gene present with earlier age of onset and often multiple tumours.[1] This pattern is discovered by studying the incidence of the disease in the population and identifying family clustering. However, so far, no classical linkage analysis, which correlates incidence of the disease with the inheritance of genetic markers, has been reported for lung cancer. The high incidence of smoking is a confounding factor in the interpretation of the results of such studies.

There are many types of genes which might be involved in predisposition to lung cancer. It is known that most of the compounds in cigarette smoke exert their carcinogenic effect after being metabolised to a more active form, and that there is inherent variation between individuals in the activity of the enzymes involved in these processes. Individuals who most successfully activate the carcinogen might thus be genetically predisposed to lung cancer development. The original carcinogenic insult to the DNA must be inherited in the population of cells at risk to be effective. Thus any reduction in efficiency of DNA repair pathways would similarly lead to an increased susceptibility to tumour development by perpetuating damaged DNA.

Evidence from breeding studies, involving mice with inherent high and low incidence of lung cancer, predicts the presence of 3 major susceptibility genes in mouse, of which one has been mapped to mouse chromosome 6.[2] The isolation of this gene will allow its human homologue to be characterised and this may prove the most accessible route to the study of human genetic predisposition to lung cancer.

In contrast to the genes which predispose to the inheritance of lung cancer, those genes actually involved in the development of the tumour itself are much better characterized.

METHODS OF DETECTION OF SOMATIC GENETIC CHANGES

Lung tumours are favourable for the study of somatic genetic changes for two reasons. Firstly, tumour samples are readily available in the form of operative specimens from patients with limited stage non small cell lung cancer (NSCLC), or as biopsy material from metastatic small cell lung cancer (SCLC). Secondly, lung cancer cells are readily established as immortal cell lines of which many hundreds are now available. Cell lines are of particular benefit when the genome is studied using cytogenetic analysis as chromosomes of much better quality can be prepared from this source than from direct preparations of biopsy material. The early chromosomal analyses of tumour samples relied on the ability to recognise chromosomes by producing a chromosome specific banding pattern after staining. Solid tumours, in general, have very complex karyotypes with severe aneupoidy and many aberrant chromosomes due to various rearrangements such as translocation and deletion. In addition, there are many 'scrambled' fragments of chromosomes, referred to as markers, because they occur consistently in different chromosomal spreads of the same sample, but whose banding pattern is so unusual that the original contributing chromosomes cannot be determined.

More recently chromosome specific 'paints' have been produced which, among their many uses, allow these highly aberrant chromosomes to be analysed. These paints are made by separating chromosomes by flow cytometry and amplifying the chromosome specific DNA, while simultaneously incorporating a fluorescent component.[3] The fluorescent 'paint' is hybridised to a normal chromosome spread to confirm that the anticipated paint has been produced, then it is used on chromosomes prepared from a tumour source and 'lights up' the distribution of that chromosome within the tumour karyotype (*see* Fig. 1). These techniques are, of course, at present confined to the research laboratory, but chromosome paints can be obtained commercially and may allow this type of analysis to have a place in diagnostic laboratories in the future.

When chromosome paints were first applied to interphase nuclei, it was surprising to see that it was still possible to detect specific regions within the nucleus. It appears that chromosomes occupy domains within the nuclei, rather than being totally dispersed throughout the nucleus as had originally been imagined.[4] The definition is obviously not as good as with metaphase chromosomes and thus when nuclei are used as targets for *in situ* hybridisation, the probes need to correspond to much smaller regions of the chromosome. This approach has now been developed to identify trisomy 21 in fetuses suspected of carrying Down's syndrome, obviating the need for growth of fetal cells in culture, thus allowing diagnosis to be made earlier in pregnancy.[4] The detection of specific chromosomal abnormalities already play a role in the diagnosis of haematological malignancies,[5] but the more complex karyotypes of the solid tumours will require a technique such as chromosome painting to provide the reliability essential for diagnostic purposes.

In parallel with the development of these more advanced types of cytogenetic analysis it has been possible to detect somatic genetic changes in tumour samples by studying the DNA directly. This has meant that cell lines are not required and that biopsy material can be used. In contrast to cytogenetics, which gives an overall picture, the study of somatic genetic changes represents a 'candidate' approach to studying the genome in that specific probes of known chromosomal location are used which target particular genes or defined regions of the genome, asking whether or not genes (or regions) are amplified or lost. Often the particular somatic genetic changes studied have been guided by earlier cytogenetic observations.

In the last few years, interest has centred around areas of genetic loss using probes which identify heterozygosity and are thus able to distinguish two chromosomal homologues. When genetic loss occurs in a tumour, it is usually from one rather than both homologues and this loss of heterozygosity (LOH)/reduction to homozygosity (more strictly, hemizygosity) can be detected. Heterozygosity can be due to a number of polymorphic variations within the DNA. Both restriction fragment length polymorphism (RFLP) and variations in the number of tandem repeats in an array are suitable sources of DNA polymorphism. Originally, these analyses were made by Southern blotting, but more recently the technique has been modified for use by the polymerase chain reaction (PCR).[6] This has been particularly important in the study

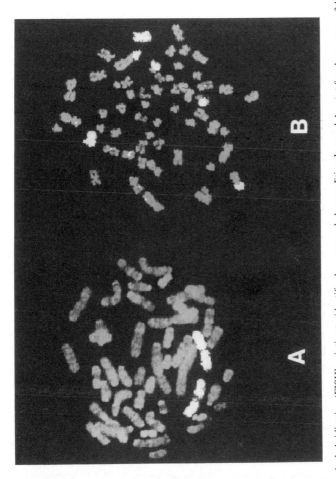

Fig. Fluorescent *in situ* hybridisation 'FISH' painting to identify chromosomal abnormalities. In panel A paint for chromosome 3 has been hybridised to normal chromosomes and two chromosome 3 can be seen fluorescing brightly. In panel B paint for chromosome 3 has been hybridised to chromosomes prepared from tumour cells and the hybridisation signal is detected on several different chromosomes including translocations.

of somatic genetic changes in very small specimens, such as in pre-invasive lesions where the quantity of DNA is so small that PCR is a prerequisite of analysis.[7]

SOMATIC GENETIC CHANGES IN MALIGNANT LUNG TUMOUR

Oncogenes

Mutated oncogenes are genetically dominant, that is, only the allele on one of the two chromosomes needs to be altered in order for the onco-gene to have a phenotypic effect. The genetic alterations which result in activation can be gene amplification or point mutation. Lung tumours have been shown to have amplified oncogenes, in particular members of the *myc* family. In fact, the L *myc* oncogene was first discovered, amplified and expressed in cell lines derived from small cell carcinomas of the lung.[8] However, when biopsies, rather than cell lines, were used as the source of lung tumour material, the proportion of samples that showed involvement of *myc* genes was reduced;[9] the cell lines probably showed disproportionate involvement because the expression of these genes facilitated the establishment of biopsy samples in tissue culture.

Members of the *ras* famiy of genes are often found activated in ade-nocarcinomas from various types of tissue; the activation being due to mutation rather than gene amplification. Of the 3 *ras* oncogenes, Kirsten (K) *ras* is by far the most frequently involved in lung tumours. Unlike mutations in the p53 gene (*see below*), where many different point mutations have been found, only 3 codons ever carry mutations. *ras* mutations occur in about one third of lung tumours and, although there are some conflicting data concerning the relationship between K-*ras* mutation incidence and tumour histology,[10] it is agreed that patients with tumours carrying a K-*ras* mutation have a significantly poorer prognosis than patients with K-*ras* negative tumours.[11]

Deletions in chromosome 3

Early in the 1980s a large number of SCLC cell lines were subjected to complete karyotype analysis with the unexpected observations that all the samples showed deletions to the short arm of chromosome 3.[12] However, a subsequent study of a large series of SCLC karyotypes was unable to confirm this observation.[13] The cytogenetic studies which followed tended to find that 3p loss was involved in most, but not all, SCLC tumours. In 1987, several reports using RFLP analysis to detect LOH confirmed that genetic loss on chromosome 3 was a uni-versal feature of SCLC.[14] From study of loss of heterozygosity at loci on both the short and the long arm of chromosome 3, it is clear that sometimes allele loss involves a complete chromosome rather than interstitial deletion. Duplication of the remaining homologue is a frequent event after non-disjunction. Cytogenetically such samples would appear normal with respect to chromosome 3. This explains how RFLP analysis can indicate that all SCLC have allele loss on chromosome 3, yet cytogenetic analysis does not always detect this.[15] NSCLC also carry genetic damage to chromosome 3, and all histologies have been implicated. The incidence within different histological subtypes varies in different studies; squamous cell carcinoma (SQC)[16] clearly have the highest incidence and in one report 100% of SQC showed 3p loss.

Regions of genetic loss identified by cytogenetic or molecular genetic analysis (or more usually both) have been of great interest recently as they have been important in the isolation of tumour suppressor genes. Mutations in suppressor genes, in contrast to oncogenes, are recessive. Thus, both copies of the gene must usually be inactivated for there to be a phenotypic effect. Following the clear demonstration of loss of alleles from 3p in lung tumours there have been several deletion mapping studies which have attempted to define the minimum region involved, as a prerequisite for gene isolation. Conflicting results were resolved by the realisation that at least 2, and possibly 3, different regions of 3p are involved in lung tumours, suggesting that several genes involved in the development of lung cancer are located on 3p.[17] If more than one of these genes must be inactivated for expression of the fully malignant phenotype, this might explain why deletions and whole homologue loss are so common in lung tumours. Two genes can be inactivated by one single chromosomal event, whereas inactivation of both genes by point mutation would require two independent events.

Over the last few years, and since the time of the early molecular analysis of allele loss on chromosome 3, the large number of polymorphic loci identified has allowed the deletion mapping studies to be much more detailed. For the 3p21 region, this approach has resulted in the identification of a minimum region of hemizygous deletion of 5 Mb (million base pairs). Once such a small region is identified, alternative methods can be used to study the region in more detail. Of particular importance is the discovery of a region of homozygous loss, i.e. loss on both chromosome homologues within the minimal hemizygously deleted region. Within a 5 Mb minimal deleted region on 3p21, homozygous deletion of about 1Mb has been detected.[18] DNA corresponding to the homozygously deleted region is presently being intensely analyzed for the presence of transcribed sequences, and any such sequences found are evaluated as a potential tumour suppressor gene.

The p53 gene

The observation of LOH on 17p did not require extensive deletion mapping to identify a candidate tumour suppressor gene, as the p53 gene was an obvious candidate. Mutations in the p53 gene are very common in SCLC,[19] and less common, but still very frequent, in NSCLC[20] (particularly SQC). Around 90 distinct mutations have been observed in the p53 gene from lung cancers; the most common mutations are the 'missense', involving the substitution of a nucleotide that results in an amino acid change in the protein. The substitution of guanine for thymidine is very frequent, and is believed to be a direct result of the chemical carcinogens in cigarette smoke several of which are known to mutate guanine residues preferentially.[21] Mutations are concentrated within 4 of the 5 evolutionarily conserved regions of the protein but no distinctive 'hot spots' have emerged which would permit a screening strategy for the early detection of lung cancer.

Mutations in the p53 gene have been identified in a wide range of tumour types and the function of both the mutated and wild type protein have been the subject of intensive research over the last few years. Transgenic mice which carry a mutant p53 gene,[22] and mice which are null for p53,[23] have been bred. The p53 transgenic mice carrying multiple copies of mutant p53 develop tumours after a long latency, and, unexpectedly, lung adenocarcinomas are the most commonly detected tumour. The long latency suggests that other genetic events are required for tumour progression and thus these mice may be useful models of human lung tumour development. Most surprisingly, the p53 null mice develop normally until about 6 months of age which suggests that the p53 protein is not required for normal cell function. At around 6 months, tumours, most frequently lymphomas, begin to develop. This, together with other observations, has led to the suggestion that p53 expression occurs in response to DNA damage and slows cell cycling in order to permit DNA repair[24] (see chapter by David Lane). Mutant p53 is predicted to be unable to delay transit through the cell cycle with the result that damaged DNA is reproduced in daughter cells. The occurrence of mutant p53 can, therefore, be seen as a flag of genome instability and, because of this might be expected to be associated with more aggressive tumour development and a poor prognosis. Attempts to correlate p53 mutation with prognosis have met with inconsistent results. A possible confounding factor in these analyses is that structurally normal proteins are inactivated by mechanisms other than mutation, for example binding to viral proteins, and these would be scored incorrectly as 'normal' in these studies of prognostic indicators.

The retinoblastoma gene

Although the most usual way of obtaining a 'global picture' of the genome is by karyotype analysis, it is possible to use molecular approaches for this task by analysing for LOH at several loci on every chromosome arm. It was by this means that deletions in the long arm of chromosome 13 were detected in SCLC.[25] Phenotypically, SCLC resembles retinoblastoma (Rb), so that the Rb gene seems a likely candidate for involvement in SCLC. A more detailed analysis of the Rb region in SCLC detected structural abnormalities even when gross deletions could not be found. In a further study even SCLC cell lines producing apparently normal mRNA were shown to have antigenically abnormal protein as a result of point mutations.[26] Overall, the retinoblastoma gene is disabled in over 90% of SCLC. NSCLC tumours also have abnormalities of the Rb gene, although less commonly.

Inactivation of the Rb gene has been detected in tumours other than retinoblastoma, particularly osteosarcomas and breast tumours. Patients who are successfully treated for retinoblastoma often develop osteosarcoma and also have a 15-fold increased risk of lung cancer. Although the Rb protein has been shown to be involved in the control of cell division, so far there is no explanation as to what is the common pathway of tumour development which links the variety of tumours which show abnormal Rb gene function.

Other somatic genetic changes in lung tumours

The extremely complex karyotypes of lung cancer make it likely that almost any chromosomal abnormality will be detected in at least some tumours. Therefore, to be confident of the significance of somatic genetic changes, they should either occur in the majority of tumours (such as the 3p deletion) or there should be molecular evidence of mutation underlying the chromosomal abnormality (such as there is for the p53 and Rb genes). Moderately frequent chromosomal abnormalities such as 11p and 5p loss, isochromosome 8 and increased copy number of chromosome 7, which are found in variable numbers of lung tumours, are difficult to evaluate. Chromosomal abnormalities of 9p have been frequently reported in NSCLC and deletion analysis with DNA markers implicates band 9p21 as the minimal region. Several tumours have been identified to have homozygous loss of markers in the region which includes the interferon gene cluster.[27] To date, no candidate tumour suppressor gene has been described, but since the region is also involved in haematological malignancies, gliomas and melanoma, it will be the subject of further intensive study.

PRE-MALIGNANT DISEASE

The sequential somatic genetic changes underlying the morphological changes in the development of colon cancers have been elucidated, and this has stimulated interest in studying other tumours in the same way.[28] The ability to do this is limited by the extent to which pre-malignant stages can be recognised. A number of pre-invasive abnormal bronchial epithelial lesions have been identified which co-exist with lung tumours (particularly SQC); and circumstantial evidence, although no longitudinal studies, suggests that these may be preneoplastic lesions. Somatic genetic changes involving chromosome 17 (the p53 gene) and chromosome 3 have been detected in such lesions isolated from the bronchus of patients with lung tumours, and also in a few instances in patients with no detectable invasive disease.[7] These studies have mainly been performed by isolating DNA from fixed material and analysing genotypes after PCR, but occasionally it has also been possible to establish short term cultures from bronchial biopsies, which have shown chromosomal changes characteristic of lung cancer but against a background of a karyotype which resembles normality.[29] To date however, no sequential order of changes has been established. This may be difficult to determine for lung tumour development, as different genetic changes may substitute each other and result in the same malignant phenotype.

CLINICAL IMPLICATIONS

It is hoped that it will be possible to use the information about the biological basis of cancer to design treatment. Somatic genetic changes are particularly attractive in this regard, as not only are they fundamental to the development of the tumour, but they distinguish tumour and normal cells absolutely. Thus, they have the potential to be used not only in the early detection of the disease but as new targets for therapeutic intervention.

REFERENCES

1 Ponder BAJ. Inherited predisposition to cancer. Trends Genet 1990; 6: 213–218.
2 Gariboldi M, Manenti G, Canzian F et al. A major susceptibility locus to murine lung carcinogenesis maps on chromosome 6. Nature Genet 1993; 3: 132–136.
3 Telenius H, Pelmear AH, Tunnacliffe A et al. Cytogenetic analysis by chromosome painting using DOP–PCR amplified flow-sorted chromosomes. Genes Chromosom Cancer 1992; 4: 257–263.
4 Trask B. Fluorescence in situ hybridisation: Application in cytogcnetics and gene mapping. Trends Genet 1991; 7: 149–154.
5 Chaganti RSK, Klein EA. The cytogenetic basis for molecular analysis of leukaemia, lymphoma and solid tumours. In: Cossman J ed. Molecular genetics in cancer diagnosis. New York: Elsevier, 1990; 73–97.
6 Ganly PS, Jarad N, Rudd RM, Rabbitts PH. PCR-based RFLP analysis allows genotyping of the short arm of chromosome 3 in small biopsies from patients with lung cancer. Genomics 1992; 12: 221–228.

7   Sundaresan V, Ganly P, Hasleton P et al. p53 and chromosome 3 abnormalities, characteristic of malignant lung tumours, are detectable in preinvasive lesions of the bronchus. Oncogene 1992; 7: 1989–1997.

8   Nau M, Brooks B, Battey J et al. L-myc a new myc-related gene amplified and expressed in human small cell lung cancer. Nature 1985; 318: 69–73.

9   Wong A, Rupper J, Eggleston J, Hamilton S, Baylin S, Vogelstein B. Gene amplification of C-myc in small cell carcinoma of the lung. Science 1986; 233: 461–465.

10 Rosell R, Li S, Skacel Z et al. Prognostic impact of mutated K-ras gene in surgically resected non-small cell lung cancer patients. Oncogene 1993; 8: 2407–2412.

11 Slebos RJC, Kibbelaar RE, Dalesio O et al. K-ras oncogene activation as a prognostic marker in adenocarcinoma of the lung. N Engl J Med 1990; 323: 561–565.

12 Whang-Peng J, Bunn Jnr PA, Kao-Shan CS et al. A non-random chromosomal abnormality, del 3p (14–23) in human small cell lung cancer (SCLC). Cancer Genet Cytogenet 1982; 6: 119–134.

13 Wurster-Hill DH, Cannizzaro LA, Pettengil OS, Sorenson GD, Cate CC, Maurer LH. Cytogenetics of small cell carcinoma of the lung. Cancer Genet Cytogenet 1984; 13: 303–330.

14 Kok KJ, Osigna B, Carritt MB et al. Deletion of a DNA sequence at the chromosomal region 3p21 in all major types of lung cancer. Nature 1987; 330: 578–581.

15 Rabbitts P, Bergh J, Douglas J, Collins F, Waters J. A submicroscopic homozygous deletion in the D3S3 locus in a cell line isolated from a small cell lung carcinoma. Cancer Genet Cytogenet 1990; 2: 231–238.

16 Houle B, Leduc F, Bradley WEC. Implication of RARB in epidemoid (squamous) lung cancer. Genes Chromosom Cancer 1991; 3: 358–366.

17 Hibi K, Takahashi T, Yamakawa K et al. Three distinct regions involved in 3p deletion in human lung cancer. Oncogene 1992; 7: 445–449.

18 Yamakawa K, Takahashi T, Horio Y et al. Frequent homozyous deletions in lung cancer cell lines detected by a DNA marker located at 3p21.3–3–p22. Oncogene 1993; 8: 327–330.

19 Takahashi T, Takahashi H, Suzuki H et al. The p53 gene is very frequently mutated in small-cell lung cancer with a distinct nucleotide substitution pattern. Oncogene 1991; 6: 1775–1778.

20 Chiba I, Takahashi T, Nau MM et al. Mutations in the p53 gene are frequent in primary, resected non-small cell lung cancer. Oncogene 1990; 5: 1603–1610.

21 Harris CC, Hollstein M. Clinical implication of the p53 tumour suppressor gene. N Engl J Med 1993; 329: 1318–1327.

22 Lavigueur A, Maltby V, Mock D, Rossant J, Pawson T, Bernstein A. High incidence of lung, bone, and lymphoid tumors in transgenic mice overexpressing mutant alleles of the p53 oncogene. Mol Cell Biol 1989; 9: 3982–3991.

23 Donehower LA, Harvey M, Slagle BL et al. Mice deficient for p53 are developmentally normal but susceptible to spontaneous tumours. Nature 1992; 356: 215–221.

24 Lane D. p53, guardian of the genome. Nature 1992; 358: 15–16.

25 Yokota J, Wada M, Shimosato Y, Terada M, Sugimura T. Loss of heterozygosity on chromosomes 3, 13 and 17 in small-cell carcinoma and on chromosome 3 in adenocarcinoma of the lung. Proc Natl Acad Sci USA 1987; 84: 9252–9256.

26 Yokota J, Akiyama T, Fung Y et al. Altered expression of the retinoblastoma (RB) gene in small-cell carcinoma of the lung. Oncogene 1988; 3: 471–475.

27 Olopade OI, Buchhagen DL, Malik K et al. Homozygous loss of the interferon genes defines the critical region on 9p that is deleted in lung cancers. Cancer Res 1993; 53: 2410–2415.

28 Vogelstein BER, Fearon SR, Hamilton SE et al. Genetic alterations during colorectal tumor development. N Engl J Med 1988; 319: 525–532.

29 Sozzi G, Miozzo M, Donghi R et al. Deletions of 17p and p53 mutations in preneoplastic lesions of the lung. Cancer Res 1992; 52: 6079–6082.

British Medical Bulletin (1994) Vol. 50, No. 3, pp. 698–707
© The British Council 1994

Genetics of urological cancers

E R Maher

University of Cambridge, Cambridge, UK

Investigations into inherited susceptibility to urological cancers have provided new insights into the clinical and molecular genetics of urological neoplasia. This review focuses on current knowledge of the genetics of renal, bladder, prostate and testicular neoplasia. Recent advances include (i) the isolation of the von Hippel-Lindau disease gene which is involved in the pathogenesis of familial and nonfamilial renal cancer, (ii) elucidation of the mechanism of multicentricity in bladder cancer, (iii) evidence that a significant proportion of early onset prostate cancer may be attributable to dominantly inherited susceptibility gene (or genes), and (iv) identification of specific cytogenetic and molecular events in the pathogenesis of testicular germ cell tumours.

KIDNEY

Although familial renal cell carcinoma (RCC) is rare (approximately 1% of all cases), failure to recognise such cases results in avoidable morbidity and mortality. The most common cause of inherited RCC is von Hippel-Lindau (VHL) disease.[1] This is a multi-system dominantly inherited familial cancer syndrome with an incidence of 1 in 36000.[2] Affected individuals are predisposed to a wide variety of tumours including retinal and central nervous system haemangioblastomas, RCC, phaeochromocytoma and pancreatic APUDomas.[3] In addition, multiple cysts of the kidneys, pancreas and epididymis are frequent. Although RCC is the presenting feature in only 10% of patients with VHL disease, it is the most common cause of death and the risk of an affected patient developing renal cell carcinoma increases to 70% by age 60 years (*see* Fig.).[3] RCC in patients with VHL disease occurs at a younger age than in sporadic cases (as young as 16 years, but on average 44 years compared to 59 years in sporadic cases), and is frequently bilateral and multicentric. The expression of VHL disease is very variable.

Onset is usually between the ages of 10 and 30 years with retinal angiomatosis and cerebellar haemangioblastoma the most common initial features. However onset may be in infancy or in the seventh decade. Phaeochromocytoma occurs in less then 10% of patients but there are interfamilial differences in predisposition to phaeochromocytoma and in some families this is the most common complication.[3] Although occasional families may have a low incidence of RCC, there is little evidence to suggest that there is an inverse relationship between predisposition to phaeochromocytoma and RCC and all VHL families should be considered to be at risk for RCC. Morbidity and mortality from VHL disease may be reduced by early detection and treatment of complications, particularly RCC and retinal angiomatosis. Systematic screening of affected patients and at risk relatives is indicated (*see* Table), and it is important that asymptomatic at risk relatives of affected patients are carefully screened as subclinical evidence of VHL disease is often found.[4] The detection of RCC in the presence of multiple renal cysts can be difficult, and renal cysts in VHL disease frequently show regions of atypical epithelial hyperplasia and carcinoma *in situ*. Although it has been suggested that RCC may arise from renal cysts, this is not yet proven.[5] The management of VHL patients with bilateral RCC is controversial. As there is a high likelihood of further primary renal tumours bilateral nephrectomy and renal replacement therapy has been advocated. An alternative approach is nephron sparing surgery with local resection, however this may be associated with a high risk of local recurrence and the optimal strategy has not yet been defined.[6]

The mapping of the VHL gene to the short arm of chromosome 3 in 1988 was followed 5 years later by the isolation of the VHL gene.[7] The VHL gene was identified by a positional cloning (reverse genetics) approach in which the position of the VHL gene was initially established by family linkage studies. Approximately 3% of VHL patients were found to have large (> 50 kb) germline deletions and this finding was crucial to the isolation of the gene.[7] Analysis of the incomplete predicted protein sequence (the full coding sequence has not yet been isolated) has not defined the precise function of the VHL gene product, although there is evidence for a membrane binding domain.[7] Mutational analysis of VHL patients reveals that up to 20% of patients have germline deletions detectable on routine Southern analysis,[7] (Maher unpublished observations). This finding allows a specific molecular diagnosis to be made and the status of at risk family members to be established. Individuals who are demonstrated not to have inherited the VHL gene mutation can be reassured and released from repeated screening. Nondeletion cases may be screened for small intragenic deletions, insertions and point mutations but there is considerable heterogeneity

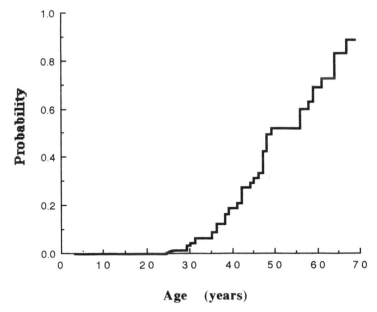

Age   (years)

Figure Cumulative probability of developing renal cell carcinoma with age in von Hippel-Lindau disease.

in VHL disease mutations. Presymptomatic diagnosis with intragenic and closely linked DNA markers can be performed in families with a suitable structure in which the VHL gene mutation has not been identified. The VHL gene functions as a tumour suppressor gene and the mechanism of tumourigenesis in VHL disease appears to be similar to that in inherited retinoblastoma (*see* Birch, this issue) with RCC resulting from inactivation or loss of both alleles of the VHL gene. The molecular pathogenesis of renal cysts in VHL disease has not yet been defined. Studies of sporadic RCC cell lines and primary tumours have implicated somatic VHL gene mutations in the pathogenesis of sporadic RCC similar to the involvement of RB gene mutations in nonfamilial retinoblastoma,[7] (Maher unpublished observations). Most nonpapillary renal cell carcinomas have evidence of chromosome 3p allele loss, but, in addition to the VHL gene, putative tumour suppressor genes mapping to chromosome 3p21 and 3p14 have been implicated in the pathogenesis of sporadic RCC.[8] The chromosome 3p14 gene may be the familial RCC gene (*see below*). The isolation of inherited RCC genes will be a major step forward in attempts to understand the molecular events in the pathogenesis of sporadic RCC.

Table Cambridge screening protocol for von Hippel-Lindau disease in affected patients and at risk relatives. For full details *see* Maher et al[3]

Affected patient
1. Annual physical examination and urine testing.
2. Annual direct and indirect ophthalmoscopy with fluoroscein angioscopy or angiography (*see text*).
3. MRI (or CT) brain scan every 3 years to age 50 and every 5 years thereafter.
4. Annual renal ultrasound scan, with CT scan every 3 years (more frequently if multiple cysts present).
5. Annual 24 h urine collection for VMAs.

At risk relative
1. Annual physical examination and urine testing.
2. Annual direct and indirect ophthalmoscopy from age 5. Annual fluoroscein angioscopy or angiography from age 10 until age 60.
3. MRI (or CT) brain scan every 3 years from age 15 to 40 years and then every 5 years until age 60 years.
4. Annual renal ultrasound scan, with abdominal CT scan every 3 years from age 20 to 65 years.
5. Annual 24 h urine collection for VMAs.

Familial renal cell carcinoma without features of VHL disease is rare but is usually inherited as an autosomal dominant trait.[1] The mean age at diagnosis of inherited RCC is similar to that in VHL disease, but renal cystic disease is less frequent. One large RCC family originally reported in 1979 by Cohen et al[9] has been the subject of extensive investigation because of the association of RCC with a balanced 3:8 translocation segregating in the family. 10 family members developed RCC and it was estimated that translocation carriers had a 87% risk of RCC by age 60 years. Follow-up of the family has demonstrated that affected family members were at risk for multiple RCC and that papillary thyroid carcinoma may also occur.[10] The mean age at onset of RCC in this family was similar to that in VHL disease, so that chromosome 3:8 translocation carriers are predisposed to early onset and multiple RCC. The chromosome 3 and 8 translocation breakpoints map to 3p14.2 and 8q24.1 respectively. Reports of a patient with a chromosome 3:6 translocation and multifocal RCC[11] and the observation of chromosome 3p14 allele loss in sporadic RCC[8] suggested that there is a RCC susceptibility gene in proximal chromosome 3p. Recently Boldog et al[12] have reported the isolation of a gene (HRCA1) which maps immediately adjacent to the 3:8 translocation breakpoint on chromosome 3p. The HRCA1 gene is a candidate tumour suppressor gene and further investigation will elucidate the possible role of HRCA1 mutations in the pathogenesis of familial and sporadic RCC.

BLADDER

Environmental factors including tobacco, occupational exposure to aromatic amine compounds and schistosomiasis have been implicated in bladder tumourigenesis. In addition, genetic factors may be relevant. There is an increased risk of bladder cancer in patients with constitutional retinoblastoma gene mutations and carcinoma of the ureter and other urological cancers may be an integral part of the cancer predisposition in some families with the Lynch II family cancer syndrome.[13] Although these groups of patients would account for only a small number of patients with bladder cancer, inherited variations in the metabolism of environmental carcinogens could represent a more frequent explanation for interindividual differences in susceptibility to bladder carcinogens. A link between bladder cancer and individuals with a slow acetylator phenotype (N-acetyltransferases) has been detected in patients with arylamine exposure but not convincingly in non-exposed patients.[14] Debrisoquine hydroxylation phenotype has been extensively studied in patients with lung cancer, and it has been suggested that individuals with poor debrisoquine metaboliser phenotype are at reduced risk of bladder cancer.[15] The definition of the molecular basis for metabolic polymorphisms of the cytochrome P450 enzyme CYP2D6, N-acetyltransferase and glutathione S-transferase (GSTM1) makes it possible for these associations to be investigated by molecular genetic techniques. Recently Daly et al[16] have reported that deletion of the GSTM1 gene is more common among bladder tumour patients than controls. Although the GSTM1 pathway is thought to be involved in the metabolism of tobacco carcinogens, there was no difference in the GSTM1 genotypes between smokers and nonsmokers with bladder cancer. Furthermore, Zhong et al[17] found no association between GSTM1 genotype and bladder cancer. Attempts to replicate these findings and investigation of the role of other candidate inherited metabolic variants, would provide a clearer picture of the relevance of inherited factors in susceptibility to environmental carcinogens in the pathogenesis of bladder cancer.

A notable feature of urothelial cancer is the frequent occurrence of multicentric tumours. Recent molecular genetic investigations suggest that multiple tumours are monoclonal in origin and result from spread from a single transformed cell rather than a 'field defect' in which there would be independent transformation of cells at several sites.[18] Under this model of tumourigenesis, inactivation of a tumour suppressor gene on chromosome 9 appears to be an early and critical event which precedes the spread of malignant cells along the urothelium. Later mutational events including loss of tumour suppressor genes on chromosomes 13 (retinoblastoma gene), 17 (p53) and 18, which may determine cancer invasiveness.[18,19]

PROSTATE

Prostate cancer is the most common cancer and the second cause of cancer death in North American men. The aetiology of prostate cancer is unknown. Environmental (eg high fat diet) and genetic factors have been implicated.[20] Evidence for a genetic contribution was provided by genetic epidemiological studies in Mormon families which suggested that the inheritability of prostate cancer was greater than that of breast or colorectal cancers.[21] A case control study by Steinberg et al[22] found 15% of prostate cancer patients had an affected father or brother compared to 8% of controls. Furthermore the relative risk increased: (i) with the number of affected relatives such that men with 1–3 affected first degree relatives were at 2-, 5- and 11-fold increased risk for developing prostate cancer respectively, and (ii) with younger age at onset of prostate cancer in the proband. Meikle and Smith[23] reported a 17-fold increase in relative risk of prostate cancer in the brothers of men developing prostate cancer between 45 and 50 years of age. Segregation analysis of the family histories of 740 prostate cancer patients suggested that familial clustering of prostate cancer could be caused by a rare highly penetrant dominantly inherited predisposition gene.[24] Under the most likely genetic model, 43% of early onset prostate cancer (age < 55 years) would occur in gene carriers but only 9% of cases aged < 85 years. This model of a rare dominant predisposing gene (or genes) is similar to that proposed for breast cancer. Further evidence for such a model would be the mapping of predisposing genes by genetic linkage studies in affected families, but significant linkage has not yet been reported. There is an increased risk of prostate cancer among relatives of women with breast cancer and familial breast cancer genes may predispose male heterozygotes to prostate cancer.[25,26] Clues to candidate regions for inherited prostate cancer genes might be provided by molecular genetic analysis of prostate cancers. The most frequent regions of allele loss are on chromosomes 16q, 10q and 8p,[27,28] and a gene on chromosome 11 has been implicated as a metastasis suppressor gene in prostate cancer.[29] The mapping of prostate cancer susceptibility genes would be a major advance towards the prospect of identifying high risk individuals who could be offered regular screening for this common cancer.

TESTIS

Testicular cancer is the most frequent cancer in men aged between 15 and 35 years of age. Most tumours are of germ cell origin (seminoma,

teratoma) but some arise from stroma (Sertoli cell), and gonadoblas-
tomas contain both germ cell and stromal elements. A genetic predisposition may be present in about 2% of all testicular tumours.[30,31] In a
recent review of the literature, it was noted that in 12 pairs of identical
twins with testicular cancer the tumours were of the same histological
type in 70% of cases, but the histology was mostly different in other
affected relative pairs.[30] Forman et al[31] found that brothers of men with
testicular cancer had a 2% risk of developing testicular cancer by age
50 years, which corresponds to a 10-fold increase in relative risk. In
families where there appears to be a significant inherited predisposition
to testicular cancer the most likely mode of transmission is dominant
inheritance with sex-limited expression. The mean age at diagnosis in
familial cases is slightly younger than in nonfamilial cases 29 years
versus 32.5 years).[31] Testicular tumours are bilateral in about 4% of
patients, which is suggestive of a genetic basis.[30] Although various
associations between HLA haplotypes and bilateral testicular germ cell
tumours has been reported,[32] HLA Class I analysis of affected sib pairs
has provided no evidence of a HLA linked gene predisposing to testicular cancer.[31]

Epidemiological studies have suggested that gonadal hormone drive
is a major factor in the development of germ cell tumours.[33] The principal risk factor for testicular cancer is cryptorchidism. This and other
conditions associated with increased risk (eg orchitis, infertility) are
associated with reduced testicular function producing an increased go-
nadotrophin drive to the testicles. Genetic factors have been implicated
in cryptorchidism, as up to 14% of cryptorchid males have an affected
relative, but it is unclear to what extent this might explain familial
occurrence of testicular tumours. Forman et al[31]found no difference
in the prevalence of cryptorchidism between familial and nonfamilial testicular cancer cases. A number of genetic disorders associated
with hypogonadism are associated with a predisposition to testicular
tumours. The risk of testicular cancer (seminoma, Sertoli cell, terato-
carcinoma and embryonal cell carcinoma) is unequivocally increased
in patients with the testicular feminization syndrome, and prophylactic
gonadectomy is usually performed after pubertal growth. Gonadoblastoma occurs in XY gonadal dysgenesis and in patients with the WAGR
syndrome. The risk of germ cell tumours in gonadal dysgenesis is associated with the presence of Y chromosome material. Girls with Turner
syndrome and 45X, 45X, 46XX or 46X, del(X) are not at increased risk
of germ cell tumours, but up to 20% of patients with gonadal dysgenesis
and 45X/46XY or other karyotypes with Y chromosome material may
develop gonadoblastoma.[34] Patients with X-linked ichthyosis (steroid-
sulphatase deficiency) appear to be at increased risk of cryptorchidism

and testicular tumours,[35] and an increased incidence of benign testicular tumours has been reported in congenital adrenal hyperplasia.[36] Although germ cell tumours have been reported in families with Li-Fraumeni syndrome,[37] there is no evidence to suggest that germline p53 mutations are a frequent cause of familial testicular tumours.[38]

Cytogenetic analysis of human germ cell tumours reveals a specific abnormality, an isochromosome of the short arm of chromosome 12, in more than 80% of tumours.[39] Isochromosome 12p is found in all major types of germ cell tumours including seminoma, teratoma and embryonal carcinoma, and in both gonadal and extragonadal tumours. Molecular cytogenetic studies with fluorescent *in situ* hybridisation techniques are more sensitive than conventional studies and suggest that an even higher proportion of germ cell tumours have an isochromosome of 12p. This specific cytogenetic finding can be used as a diagnostic aid in investigating the histological type of undifferentiated carcinomas of unknown primary site. Molecular genetic analysis has suggested that loss of tumour suppressor genes on the long arm of chromosome 12 is a critical early event in male germ cell tumourigenesis.[40] The formation of an isochromosome 12p and the chromosome 12q deletions appear to be aetiologically independent.

The occurrence of testicular tumours in high-risk individuals can be prevented by appropriate measures. Early correction of cryptorchidism may reduce the risk of testicular tumours. Non-functioning testes which present a significant risk for tumourigenesis (as in the testicular feminization syndrome or intersex states), should be removed. Individuals thought to be at high risk of familial testicular tumours can be monitored by regular self examination and ultrasonography.

REFERENCES

1 Maher ER, Yates JRW. Familial renal cell carcinoma - clinical and molecular genetic aspects. Br J Cancer 1991; 63: 176–179.
2 Maher ER, Iselius L, Yates JRW et al. Von Hippel-Lindau disease: A genetic study. J Med Genet 1991; 28: 443–447 .
3 Maher ER, Yates JRW, Harries R, Benjamin C, Harris R, Ferguson-Smith MA. Clinical features and natural history of von Hippel-Lindau disease. Q J Med 1990; 77: 1151–1163.
4 Moore AT, Maher ER, Rosen P, Gregor Z, Bird AC. Ophthalmological screening for von Hippel-Lindau disease. Eye 1991; 5: 723–728.
5 Choyke PL, Glenn GM, Walther MM et al. The natural history of renal lesions in von Hippel-Lindau disease: A serial CT study in 28 patients. Am J Radiol 1992; 159: 1229–1234.
6 Novick AC, Streem S. Long-term follow-up after nephron sparing surgery for renal cell carcinoma in von Hippel-Lindau disease. J Urol 1992; 147: 1488–1490.
7 Latif F, Tory K, Gnarra J et al. Identification of the von Hippel-Lindau disease tumour suppressor gene. Science 1993; 260: 1317–1320.

8 Yamakawa K, Morita R, Takahashi E, Hori T, Ishikawa J, Nakamura Y. A detailed deletion mapping of the short arm of chromosome 3 in sporadic renal cell carcinoma. Cancer Res 1991; 51: 4707–4711.

9 Cohen AJ, Li FP, Berg S et al. Hereditary renal cell carcinoma associated with a chromosomal translocation. N Engl J Med 1979; 301: 592–595.

10 Li FP, Decker HJ, Zbar B et al. Clinical and genetic studies of renal cell carcinomas in a family with a constitutional chromosome 3:8 translocation. Ann Intern Med 1993; 118: 106–111.

11 Kovacs G, Brusa P, De Rieses W. Tissue-specific expression of a constitutional 3:6 translocation: development of multiple bilateral renal-cell carcinomas. Int J Cancer 1989; 43: 422.

12 Boldog FL, Gemmill RM, Wilke CM et al. Positional cloning of the hereditary renal carcinoma 3:8 translocation breakpoint. Proc Natl Acad Sci USA 1993; 90: 8509–8513.

13 Hodgson SV, Maher ER. A Practical Guide to Human Cancer Genetics. Cambridge: Cambridge University Press, 1993.

14 Wolf CR. Metabolic factors in cancer susceptibility. Cancer Surv 1990; 9: 437–474.

15 Kaisary A, Smith P, Jacqz E et al. Genetic predisposition to bladder cancer: ability to hydroxylate debrisoquine and mephynytoin as risk factors. Cancer Res 1987; 47: 5488–5493.

16 Daly AK, Thomas DJ, Cooper J, Pearson WR, Neal DE, Idle JR. Homozygous deletion of the gene for glutathione S-transferase M1 in bladder cancer. BMJ 1993; 307: 481–482.

17 Zhong S, Wyllie AH, Barnes D, Wolf CR, Spurr NK. Relationship between the GSTM1 genetic polymorphism and susceptibility to bladder, breast and colon cancer. Carcinogenesis 1993; 14: 1821–1824.

18 Sidransky D, Frost P, Von Eschenbach A, Oyasu R, Preisinger AC, Vogelstein B. Clonal origin of bladder cancer. N Eng J Med 1992; 326: 737–740.

19 Habuchi T, Ogawa O, Kakehi Y et al. Accumulated allelic losses in the development of invasive urothelial cancer. Int J Cancer 1993; 53: 579–584.

20 Pienta KJ, Esper PS. Risk factors for prostate cancer. Ann Int Med 1993; 118: 793–803.

21 Cannon L, Bishop DT, Skolnick M, Hunt S, Lyon JL, Smart CR. Genetic epidemiology of prostate cancer in the Utah Mormon genealogy. Cancer Surv 1982; 1: 47–69.

22 Steinberg GS, Carter BS, Beaty TH, Childs B, Walsh PC. Family history and the risk of prostate cancer. Prostate 1990; 17: 337–347.

23 Meikle AW, Smith JA. Epidemiology of prostate cancer. Urol Clin N Am 1990; 17: 709–718.

24 Carter BS, Beaty TH, Steinberg GD, Childs B, Walsh PC. Mendelian inheritance of familial prostate cancer. Proc Nat Acad Sci USA 1992; 89: 3367–3371.

25 Arason A, Barkardottir RB, Egilsson V. Linkage analysis of chromosome 17q markers and breast-ovarian cancer in Icelandic families, and possible relationship to prostatic cancer. Am J Hum Genet 1993; 52: 711–717.

26 Tulinius H, Egilsson V, Olafsdottir GH, Sigvaldason H. Risk of prostate, ovarian, and endometrial cancer among relatives of women with breast cancer. BMJ 1992; 305: 855–857.

27 Bergerheim US, Kunimi K, Collins VP, Ekman P. Deletion mapping of chromosomes 8, 10, and 16 in human prostatic carcinoma. Genes Chromosom Cancer 1991; 3: 215–220.

28 Carter BS, Ewing CM, Ward WS, Treiger BF, Aalders TW, Schalken JA, Epstein JI, Isaacs WB. Allelic loss of chromosomes 16q and 10q in human prostate cancer. Proc Nat Acad Sci USA 1990; 87: 8751–8755.

29 Ichikawa T, Ichikawa Y, Dong J et al. Localization of metastasis suppressor gene(s) for prostatic cancer to the short arm of human chromosome 11. Cancer Res 1992; 52: 3486–3490.

30 Patel SR, Kvols LK, Richardson RL. Familial testicular cancer: report of six cases and review of the literature. Mayo Clin Proc 1990; 65: 804–808.
31 Forman D, Oliver RTD, Brett AR et al. Familial testicular cancer: a report of the UK family register, estimation of risk and an HLA class 1 sib pair analysis. Br J Cancer 1992; 65: 255–262.
32 Kratzik C, Aiginger P, Kuber W et al. Risk factors for bilateral testicular germ cell tumors. Does heredity play a role?. Cancer 1991; 68: 916–921.
33 Oliver RT. Atrophy, hormones, genes and viruses in aetiology germ cell tumours. Cancer Surv 1990; 9: 263–286.
34 Verp MS, Simpson JL. Abnormal sex differentiation and neoplasia. Cancer Genet Cytogenet 1987; 25: 191–218.
35 Lykkesfeldt G, Bennett P, Lykkesfeldt AE et al. Testis cancer. Ichthyosis constitutes a significant risk factor. Cancer 1991; 67: 730–734.
36 Cunnah D, Perry L, Dacie JA et al. Bilateral testicular tumours in congenital adrenal hyperplasia: a continuing diagnostic and therapeutic dilemma. Clin Endocrinol 1989; 30: 141–147.
37 Hartley AL, Birch JM, Kelsey AM, Marsden HB, Harris M, Teare MD. Are germ cell tumors part of the Li-Fraumeni cancer family syndrome? Cancer Genet Cytogenet 1989; 42: 221–226.
38 Heimdal K, Lothe RA, Lystad S, Holm R, Fossa SD, Borresen AL. No germline TP53 mutations detected in familial and bilateral testicular cancer. Genes Chromosom Cancer 1993; 6: 92–97.
39 Chaganti RS, Rodriguez E, Bosl GJ. Cytogenetics of male germ-cell tumors. Urol Clin N Am 1993; 20: 55–66.
40 Murty VV, Houldsworth J, Baldwin S et al. Allelic deletions in the long arm of chromosome 12 identify sites of candidate tumor suppressor genes in male germ cell tumors. Proc Natl Acad Sci USA 1992; 89: 11006–11010.

British Medical Bulletin (1994) Vol. 50, No. 3, pp. 708–717
© The British Council 1994

Cancer and DNA processing disorders

A M R Taylor
C M McConville
P J Byrd

CRC Department of Cancer Studies, The Medical School, University of Birmingham, Birmingham, UK

Defects in cloned DNA repair genes are now associated with particular human disorders in which an important feature is a predisposition to cancer. Recently some repair genes have been implicated in other aspects of DNA metabolism such as transcription initiation. In addition mutations in a single gene can give rise to phenotypes recognised clinically as different disorders. These newly appreciated complexities, amongst others, will eventually help us to understand the development of the complete clinical phenotype in a range of 'DNA processing disorders'.

The involvement of defective DNA repair in the development of some cancers is now well established, particularly from studies on patients with the disorder Xeroderma Pigmentosum (XP). There are several other disorders, Cockayne's syndrome (CS), Trichothiodystrophy (TTD), Fanconi's Anaemia (FA), Bloom's syndrome (BS), Ataxia Telangiectasia (A–T), Nijmegen Breakage syndrome (NBS) and the individual 46BR in which patients show an unusual sensitivity to environmental agents. There is an increased predisposition to cancer in all of these disorders with the apparent exception of Cockayne's syndrome and Trichothiodystrophy. Several of these disorders have, alternatively, been grouped together as chromosome instability syndromes. They should, perhaps, now better be considered as all having a defect in the processing of DNA. Defective genes may include those whose products normally control replicative DNA synthesis, DNA repair synthesis, recombination, transcription or combinations of these functions. The disorders are considered below in 4 separate groups; a clinical description is provided for each and the relationship of the DNA processing defect to cancer development is discussed. The Table summarizes some features of these disorders.

Table Human DNA processing genes

Disorder/group/clone gene	Predisposition to cancer	Gene location
Group 1 – Disorders unusually sensitive to UV light		
XP/A [a]	Skin	9q34
XP/B (ERCC3)		2q21
XP/C [a]	Skin	?
XP/D (ERCC2)	Skin	19q13.2
XP/E		?
XP/F		?
XP/G (ERCC5)		13q32–33
XP/V	Skin	?
CS/A	No skin cancer	?
CS/B (ERCC6)	No skin cancer	10q11–21
TTD/XPD	No skin cancer	19q13
TTD/2	No skin cancer	?
Group 2 – Disorders unusually sensitive to IR		
A-T/A, C, D, E	Lymphoma/leukaemia	11q22–23
NBS/V1, V2	Lymphoma	?
Group 3 – Disorders unusually sensitive to crosslinking agents		
FA/A	AML	?
FA/B	AML	?
FA/C [b]	AML	9q22.3
FA/D	AML	?
Group 4 – Disorders unusually sensitive to alkylating agents		
BS	Lymphoma/leukaemia/carcinoma	?
46BR	Lymphoma	19q13

[a]XPA and XPC are the most common groups followed by XPD and XPV; [b]There is evidence for linkage of a Franconi anaemia gene to chromosome 20q.[25]

XERODERMA PIGMENTOSUM, COCKAYNE'S SYNDROME, TRICHOTHIODYSTROPHY – Disorders showing an unusual sensitivity to UV light

Patients whose cells in culture can be shown to have an unusual sensitivity to the killing effects of UV light have been diagnosed as having one of the 3 disorders: Xeroderma Pigmentosum, Cockayne's syndrome, or Trichothiodystrophy.[1]

XP patients clearly have an increased sensitivity to sunlight, although the degree depends on the level of exposure and also on the particular mutation they have.[1] They also show an increased likelihood of developing tumours, early in life, on sun exposed areas of the skin. Tumour types include basal and squamous cell carcinomas and malignant melanomas. Some patients also show neurological abnormalities. Skin fibroblast cultures from most XP patients show a defect in nucleotide excision repair (NER) which can, for example, be conveniently measured as unscheduled DNA synthesis (UDS) by autoradiograghy. The precise nature of the repair defect in XP cells remains unknown but is believed to be in either the initial incision step or in a step preceding this.[1] The repair defect is also in a process that affects the whole of the genome irrespective of transcriptional state. At least 7 different complementation groups, which are deficient in excision repair, have been identified by cell fusion studies. These are designated XPA–XPG.[1,2] The level of measurable repair varies between these complementation groups. One additional group (XP variants) has normal levels of NER but a less well defined defect in daughter strand gap repair. Most XP patients fall into complementation groups A and C and groups B, E, F and G are rare. XP is also a multilocus disorder and gene localisations are given in the Table.

Whereas the major clinical features of XP are associated with the skin, Cockayne's syndrome patients show a quite different clinical phenotype. Although there is also sun sensitivity the major features are dwarfism, mental retardation, microcephaly and retinal and skeletal abnormalities.[2] Some patients with TTD also show unusual sun sensitivity, but the major features of this disorder are mental and physical retardation, sulphur deficient brittle hair and ichthyotic skin.[1,3] The term PIBIDS, an acronym for Photosensitivity, Ichthyosis, Brittle hair, Impaired intelligence, Decreased ferility, and Short stature is sometimes used for these patients.

There is no evidence for the same predisposition to skin cancer in Cockayne's syndrome and Trichothiodystrophy that is seen in XP. In classical CS patients the excision defect is preferentially in the ability of their cells to repair damage in actively transcribing genes.[4] This contrasts with the defect across the whole genome (overall genome) in XP cells. Since repair of actively transcribing regions makes a small contribution to total repair in the cell, CS cells show a normal level of UDS. A readily measurable result of the defect in repairing transcribed genes in CS cells, however, is the failure of the rapid recovery of RNA synthesis following UV exposure.[5] Using an assay based on this observation most CS patients can be assigned to one of two complementation groups (CS-A and CS-B).[1]

The close genetic relationship between XP and CS is shown by the reports of 2 patients who simultaneously displayed features of both XP and CS. These patients are firstly, the sole representative of XP group B and secondly, a patient from XP group D.[1] Recently patients with CS have been shown to have the biochemical defect of XPG.[2] 2 of the 7 NER genes which can cause XP alone (XPD and XPG) can, therefore, also result in partial or complete CS.

In TTD there is heterogeneity in the biochemical defect. Some patients have no defects in excision repair but others have a severe defect in this repair pathway. In most patients of this latter group the defect has been assigned to XP complementation group D.[3] Defects in the *XPD* gene can therefore be found in patients with XP, or XP/CS or TTD. A second excision repair complementation group has recently been described in TTD.[6]

In addition to the human genes identified by complementation analysis of cells from XP, CS and TTD patients another approach has also identified human repair genes. Rodent cells mutated to be hypersensitive to the killing effects of UV can be corrected to normal UV sensitivity by transfection of normal human DNA.[1] The cloned human genes conferring this normal phenotype are designated *ERCC1-ERCC3, 5* and *6* (Excision Repair Chinese hamster Complementing). Most of these genes also have identified yeast homologues. No human disorder has so far been identified in which *ERCC1* is deficient but *ERCC2, 3, 5* and *6* have now been found to correct the defects in XPD, XPB, XBG and CSB respectively.[7–10] The precise functions of these genes are currently being investigated. *ERCC3*, for example, the repair gene defective in the complex XPB patient, is believed to have a DNA unwinding function (helicase) on the basis of its amino acid sequence. The product of this gene has also recently been reported to be part of the basal transcription factor TFIIH.[11] This single protein may be involved in 2 different aspects of 'DNA processing' viz transcription initiation and DNA repair. In the sole XPB individual a very rare mutation in *ERCC3* causing a subtle defect in both gene expression and in NER may result in the complex XP/CS phenotype. Other repair proteins that may have a similar role as part of a transcription initiation complex include the ERCC2 protein that complements XPD and which is a known DNA helicase, and possibly ERCC5. The second complex patient with features of both XP and CS is in complementation group D and patients in XP group G have been described with CS. Rare mutations in genes coding for proteins with more than one function in DNA processing might give rise to these unusual complex phenotypes. It is also possible that mutations in different domains of the same gene (eg *XPD*) might give rise to clinically distinct disorders depending on how much the efficiency of one process, compared with another, is affected. Proneness to skin cancer appears to be more associated with the common XP groups A and C. The relationships between complementation group, type and level of repair defect, and cancer proneness are still not understood.

ATAXIA TELANGIECTASIA AND NIJMEGEN BREAKAGE SYNDROME – Disorders showing an increased radiosensitivity

The clinical phenotypes of these 2 disorders are quite different. A–T patients show a progressive cerebellar ataxia, oculomotor dyspraxia, and dysarthria.[12] A–T is also the commonest immunodeficiency disorder. The resulting predisposition to infection, however, is very variable across the range of patients. Approximately 10% of all A–T patients develop a malignancy in childhood or early adulthood.[13] A minority of tumours are epithelial in origin but the majority are lymphoid leukamias or lymphomas. A greater proportion of A–T patients with leukaemia compared with patients in the non A–T population, have T cell tumours which may be either T cell lymphoma, T-ALL or T-PLL.[13]

An important cellular feature in A–T which is not observed in the UV sensitive disorders is the spontaneous occurrence of specific chromosome translocations in the peripheral lymphocytes of these patients.[13] The majority of translocations have both breakpoints apparently involving T cell receptor genes, eg t(7;14)(q35;q11). There is no evidence that cells with these particular translocations have a malignant potential. Other cells, however, containing translocations involving only one TCR gene and an unknown gene often at 14q32, eg inv(14)(q11q32), t(14;14)(q11;q32) and t(X;14)(q28;q11) can proliferate to produce clones as large as 90% of the circulating T cells. These cells also have a leukaemic potential.

Patients with Nijmegen Breakage syndrome show microcephaly, short stature, a bird-like face, immunodeficiency, *café au lait* spots[14] and a predisposition to lymphoid tumours. It is not clear whether the lymphomas are T or B cell tumours. There appears to be some clinical heterogeneity but cerebellar degeneration is not part of the disorder. Translocations occur in T lymphocytes between chromosomes 7 and 14 at the same breakpoints as seen in A–T. No inv(14)(q11q32) inversions have been observed in the lymphocytes of NBS patients, t(14;14)(q11;q32) translocations are rare and there are no reports of very large translocation clones. This is interesting as both of these rearrangements and large clones are associated with the development of T cell leukaemia in A–T patients.

Cells from both A–T and NBS patients show an unusual sensitivity to the killing effects of ionising radiation and chromosomally radiomimetic drugs.[13,15] An increased chromosomal radiosensitivity is also observed in both disorders. In addition there is a lack of inhibition of DNA synthesis in both A–T and NBS cells following exposure of cells to either gamma-rays or radiomimetic drugs.

There is good evidence for 4 complementation groups in A–T [16] but not that it is a multilocus disorder like XP. On the contrary, results from genetic studies are consistent with the existence of a single A–T locus, or a cluster of tightly linked loci, since there is strong evidence that A–T complementation groups A, C, D, and possibly E all map to chromosome region 11q22-23.[17] NBS patients have been assigned to one of two complementation groups, V1 or V2, different to those of A–T but the gene location remains unknown. Twins have been described with the features of both A–T and NBS and assigned to NBS complementation group V1.[18] Are these rare individuals analogous to the rare XP/CS patients described above? It is intriguing that patients with A–T and NBS show very similar cellular features of increased radiosensitivity and similarities in some clinical features although the major diagnostic features are quite different.

The precise function of the A–T gene(s) remains unknown. There is evidence at the cellular level of a defect in DNA repair.[19] The presence of spontaneously occurring chromosome translocations suggests a defect in some form of recombination. There is also an increased frequency of T cell receptor hybrid genes formed by interlocus recombination in A–T lymphocytes compared with normals.[20] Greatly increased spontaneous intrachromosomal recombination rates were also found in transformed A–T fibroblasts compared with normal cells.[21] In addition to these, other cellular features of A–T cells include a lack of inhibition of DNA synthesis following exposure of cells to ionising radiation and a tendency for chromosomes in A–T lymphocytes to form telomeric fusions possibly indicating a defect in telomere formation. One can perhaps predict that, like the products of some XP genes, the A–T gene product(s) will be shown to be involved in several quite different aspects of DNA processing.

One consequence of the mutant gene product is to allow the formation of a much higher levels of chromosome translocations involving the incorrect rejoining of TCR genes in T lymphocytes than occurs in non A–T patients. In some A–T patients a translocation which affects a gene at the top of the regulatory cascade will be associated with the development of T-ALL; in other patients the translocation may activate a gene which allows a steady proliferation of lymphocytes in which further mutational events accumulate to give eventual transformation to, say T-PLL, which is observed in older patients.

The abnormally high levels of serum AFP, the presence of thymic hypoplasia, hypogonadism and growth retardation may be the consequences of a failure of control of gene transcription/expression mediated by the same product.

FANCONI'S ANAEMIA

Fanconi's anaemia is a recessively inherited disorder in which patients present with short stature, a pancytopaenia which develops between the ages of 5 and 10 years and the presence of some dysmorphic features, the most prominent of which are dysplastic or absent thumbs and/or radii. In addition there may be skin hyperpigmentation, growth retardation, deafness and genital, ocular, renal and cardiac defects.[12] There is, however, considerable clinical heterogeneity in presentation of the disorder and it may not always be readily recognised since some patients may show a minimal number of these features.[12] Most but not all patients show an elevated level of chromosome breakage which is quite different from the specific translocations observed in A–T patients. They also have a predisposition to the development of acute myelogenous leukaemia.

FA cells are characterised by an increased sensitivity to bifunctional cross-linking agents (such as nitrogen mustard, mitomycin C, and diepoxybutane) as shown by colony forming assays on cultured skin fibroblasts or on lymphocyte chromosomes.[12] A defect in DNA-DNA crosslink repair has been suggested for FA but the precise gene defect remains unknown. The presence of clinical heterogeneity might predict the presence of genetic complementation in FA and there is evidence for at least 4 groups,[22] designated FA(A)-FA(D). The cDNA defective in group FA(C) has been cloned and complements the increased cellular sensitivity to DEB and MMC in the group C cells.[23] One patient was found to be heterozygous for the mutation L553P which was also shown to be maternally inherited. In a further 2/4 unclassified FA cell lines the same single base deletion was seen in one allele. No other mutations were detected in the coding region for the other allele.[23] More recently a patient has been described with a homozygous mutation (R185X) that would prevent the production of any normal FACC protein.[24] This adds to the evidence that mutation in the FACC gene can produce the FA phenotype. No homology to known proteins has been reported and no functional domains have been recognised.

The FACC gene has been localised to chromosome 9q22.3.[22] There is also a report of linkage of a FA gene on chromosome 20q.[25] These observations, while requiring confirmation, might suggest that FA like

XP is a multilocus disorder. It is intriguing that other disease assignments to chromosome 9q22.3 include Xeroderma Pigmentosum group A (XPA), multiple self-healing squamous cell epithelioma (ESSI), and nevoid basal cell carcinoma syndrome (NBCCS).

BLOOM'S SYNDROME AND 46BR

Bloom's syndrome patients are characterised by their small birth size, growth retardation, narrow face and telangiectasia in the butterfly area of the face. They are also immunodeficient.[12] A major feature of the disorder is the high frequency of malignant disease with about a quarter of patients developing cancer early in life. Unlike the other disorders described above, BS is remarkable for the variety of histological types of tumour including acute leukaemia, lymphoma and various carcinomas.[12]

BS patients also show a spontaneous chromosome breakage similar to that in Fanconi's Anaemia with the important difference that the characteristic interchanges tend to occur between homologous chromosomes. The most striking and unique chromosomal feature of BS is the large increased frequency of sister chromatid exchanges (SCE).[12] BS cells appear to be unusually sensitive to the killing effects of simple alkylating agents such as EMS and N-ethyl-N-nitrosourea.[12,26]

The single patient 46BR showed dwarfism, a profound immunodeficiency resulting in recurrent serious chest infection and a slow growing lymphomatous liver infiltration. She died at the age of 19 years from acute pulmonary infection. Cultured cells from this patient showed an increased sensitivity to different alkylating agents, UV light and ionising radiation. The level of SCE in her cells was slightly higher than normal but much lower than levels seen in BS patients. Patient 46BR appeared, therefore, to be quite distinct from BS patients.[26] Cellular defects in BS cells include delayed joining of large DNA replication intermediates and a reduced rate of progression of replication forks. In contrast the major feature of 46BR cells was the retarded rate of rejoining of Okazaki fragments during DNA replication and the greatly reduced rate of DNA single strand rejoining following exposure of cells to DNA damaging agents.[26] It is clear that both disorders might have a defect in DNA ligase. Indeed partially purified DNA ligase 1 fractions from BS cells showed altered biochemical properties.[27] A search was made in 46BR cells and BS cell lines for mutations in the structural gene coding for DNA ligase 1. No coding mutations were found in DNA ligase 1 in several BS lines in two studies[26,28] but two missense mutations occurring in different alleles of the DNA ligase gene were found in patient 46BR.[26] At the biochemical level, in 46BR cells, there is a strongly reduced ability of DNA ligase 1 to form a labelled enzyme-adenylate intermediate. 46BR appears, therefore, to represent the phenotype caused by coding changes in the DNA ligase 1 gene. It is not known what the basis is of the altered DNA ligase activity in BS cells.

SUMMARY

Studies of these disorders will help our understanding of the cells response to various types of environmental damage. Much remains to be learned about the roles of single gene products in the various aspects of DNA metabolism and how in some instances this can result in cancer. The effects on development of mutations in *ERCC2*, which in man can give rise to XP, CS or TTD, can be studied by the construction of mouse models using different mutations in the gene. It will be interesting to know what the equivalent mouse phenotypes will be. The A–T gene also gives a complex clinical phenotype and will undoubtedly contribute to our understanding of the relationships between different aspects of DNA processing, which are defective in this disorder, and their roles in development.

ACKNOWLEDGEMENTS

We thank the Cancer Research Campaign for continued support; the Medical Research Council, the A–T Society, the A–T Medical Research Trust and the A–T Research and Support Trust for financial help.

REFERENCES

1 Hoeijmakers JHJ. Nucleotide excision repair II: from yeast to mammals. Trends Genet 1993; 9: 211–217.
2 Vermeulen W, Jaeken NG, Jaspers NGJ, Bootsma D, Hoeijmakers JHJ. Xeroderma pigmentosum complementation group G associated with Cockayne syndrome. Am J Hum Genet 1993; 53: 185–192.
3 Stefanini M, Giliani S, Nardo T et al. DNA repair investigations in nine Italian patients affected by Trichothiodystrophy. Mutat Res 1992; 273: 119–125.
4 Venema J, Mullenders LHF, Natarajan AT, Van Zeeland AA, Mayne LV. The genetic defect in Cockayne syndrome is associated with a defect in repair of UV-induced DNA damage in transcriptionally active DNA. Proc Natl Acad Sci USA 1990; 87: 4707–4711.
5 Mayne LV, Lehmann AR. Failure of RNA synthesis to recover after UV irradiation: an early defect in cells from individuals with Cockayne's syndrome and xeroderma pigmentosum. Cancer Res 1982; 42: 1473–1478.
6 Stefanini M, Vermeulen W, Weeda G et al. A new nucleotide-excision-repair gene associated with the disorder Trichothiodystrophy. Am J Hum Genet 1993; 53: 817–821.
7 Fletjer WL, McDaniel LD, Johns D, Friedberg EC, Schultz RA. Correction of xeroderma pigmentosum complementation group D mutant cell phenotypes by chromosome and gene transfer: involvement of the human ERCC2 DNA repair gene. Proc Natl Acad Sci USA 1992; 89: 261–265.
8 Weeda G, van Ham RCA, Vermeulen W, Bootsma D, van der Eb AJ, Hoeijmakers JH. A presumed DNA helicase encoded by the excision repair gene ERCC-3 is involved

in the human repair disorders xeroderma pigmentosum and Cockayne's syndrome. Cell 1990; 62: 777–791.

9 O'Donovan A, Wood RD. Identical defects in DNA repair in xeroderma pigmentosum group G and rodent ERCC group 5. Nature 1993; 363: 185–188.

10 Troelstra C, van Gool A, de Wit J, Vermeulen W, Bootsma D, Hoeijmakers JHJ. ERCC6, a member of a subfamily of putative helicases, is involved in Cockayne's syndrome and preferential repair of active genes. Cell 1992; 70: 939–953.

11 Schaeffer L, Roy R, Humbert S et al. DNA repair helicase: A component of BTF2 (TFIIH) basic transcription factor. Science 1993; 260: 58–63.

12 Taylor AMR, McConville CM. Chromosome breakage disorders. In: Brock JH, Rodeck CH, Ferguson-Smith MA, eds. Prenatal Diagnosis and Screening. Edinburgh: Churchill Livingstone, 1992: pp 405–421.

13 Taylor AMR. Ataxia telangiectasia genes and predisposition to leukaemia, lymphoma and breast cancer. Br J Cancer 1992; 66: 5–9.

14 Weemaes CMR, Hustinx JWJ, Scheres JMJG et al. A new chromosomal instability disorder. The Nijmegen breakage syndrome. Acta Paed Scand 1981; 70: 557–564.

15 Taalman RDFM, Jaspers NGJ, Scheres JMJC, de Wit J, Hustinx JWJ. Hypersensitivity to ionising radiation in vitro in a new chromosome breakage disorder, the Nijmegen breakage syndrome. Mutation Res 1983; 112: 23–32.

16 Jaspers NGJ, Gatti RA, Baan C, Linssen PCML, Bootsma D. Genetic complementation analysis of ataxia telangiectasia and Nijmegen Breakage syndrome: a survey of 50 patients. Cytogenet Cell Genet 1988; 49: 259–263.

17 McConville CM, Byrd PJ, Ambrose HJ et al. Paired STSs amplified from radiation hybrids, and from associated YACs, identify highly polymorphic loci flanking the ataxia telangiectasia locus on chromosome 11q22-23. Hum Mol Genet 1993; 2: 967–974.

18 Curry CJR, Tsai J, Hutchinson HT, Jaspers NGJ, Wara D, Gatti RA. A–T FRESNO: a phenotype linking ataxia telangiectasia with the Nijmegen breakage syndrome. Am J Hum Genet 1989; 45: 270–275.

19 Cox R. A cellular description of the repair defect in ataxia telangiectasia. In: Bridges BA, Harnden DG, eds. Ataxia telangiectasia: A cellular and molecular link between cancer, neuropathology and immune deficiency. Chichester: Wiley, 1982: pp 141–153.

20 Lipkowitz S, Stern M-H, Kirsch IR. Hybrid T cell receptor genes formed by interlocus recombination in normal and ataxia telangiectasia lymphocytes. J Exp Med 1990; 172: 409–418.

21 Meyn MS. High spontaneous intrachromosomal recombination rates in ataxia telangiectasia. Science 1993; 260: 1327–1330.

22 Strathdee CA, Duncan AMV, Buchwald M. Evidence for at least four Fanconi anaemia genes including FACC on chromosome 9. Nature Genet 1992; 1: 196–198.

23 Strathdee CA, Gavish H, Shannon WR, Buchwald M. Cloning of cDNAs for Fanconi's anaemia by functional complementation. Nature 1992; 356: 763–767.

24 Gibson RA, Hajianpour A, Murer-Orlando M, Buchwald M, Mathew CG. A nonsense mutation and exon skipping in the Fanconi anaemia group C gene. Hum Mol Genet 1993; 2: 797–799.

25 Mann WR, Venkatraj VS, Allen RG et al. Fanconi Anaemia: Evidence for linkage heterogeneity on chromosome 20q. Genomics 1991; 9: 329–337.

26 Barnes DE, Tomkinson AE, Lehmann AR, Webster ADB, Lindahl T. Mutations in the DNA ligase 1 gene of an individual with immunodeficiencies and cellular hypersensitivity to DNA-damaging agents. Cell 1992; 69: 495–503.

27 Willis AE, Weksberg S, Tomlinson S, Lindahl T. Structural alterations of DNA ligase 1 in Bloom syndrome. Proc Natl Acad Sci USA 1987; 84: 8016–8020.

28 Petrini JM, Huwiler KG, Weaver DT. A wild type DNA ligase 1 gene is expressed in Bloom's syndrome cells. Proc Natl Acad Sci USA 1991; 88: 7615–7619.

British Medical Bulletin (1994) Vol. 50, No. 3, pp. 718–731
© The British Council 1994

Metabolic polymorphisms in carcinogen metabolising enzymes and cancer susceptibility

C R Wolf
C A D Smith*

Imperial Cancer Research Fund, Molecular Pharmacology Unit, Biomedical Research Centre, Ninewells Hospital and Medical School, Dundee, UK
Present address: Department of Pathology, University of Edinburgh, Medical School, Edinburgh, UK

D Forman
Imperial Cancer Research Fund, Cancer Epidemiology Unit, Radcliffe Infirmary, Oxford, UK

Molecular genetic analysis is providing us with enormous advances in understanding the pathogenesis of human diseases such as cancer. The study of familial disease and the subsequent mapping and identification of the mutations which contribute to disease susceptibility, is not only providing insights into the factors involved in the pathogenesis of the disease but also identifying new targets for therapy.

It is now clear that human tumours result from a complex sequence of mutation events. Each individual step makes the mutated cell more independent of its normal growth regulatory processes, eventually resulting in the formation of a metastatic tumour. There are a multitude of biochemical changes that these mutations confer, which provide preneoplastic cells with a selection advantage. In addition to an increased rate of cell division, such changes may make the cells resistant to cytotoxic insult or to programmed cell death. They can also confer an increased ability to survive independent of a normal hormonal environment. It is now clear that all these types of change may contribute to tumour cell progression.

In recent years, there has been an intense effort directed to identifying the sequence of molecular changes that result in cancer. Of particular interest has been attempts to relate environmental agents to specific mutation events.[1] Thus, for example, the pattern of mutations observed in the tumour suppressor gene p53 differs in characteristic ways in lung, skin and liver cancers.[2] These patterns can be frequently associated with the action on DNA of major environmental risk factors for these three cancers: cigarette smoke, ultra-violet light and aflatoxin, respectively. This research provides a direct connection between classical epidemiology, which has provided unequivocal evidence for the environmental causes of disease, and molecular biology. The analysis of mutation spectra in other genes and in other types of cancer, has demonstrated a likely role for environmental mutagens even when specific agents have not been identified. Molecular analysis is, therefore, confirming the importance of environmental agents in the pathogenesis of many important cancers.

All higher organisms have evolved a complex spectrum of mechanisms which protect them from the toxic effects of environmental insults. In many cases this provides a selective advantage and allows them to survive in an environment hostile to others. In many instances the ability to metabolise and detoxify the environmental agent provides the primary mechanism of resistance.[3] On the basis of the above discussion it would be predicted that genetic polymorphisms which affect the function of the enzymes involved in these processes will result in altered susceptibility to cancer. Indeed, polymorphism in these enzyme systems may be a susceptibility factor in a wide range of human diseases where exposure to toxic environmental agents has been implicated.

Of the enzymes involved in detoxification, the cytochrome P450-dependent monooxygenases play a pivotal role. These hemoproteins have evolved because of their ability to insert an atom of molecular oxygen into a lipophilic organic substrate. In most cases this reaction results in chemical inactivation, increased water solubility and excretion from the cell. Unfortunately and counter-productively, in mammals, P450-mediated oxidation can also result in the formation of chemically reactive electrophilic products. These intermediate compounds are often mutagenic and will bind to DNA to induce mutations resulting in the activation of oncogenes or in the inactivation of tumour suppressor genes.[4] This is the initiating event in the action of almost all known environmental carcinogens (Fig. 1).

The cytochrome P450 system, like many other similar enzyme systems, has diversified into a series of multigene families of proteins, with each individual enzyme having a unique spectrum of activity. The sensitivity of an individual to a toxin or carcinogen would, at least in

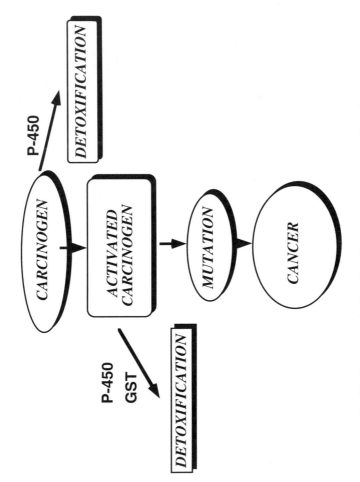

Fig. 1 Initiating event in the action of most known environmental carcinogens.

part, be determined by the balance between the P450 forms involved in chemical activation versus inactivation. There is no doubt that there is extensive genetic variation in the cytochrome P450 system which can lead to profound differences in response to pharmaceutical drugs. There is, therefore, a good *a priori* rationale for anticipating that a similar variability in the response to chemical carcinogens may be a factor in cancer susceptibility.

In addition to the cytochrome P450 system, a variety of other drug metabolising enzymes are important in determining the potency of chemical carcinogens. The glutathione S-transferases (GST) play a central role in these effects. The ability of GSTs to protect a wide range of organisms – including plants, prokaryotes and insects from chemical toxins – is unequivocal.[5] The GST enzymes are a multigene family of proteins whose primary role is the detoxification of toxic and mutagenic electrophiles. In mammals, 5 glutathione S-transferase gene families have been identified. Of these 4 – GSTA, GSTM, GSTP and GST T – are cytosolic and one is membrane bound.[5] These enzymes all catalyse the conjugation of glutathione to a substrate resulting in its inactivation and subsequent excretion. As with the cytochrome P450 system, in certain cases, GST-mediated conjugation reactions can lead to activation to a mutagenic product. This is particularly the case for halogenated hydrocarbon substrates, where GST-mediated metabolism is an important component of the activation pathway. The role of the GST in protecting against carcinogens is best illustrated by the effects of modulating GST levels on carcinogen potency. In the case of aflatoxin b_1-induced liver tumours in rats, for example, it has been shown that the profound chemoprotective effects of certain antioxidants, such as butylated hydroxy anisole,[6] can be ascribed to the induction of specific GSTs which detoxify the mutagenic aflatoxin b_1 epoxide.[7]

A further group of conjugation enzymes involved in carcinogen metabolism and studied in relation to cancer susceptibility are the N-acetyl transferases (NAT). Acetylator polymorphisms have been well documented, 40–70% of Caucasians are of the slow acetylator phenotype and are less efficient than rapid acetylators in acetylating a range of drugs in a manner which prolongs their biological half life. A similar effect has been intimated for chemical carcinogens.[8]

The central role of the drug metabolising enzymes described above suggests that individual differences in their expression will be a factor in susceptibility to diseases such as cancer.

COMPLEXITY OF STUDY DESIGN

The majority of studies looking at genetic polymorphisms in drug metabolising enzymes and cancer susceptibility have focused on the cytochrome P450, GST and NAT enzyme systems where, in most cases, well defined polymorphisms exist. Several of the studies have produced contradictory results. In some instances this has been ascribed to difficulties with the phenotyping assays employed. Until recently, assays for polymorphic cytochrome P450 gene loci have been based on measuring either the rate of metabolism of a marker drug in vivo or the inducibility of specific P450s in activated lymphocytes.[9,10] There has been much debate about the potential shortfalls of these approaches. In the case of the lymphocyte assay the reliability and reproducibility of the assay itself has been a major concern. In the case of phenotyping using marker substrates, metabolism and excretion can be affected by factors such as drug/drug interactions, smoking status, disease state and renal impairment.[9] The standard design of such studies is to administer the marker drug to a group of cancer patients and matched controls and then to quantitate the excretion of metabolised and unmetabolised drug over a set time period. Individuals who metabolise the drug at a significantly reduced rate and excrete predominantly unmetabolised compound are assumed to be homozygous 'poor metabolisers'. The extent to which metabolised end-product is excreted can sometimes, but not always, be used to discriminate homozygous 'extensive metabolisers' from heterozygous 'intermediate metabolisers'. Such studies are, by their nature, time-consuming at both the sample collecting (controlled drug administration, urine collection) and analytical (usually HPLC) stages. This often restricts the size of such studies. In addition, any factor which affects the metabolism of the marker drug will produce a false assessment of the underlying genotype. It is essential, therefore, to control for such confounding factors in the design stage of these studies and match cases and controls extremely carefully for smoking behaviour, drug usage etc. If, as sometimes happens, the presence of cancer itself can influence drug metabolism then the interpretation of metabolic phenotyping studies can be extremely difficult.

In contrast, studies that use a genotyping assay are not only much less laborious to conduct, involving small (often pin-prick) blood samples and automated PCR technology, but are also less restrictive in design. This is because genotype assignment will not be influenced by the existence of disease, concomitant drug use, smoking status etc. Matching criteria for case-control studies using genotyping can therefore be less stringent than for studies using phenotyping. In general, this means that larger studies can be conducted more rapidly and with increased statistical power. As many of the relevant enzyme polymorphisms are relatively rare (maybe 5% or less of the population) it is of obvious importance to have large sample sizes in order to detect small differences.

Genotype studies depend on the detection of mutant alleles and the background prevalence of these may vary between populations. Other genetic polymorphisms, eg, in the HLA system, show well-defined ethnic differences in their frequency[11] and therefore in case-control studies the ethnic group will be a critical matching variable. Thus, cases and controls should always be selected from the same ethnic population. Although this may seem obvious, it may be of relevance in some studies, such as those cancers that are more common in immigrant groups. An argument has been made[12] for the consideration of matching variables apart from ethnicity, even in genotype based studies involving the P450 system. Although factors, such as age, cannot influence genotype *per se*, if a particular genotype were strongly associated with a high prevalence of a fatal disease (such as ischaemic heart disease) as a population aged the proportion of individuals with the genotype would correspondingly decrease. A failure to match on age might, therefore, result in older cases being compared with younger controls with a significant difference being observed which was purely the result of an age effect. Similarly if a specific genotype strongly influenced the desire to take up smoking, for example by being involved in nicotine metabolism, a failure to match case and controls on smoking might result in a false-positive association in a comparative study of a smoking-associated cancer. Thus the genotype might be identified more frequently among lung cancer cases than unmatched controls because of its influence on smoking uptake rather than activation of cigarette smoke carcinogens.

A further problem in genotyping studies might result from more subtle interactions. For example, the risk of cancer associated with high levels of exposure to a chemical may not be modified by polymorphisms in the relevant gene, whereas the risk associated with low or modest exposures may depend on the presence or absence of a polymorphism (see below).

It is important to ensure that no major mutant alleles are missed in screening for genetic polymorphisms as this significantly compromises the power of the statistical analysis. This requires a detailed search for the mutations in the relevant genes of individuals expressing a variant phenotype. Case-control studies using genotyping should only be conducted after such appropriate preliminary studies. In the case of drug metabolising enzymes one further possible complication is the presence of alleles which do not inactivate the enzyme concerned but change its turnover number or substrate specificity. These could give an intermediate phenotype and/or change the spectrum of compounds which the enzyme metabolises.[13] In most cases to date, only alleles which result in significantly reduced amounts (or no) gene product have been studied in relation to disease susceptibility. This is however, an important area for studies in the future.

POLYMORPHISMS AT CYTOCHROME P450 GENE LOCI IN RELATION TO CANCER SUSCEPTIBILITY

There is an increasing body of evidence demonstrating the presence of allelic variants of many different forms of human cytochrome P450. Two of these have received particular attention in relation to studies in cancer susceptibility. These are the cytochrome P450 CYP2D6 polymorphism associated with the polymorphic oxidation of a wide range of important therapeutic drugs, such as debrisoquine and sparteine,[14] and the CYP1A1 polymorphism associated with the metabolism of a wide range of environmental toxins and carcinogens.[15]

The polymorphism at the cytochrome P450 CYP2D6 gene locus has been unequivocally shown to have a profound effect on the rate of metabolism of many drugs.[14] As a consequence it has been suggested that it may also be associated with an altered rate of carcinogen metabolism and therefore be a factor in cancer susceptibility. Most of the CYP2D6 studies have been concerned with the possible association with lung cancer because of the clear role of carcinogens in the pathogenesis of this disease. It was thought that poor metabolisers (PMs) of the drugs broken down by CYP2D6 might be less able to metabolise and activate carcinogens in tobacco smoke. Hence PMs should be at a reduced risk of lung cancer.

Following the original report of Ayesh et al[16] showing a strong association between the CYP2D6 phenotype and lung cancer susceptibility, there have been at least 12 other studies summarised in Table 1 and 2. Table 1 shows the studies based on phenotyping and overall it is apparent that the PM phenotype was found significantly less frequently among lung cancer patients (4.2%) than among their matched controls (8.2%). This results in a reduced risk of developing lung cancer in those with a PM phenotype (odds ratio = 0.46, 95% confidence intervals 0.31–0.65). The PM individuals have, therefore, an approximately 50% reduction in their lung cancer risk. It is noteworthy that despite variation between the studies in the odds ratio, which is only to be expected given the size of the studies and the relative rarity of the PM phenotype, the proportion of PMs among lung cancer cases was consistently less than that among the controls. The results of 6 genotyping studies are shown in Table 2. Again the genotype associated with poor metabolism was seen less frequently among the lung cancer patients (4.1%) than among the controls (5.9%) although this difference was only of borderline significance ($P = 0.067$). The reduction in risk (odds ratio = 0.67, 8.5%

confidence intervals 0.43–1.03) was somewhat lower than that observed in the phenotype studies.

Comparison of Tables 1 and 2 shows that the difference between the two sets of data arises because of a difference in the prevalance of PMs among the controls (5.9% in the genotyping studies and 8.2% in the phenotyping studies). This might, at first sight, indicate that not all the mutant alleles have been identified for this gene and thus genotyping may be incomplete. However, studies in which the same individuals have been both genotyped and phenotyped[17,18] do not indicate the existence of other major mutations.

An alternative explanation is that a small proportion of individuals with a normal genotype fail to metabolise the drug properly as a consequence of an uncontrolled confounding factor. Such individuals could also have a compromised ability to metabolise cigarette smoke carcinogens. Finally, the difference may arise simply through the play of chance on small numbers. Clearly this discrepancy needs to be resolved as the current data beg the question about whether genotyping and phenotyping are measuring the same polymorphisms and, if not, which one is of most relevance.

What is quite clear from these results is that even among lung cancer patients, there is approximately a 4% prevalence of PMs. Given that the prevelance in the general population is unlikely to be much higher than 8% (as defined by the phenotyping studies), then the protection provided by being a poor metaboliser at best halves the risk of contracting lung cancer. The rarity of the PM polymorphism, combined with the size of the risk reduction, make the association of limited public health significance but may tell us about factors involved in the pathogenesis of the disease. What will be of interest in the future will be the assessment of the lung cancers among the PMs – for example, are they associated with very high levels of smoking or are they independent of smoking? A fascinating insight into this will be provided by the analysis of the mutation spectra in the p53 gene in tumour material from these patients.

The CYP2D6 polymorphism has also been associated with altered susceptibility to bladder cancer, but again results using phenotyping assays have not been substantiated by subsequent genotyping studies.[31] Some interesting associations between the CYP2D6 polymorphism and other cancer types (eg leukaemia and melanoma have been observed in isolated studies) but these must still be considered as preliminary and need to be substantiated.[31]

Polymorphism associated with the expression of cytochrome P450 CYP1A1 has also received particular attention in relation to cancer susceptibility. This is particularly the case because this enzyme has high

Table 1 Phenotyping studies of lung cancer and CYP2D6 polymorphism

Population	Lung cancer cases			Controls			Odds ratio	(95% CI)	P
	No.	No. PM	(%)	No.	No. PM	(%)			
UK[16]	245	4	(1.6)	234	21	(9.0)	0.17	(0.5–0.53)	0.0003
Germany[19]	270	19	(7.0)	270	30	(11.1)	0.61	(0.32–1.15)	0.100
USA[20]	130	3	(2.3)	142	9	(6.3)	0.35	(0.07–1.45)	0.107
France[21]	153	10	(6.5)	254	20	(7.9)	0.82	(0.35–1.90)	0.617
UK[22]	104	2	(1.9)	104	9	(8.7)	0.21	(0.03–1.06)	0.031
Spain[23]	85	5	(5.9)	556	34	(6.1)	0.96	(0.32–2.67)	0.933
USA[24]	89	2	(2.2)	92	12	(13.0)	0.15	(0.02–0.76)	0.007
Total	1076	45	(4.2)	1652	135	(8.2)	0.46†	(0.31–0.65)	0.000013

† Summary (M-H) OR.

Table 2 Genotyping studies of lung cancer and CYP2D6 polymorphism

Population	Lung cancer cases			Controls			Odds ratio	(95% CI)	P
	No.	No. PM	(%)	No.	No. PM	(%)			
UK[31]	361	13	(3.6)	720	36	(5.0)	0.71	(0.35–1.41)	0.297
Germany[26]	109	4	(3.7)	125	12	(9.6)	0.36	(0.09–1.25)	0.074
USA[27]	69	0	(0.0)	36	3	(8.3)	–	–	0.015
USA[28]	45	0	(0.0)	38	4	(10.5)	–	–	0.027
Finland[29]	106	1	(0.9)	122	7	(5.7)	0.16	(0.01–1.30)	0.050
Norway[30]	190	18	(9.5)	220	12	(5.5)	1.81	(0.80–4.13)	0.120
Total	880	36	(4.1)	1261	74	(5.9)	0.67[†]	(0.43–1.03)	0.067

† Summary (M-H) OR.

catalytic activity towards a wide range of known human carcinogens. It has been reported that an *Msp*1 restriction fragment length polymorphism has been linked to an amino acid substitution in the active site of this enzyme[32] which generates a protein with a higher activity than the parent enzyme. Studies in Japan have indicated that this polymorphism is associated with an increased susceptibility to diseases such as lung cancer.[33] A study in Caucasians, where this polymorphism is much rarer, has not reproduced the findings of the Japanese study.[34] In view of the potentially central role of this enzyme in carcinogen disposition, additional studies in this area may be of value. Also, the transcription factors which mediate the regulation of this protein associated with the Ah locus have been recently cloned and identified.[35,36] Studies into polymorphism in these genes and their association with cancer susceptibility are in progress.

GST M1 POLYMORPHISM

The central role of the GST in carcinogen detoxification has led to studies into the association between polymorphisms for these enzymes and cancer susceptibility. The best characterised polymorphism in this gene cluster is in the GSTM1 gene locus.[37] This gene is homozygous null, in approximately 40% of the population. There are now several independent studies which indicate that the null phenotype or genotype is associated with an increased risk of lung cancer.[38–40] The GSTM1 polymorphism has also been studied in relation to other cancer types and associations with specific types of skin cancer as well as with colon cancer have been observed.[41–43] The association with colon cancer is particularly interesting because when this disease is subdivided into disease site, almost 70% of individuals with tumours in the proximal colon were found to be homozygous null at the GSTM1 locus. This implies that the gene may play an important role in the inactivation of those environmental agents which induce tumours in this region of the colon.

NAT POLYMORPHISM

The NAT, like the P450s and GSTs, have the capacity to either activate or inactivate chemical carcinogens such as aromatic amines.[1,8] These compounds are known to cause bladder cancer in man. A genetic polymorphism at the NAT2 gene locus has been associated with susceptibility to bladder cancer with **slow** acetylators having an **increased** susceptibility to this disease.[1,8,44] These data are in contrast with other studies indicating the **slow** acetylator phenotype is associated with a **decreased** susceptibility to colon cancer. This apparent dichotomy has been ascribed to potentially different metabolic reactions being carried out in these two tissues.[1,8] Although there are now DNA based assays for identifying individuals with the slow acetylator genotype,[45,46] there are still too few studies where such assays have been used to look for associations with cancer susceptibility.

COMBINATIONS OF ALLELES OF DRUG METABOLISING ENZYMES AND CANCER SUSCEPTIBILITY

On the basis that the overall concentration of and balance between activating and inactivating enzymes are an important component in determining the susceptibility of cells to a carcinogen, there are now a number of studies which have investigated whether combinations of polymorphisms in these enzyme systems may increase cancer risk.[33] Japanese studies show that individuals with a combination of the GST GSTM1 polymorphism together with the P4501A1 genetic polymorphism may have up to a 41-fold increased risk of lung cancer.[47] Interestingly, this association was strongest for individuals with intermediate cigarette use. Combination studies are still at an early stage but identify an important area for future research. The major limitation for such studies is that for those polymorphisms which are relatively rare (between 5–10% of the population affected) individuals with both of these polymorphisms would be extremely infrequent (less than 1% of the population). Fortunately certain genetic polymorphisms in drug metabolising enzymes are much more common.

CONCLUSION

The association between genetic polymorphisms and drug metabolising enzymes is being pursued with increasing interest. As a consequence of the development of DNA based assays, a large number of patient samples can be studied, to establish whether these assays are predictive of adverse drug reactions. The importance of polymorphisms in these enzymes in determining susceptibility to cancer is still in most cases an open question. In the case of the GSTM1 there is increasing evidence indicating that it is important. For the other genes at the present time, the situation is not clear and more definitive studies are required to establish the role of these enzymes in determining cancer susceptibility.

REFERENCES

1 Wolf CR. Metabolic factors in cancer susceptibility. Cancer Surv 1990; 9: 437–474.
2 Hollstein M, Sidransky D, Vogelstein B, Harris CC. p53 mutations in human cancers. Science 1991; 253: 49–53.
3 Hayes JD, Wolf CR. Molecular mechanisms of drug resistance. Biochem J 1990; 272: 281–205.
4 Harris CC. p53: at the crossroads of molecular carcinogenesis and risk assessment. Science 1993; 262: 1980–1981.

5 Tew KD, Pickett CB, Mantle TJ, Mannervik B, Hayes JD eds. Structure and function of glutathione S-transferases. London: CRC Press, 1993.

6 Wattenberg LW. Prevention – therapy – basic science and the resolution of the cancer problem: presidential address. Cancer Res 1993; 53: 5890–5896.

7 Hayes JD, Judah DJ, McLellan LI, Kerr LA, Peacock SD, Neal GE. Ethoxyquin-induced resistance to aflatoxin B1 in the rat is associated with the expression of a novel alpha-class glutathione S-transferase subunit, Yc_2, which possesses high catalytic activity for aflatoxin B1-8,9-epoxide. Biochem J 1991; 279: 385–388.

8 Grant DM. Molecular genetics of the N-acetyltransferases. Pharmacogenetics 1993; 3: 45–50.

9 Caporaso NC, Idle JR. The rationale for case-control methodology in epidemiological studies of cancer risk. Br J Clin Pharmacol 1990; 30: 149–150.

10 Kouri RE, McKinney CE, Siomiany DJ, Snodgrass DR, Wray NP, McLemore T. Positive correlation between high aryl hydrocarbon hydroxylase activity and primary lung cancer as analyzed in cryopreserved lymphocytes. Cancer Res 1982; 42: 5030–5037.

11 Tsuji K, Aizawa M, Sasazukai T eds. HLA – 1991: Proceedings of the 11th International Histocompatible Workshop and Conference, Chapter W5. Oxford: Oxford University Press, 1992: pp 621–689.

12 Idle JE, Armstrong M, Boddy AV et al. The pharmacogenetics of chemical carcinogenesis. Pharmacogenetics 1992; 2: 246–258.

13 Lindberg R, Burkhart B, Ichikawa T, Negishi M. The structure and characterisation of type I P-450 (15) alpha gene as a major steroid 15-alpha-hydroxylase and its comparison with type II P-450 (15) alpha gene. J Biol Chem 1989; 264: 6465–6471.

14 Tucker GT. Clinical implications of genetic polymorphism in drug metabolism. J Pharmacol 1994 (in press).

15 Nebert DW, Petersen DD, Puga A. Human AH locus polymorphism and cancer: inducibility of CYP1A1 and other genes by combustion products and dioxin. Pharmacogenetics 1991; 1: 68–78.

16 Ayesh R, Idle JR, Ritchie JC, Crothers MJ, Hetzel MR. Metabolic oxidation pehnotypes as markers for susceptibility to lung cancer. Nature 1984; 312: 169–170.

17 Gough AC, Miles JS, Spurr NK et al. Identification of the primary gene defect at the cytochrome P450 CYP2D locus. Nature 1990; 347: 773–776.

18 Ingelman-Sundberg M, Johansson I, Persson I et al. Genetic polymorphism of cytochromes P450: interethnic differences and relationship to incidence of lung cancer. Pharmacogenetics 1992; 2: 264–271.

19 Roots I, Drakoulis N, Ploch M et al. Debrisoquine hydroxylation phenotype, acetylation phenotype and ABO blood groups as genetic host factors of lung cancer risk. Klin Wochenschr 1988; 66: 87–97.

20 Caporaso N, Hayes RB, Desemeci M et al. Lung cancer risk, occupational exposure and the debrisoquine metabolic phenotype. Cancer Res 1989; 49: 3675–3679.

21 Duche JC, Joanne C, Barre J et al. Lack of relationship between the polymorphism of debrisoquine oxidation and lung cancer. Br J Clin Pharmacol 1991; 31: 533–536.

22 Law MR, Hetzel MR, Idle JR. Debrisoquine metabolism and genetic predisposition to lung cancer. Br J Cancer 1989; 59, 686–687.

23 Benitez J, Laddero JM, Fernandez-Gundin JM et al. Polymorphic oxidation of debrisoquine in bladder cancer. Ann Med 1990; 22: 157–160.

24 Caporaso NE, Tucker MA, Hoover RN et al. Lung cancer and the debrisoquine metabolic phenotype. J Natl Cancer Inst 1990; 82: 1264–1271.

25 Wolf CR, Smith CAD, Bishop T, Forman D, Gough AC, Spurr NK. CYP2D6 genotyping and the association with lung cancer susceptibility. Pharmacogenetics 1994 (in press).

26 Roots I, Brockmöller J, Drakoulis N, Kerb, M. Mutant alleles of cytochrome P4502D6 in lung cancer. Clin Pharmacol Ther 1992; 51: 181.

27 Caporaso N, Shields P. Unpublished data. Cited in: Idle, JE, Armstrong M, Boddy AV et al. The pharmacogenetics of chemical carcinogenesis. Pharmacogenetics 1992; 2: 246–258.

28 Sugimura H, Caporaso NE, Shaw GL et al. Human debrisoquine hydroxylase gene polymorphisms in cancer patients and controls. Carcinogenesis 1990; 11: 1527–1530.

29 Hirvonen A, Husgafvel-Pursiainen K, Anttila S, Karjalainen A, Pelkonen O, Vainio H. PCR based CYP2D6 genotyping for Finnish lung cancer patients. Pharmacogenetics 1993; 3: 19–27.

30 Tefre T, Daly A, Armstrong M et al. Genotyping of the CYP2D6 gene in lung cancer patients and controls. J Basic Clin Phsyiol Pharmacol 1992; Suppl. 3: p. 32.

31 Wolf CR, Smith CAD, Gourgh AC et al. Relationship between the debrisoquine hydroxylase polymorphism and cancer susceptibility. Carcinogenesis 1992; 13: 1035–1038.

32 Kawajiri K, Makachi K, Imai K, Yoshii A, Shinoda N, Watanabe J. Identification of genetically high risk individuals to lung cancer by DNA polymorphisms of the cytochrome P450IA1 gene. FEBS Lett 1990; 263: 131–132.

33 Kawajiri K, Nakachi K, Imai K, Watanabe J, Hayashi S-I. Germ line polymorphisms of p53 and CYP1A1 genes involved in human lung cancer. Carcinogenesis 1993; 14: 1085–1089.

34 Tefre T, Ryberg D, Haugen A et al. Human CYP1A1 (cytochrome P_1450) gene: lack of association between the Msp1 restriction fragment length polymorphism and incidence of lung cancer in a Norwegian population. Pharmacogenetics 1991; 1: 20–25.

35 Durbach KMA, Poland A et al. Cloning of the Ah-receptor cDNA reveals a distinctive ligand-activated transcription factor. Proc Natl Acad Sci USA 1992; 89: 8185–8189.

36 Hoffman EC, Reyes H et al. Cloning of a factor required for activity of the Ah (Dioxin) receptor. Science 1991; 252: 954–958.

37 Board PG, Coggan M, Johnston P, Ross V, Suzuki T, Webb G. Genetic heterogeneity of the human glutathione transferases: a complex of gene families. Pharmacol Ther 1990; 48: 357–369.

38 Seidegard J, Pero RW, Markowitz M, Roush G, Miller WR, Beattie EJ. Isozyme(s) of glutathione transferase (class mu) as a marker for the susceptibility to lung cancer: a follow up study. Carcinogenesis 1990; 11: 33–36.

39 Nazar-Stewart V, Motulsky AG, Eaton DL et al. The glutathione S-transferase μ polymorphism as a marker for susceptibility to lung carcinoma. Cancer Res 1993; 53: 2313–2318.

40 Zhong S, Howie AF, Ketterer B et al. Glutathione S-transferase mu locus: use of genotyping and phenotyping assays to assess association with lung cancer susceptibility. Carcinogenesis 1991; 12: 1533–1537.

41 Zhong S, Wyllie AH, Barnes D, Wolf CR, Spurr NK. Relationship between the GSTM1 genetic polymorphism and susceptibility to bladder, breast and colon cancer. Carcinogenesis 1993; 14: 1821–1824.

42 Strange RC, Matharoo B, Faulder GC et al. The human glutathione S-transferases: a case-control study of the incidence of the GST1 0 phenotype in patients with adenocarcinoma. Carcinogenesis 1991; 12: 25–28.

43 Hegerty AHM, Fitzgerald D, Smith A et al. Glutathione S-transferase GSTM1 phenotypes and protection against cutaneous tumours. Lancet 1994; 343: 266–267.

44 Cartwright RA, Glashan RW, Rogers HJ et al. Role for N-acetyltransferase phenotypes in bladder carcinogens: a pharmacogenetic epidemiological approach to bladder cancer. Lancet 1982; ii: 842–845.

45 Blum M, Demierre A, Grant DM, Heim M, Meyer UA. Molecular mechanisms of slow acetylation of drugs and carcinogens in humans. Proc Natl Acad Sci USA 1991; 311: 5237–5241.

46 Hickman D, Sim E. N-Acetyltransferase polymorphism. Comparison of phenotype and genotype in humans. Biochem Pharmacol 1991; 42: 1007–1014.

47 Nakachi K, Imai K, Hayashi S, Kawajiri K. Polymorphisms of the CYPIA 1 and glutathione 5-transferase genes associated with susceptibility to lung cancer in relation to cigarette dose in a Japanese population. Cancer Res 1993; 53: 2994–2999.

British Medical Bulletin (1994) Vol. 50, No. 3, pp. 732–745
© The British Council 1994

Setting up and running a familial cancer clinic

B A J Ponder

CRC Human Cancer Genetics Research Group, Department of Pathology, Cambridge, UK

This article is based on the author's own experience of establishing and running a familial cancer clinic over the past 9 years. There are certainly other ways of doing it, depending on the clinical context – resources, involvement of colleagues from other specialities – and each clinic should be adapted to local circumstances.[1,2] As the familial component of the common cancers such as breast and colorectal cancers is increasingly recognised, and DNA-based predictive testing becomes a possibility, the future demand for genetic advice is likely to increase dramatically. This will almost certainly require a re-appraisal of the way in which familial cancer services are provided, which is discussed in the final section.

THE PURPOSE AND SCOPE OF A FAMILIAL CANCER CLINIC.

The minimal purposes of a familial cancer clinic are:

- To confirm, interpret and extend family histories of cancer
- To advise the individual and the doctor about risks and possible action to be taken
- To advise about the possibility and appropriateness of DNA-based testing and to arrange it if agreed, and to supervise the giving of results
- To provide a resource for research, including the evaluation of the clinic itself, which is important for future funding of familial cancer services.

To obtain an accurate and complete family history

Since, at present, the evaluation of risk is based almost entirely on the pattern of specific types of cancer in the family, an accurate and complete history is critical. Histories presented in referral letters have generally been obtained by non-specialists in a busy clinic, and may be no more than a general indication that there may be something to pursue. Serious inaccuracies are common (breast 'cancers' which were non-malignant lumps, 'ovarian cancers' that were hysterectomies for fibroids, affected individuals placed in the wrong generation or even on the wrong side of the family). The history may be incomplete, both in numbers of individuals affected and the ages at diagnosis of cancer. This is important, because it is the extent of the history which determines the likelihood that the family history reflects inherited predisposition rather than chance coincidence of cancers; and which family members are most at risk. The taking of the family history will be discussed in more detail.

To advise family members and their doctors about the cancer risks and possible action to be taken

The familial cancer clinic can provide risk estimates for specific family members on the basis of the family history, which should include confirmation of relevant diagnoses where possible, and communicate these risks to the individuals and their doctors. Recommendations may be made about the need for screening or preventive treatment (including prophylactic surgery), but in general, unless the clinic sets out to provide comprehensive care, clinical management and follow-up should be arranged between the individual and his or her doctor. The familial cancer clinic should remain available for consultation if requested. Most general familial cancer clinics will have neither the resources nor the expertise relevant to each cancer site, to become involved in clinical management. An exception to this principle may be the development of site-specific familial cancer clinics (see below), for example for breast cancer or colon cancer. Such clinics would be multidisciplinary – including for example surgeons, radiologists/endoscopists and specialist nurses.

To arrange DNA-based genetic testing where appropriate

Prediction of inheritance of inherited susceptibility genes either by linked genetic markers or by direct analysis of DNA for mutations is already possible for families with several of the inherited cancer syndromes. The familial cancer clinic can arrange and supervise such testing. Soon, with the cloning of susceptibility genes for the common cancers, there may be a demand for testing from individuals with only one or two affected relatives, or indeed with no family history at all. The familial clinic has a role here, too. It is important that individuals who are contemplating testing (as well as doctors who may be requesting it for their patients) understand clearly the issues involved. If testing is carried out, it is important that the implications of the result are understood by both the family member and the clinicians, and that the action which is taken is appropriate. Our experience with genetic testing in the inherited cancer syndromes indicates that at present these issues are not well understood. The familial cancer clinic can both advise when testing is appropriate, and for which individuals; and also guide clinicians and family in the use of the results.

Families will often be seen for whom genetic testing is either not possible or not appropriate now, but is likely to become so in the future. The collection and storage of DNA, either from blood or pathology blocks may be important, and someone must take responsibility for it. At present, most familial cancer clinics, being research-based, have neither the resources nor the assurance of continuity which are needed to undertake this service: but arrangements may be possible through other organisations, for example in the UK, the NHS Regional Genetics Centres.

To act as a resource for research and evaluation

There is hardly an aspect of familial cancer which does not require further research, from the description of familial patterns of cancer and the correlation of these with specific mutations, to the psychological and social aspects of giving genetic information. The familial cancer clinic, while providing a service, should nevertheless be organised to promote research, which will include the evaluation of its own activities and effectiveness. The blurred line between clinical service and research may sometimes cause difficulties with funding, but charities and government agencies in many countries are increasingly aware of the need to provide appropriate clinical resources for the evaluation of 'the new genetics'. Those who wish to start or develop a clinic may find that it is possible to bid for funds under one or another specific programme. These bids are likely to be enhanced if it can be shown that the clinic has a research element.

Familial cancer clinics for specific cancers

An alternative to the general familial cancer clinic is the clinic which focuses on cancers at a specific site – for example, breast or colorectal cancer. The advantage of these clinics is that by combining genetic and organ-specific clinical expertise, it is possible to offer a high standard of clinical assessment, screening, and specific advice on prevention or techniques such as breast self-examination, in a single visit. The clinic can be set up with preliminary evaluation by genetic nurses to allow a greater number of patients to be seen, with selection for more detailed assessment of those with more complex family histories or problems that require further investigation. The cumbersome and time-consuming procedure of evaluation in a separate genetics clinic followed by re-referral to the appropriate specialists is avoided. Such clinics are likely to be the most effective means to provide a familial cancer service for the common cancers, where a large population living local to the clinic is involved; and they should also prove a useful means of disseminating basic genetic concepts among general clinicians and nurses, as well as educating geneticists about the new diseases they are being asked to see. The need will remain, however, for the purely genetics-based familial cancer clinic to deal with more complex problems, as well as those which span several organ systems and which require coordination between several clinical specialities (for example, inherited syndromes such as neurofibromatosis).

SETTING UP A FAMILIAL CANCER CLINIC

Some of the questions to be thought about are summarised in Table 1.

Table 1 Setting up a familial cancer clinic

Which department?	Clinical genetics or other
What patient load?	Clinic space, time
What staff?	Medical; nurse/interviewers; secretarial; records; laboratory
What referral mechanism?	Through doctors only or also direct? Publicity for clinic? Minimum criteria for a 'family'?
Funding issues	Service, research Long-term responsibilities

Which department of the hospital should the clinic be in?

Clearly this will be influenced by local conditions. For a general familial cancer clinic, there are several advantages to being closely affiliated to a clinical genetics department. These include: (a) the need for skills in family history-taking, risk estimation and counselling; (b) the set-up of the clinic space, which is likely to be arranged for lengthy, undisturbed consultations in a rather informal setting, in contrast to the atmosphere of a busy surgical clinic; (c) the existence of staff such as genetic nurse-counsellors who can help with family interviewing, make home visits, explore possibly delicate family relationships, and provide an informal telephone contact person, if needed; and (d) the probability that the clinical genetics department will have its own medical record and biological specimen storage systems separate from those of the main hospital. This can provide both privacy (an increasingly sensitive issue) as well as a system geared to continuity over many years – an important consideration now that many hospitals discard records and samples within a few years.

If a cancer site-specific clinic is envisaged, it will almost certainly be necessary for it to be integrated into the appropriate department: but even in this case, a strong formal link with a clinical genetics department is recommended, for access to the resources listed above.

What patient load is envisaged?

This will determine the space, clinic time, staff and funds that are required. It will in part be determined by the criteria for clinic referral and how heavily the clinic is advertised.

General advice must always be: *start slowly*. It is surprising how much work can be involved in even an apparently simple cancer family. Each consultation requires about an hour; the preliminary correspondence, outline family history taking, and letters from the clinic are further work for the doctor and a secretary. If distant or dead relatives must be traced and diagnoses confirmed, the work will be much greater. With this in mind, a sensible starting point might be to aim at one half-day clinic a month. This will translate into about 50 new families a year. It may not sound much; but it is easier to increase the clinic frequency once the need is shown than it is to cut it back. This load should be easily within the scope of one doctor with the part-time help of a genetic nurse and secretary: but even if your resources are greater, you should begin cautiously until you have experience of the work involved. If the criteria for clinic referral are wide, and access open, as might be the case for a familial breast cancer clinic, careful assessment of the likely demand is needed. Epidemiological estimates of the number of individuals of a given age living within the catchment area of the clinic who will have a given family history (eg 2 or more close relatives with breast cancer diagnosed before age 55) may be a useful guide.

What staff will be required?

The types of staff that will be needed include:

(a) A **doctor**, able to give substantially full-time attention to familial cancer. The doctor should have experience of genetic counselling and risk estimation, familiarity with (and preferably some practical experience of) the basic molecular genetic techniques involved in DNA based prediction, and knowledge of the main clinical features of the cancers to be encountered, especially their familial associations, and the current options for screening, prophylactic surgery, and prevention. A complete formal training in clinical genetics is probably not necessary: a background in oncology with experience in cancer genetics may be appropriate.

(b) A **family interviewer/genetic counsellor**, who is most likely to be trained as a nurse, with or without additional genetics training. Such a person can make preliminary investigation of the family tree before referral to the clinic, which helps to eliminate inappropriate referrals; is an informed and available person for family members to contact if they have anxieties or need support; and most important, can deal with much of the work of tracing family members and obtaining hospital records and death certificates, that will be generated by the clinic.

(c) Access to **secretarial help** for the clinics is essential, although in the early stages much of the letter-writing and record keeping associated with family tracing can be done by the family interviewers.

(d) The help of a **laboratory technician** is also essential for the receipt, processing and storage of blood and tissue samples. It may be difficult to justify a full salary at the start, and the work can possibly be done either by the family interviewer or by arrangement with the clinical genetics laboratory.

What should be the referral mechanism for the clinic?

In the UK, most hospital clinics will not accept referral except through another doctor, usually the patient's GP. Most familial cancer clinics make an exception to this, and accept self-referrals direct from family members. The reason is that, until now, many doctors have not been aware of the potential for family susceptibility to cancer, and have tended to dismiss the idea, or provide family members with misplaced reassurance.

If self-referrals are accepted, the familial cancer clinic should keep the family doctor and any specialists already involved in the care of the patient fully informed (provided the patient agrees – this consent must be explicitly obtained). This is discussed further below. It is also prudent, with both self-referrals and medical referrals, to set some minimal criteria of family history that will justify the use of a clinic space, and to check as far as possible that these are met, before making the clinic appointment. In our experience, medical colleagues very much appreciate some guidelines for referral.

Suggested referral guidelines for a beginning family cancer clinic with modest resources are shown in Table 2. These should ensure that most of the clinic resources are spent on families where there is good *a priori* reason to think that there may be significant risk. It is difficult to formulate totally satisfactory definitions, however, and there should always be the possibility of exceptions if the patient (or the doctor!) is particularly anxious and likely to benefit from face-to-face advice. Research interests and resources will also influence the scope of the clinic, as will the possibilities for benefit (eg by screening) if the individual is found to be at risk. In cases which do not meet the criteria, advice may be given by letter or telephone and clinic referral arranged only if there is still a problem. Once again, if the contact is with the patient, it is important to keep the patient's doctor informed. A risk of excluding clinic referrals on the grounds of insufficient family history is that there may be a more extensive history which the clinic would have uncovered. The best that can be done to meet this, is to ensure (if possible) that each 'rejected' case has had a family history taken by telephone by the clinic nurse/interviewer, as part of the giving of advice outlined above.

Table 2   Referral guidelines for a new general familial cancer clinic

1	Two or more unusual cancers in the same individual or in close relatives (eg brain tumour and sarcoma).
2	Cancer in the context of an associated syndrome. eg glioma in neurofibromatosis type 1 melanoma with dysplastic naevi renal cancer with retinal angiomata (Von Hippel-Lindau)
3	Commoner cancers. (a) Three or more cancers of the same type or related types (eg breast/ovary/endometrium/colorectum/prostate) in close relatives on the same side of the family. (b) Two cancers of the same or related types in close relatives, at least one diagnosed before age 50. (c) An immediate relative (parent, sibling) with one of the common 'adult' cancers (eg breast, colorectal) diagnosed below age 40.

Note: These are guidelines for referral only. Not all cases where there is significant predisposition will fall within these groups; conversely, many individuals or families which meet these criteria will not, in fact, turn out to be predisposed. The aim is to provide a simple scheme, and to encourage clinicians to refer outline family histories in cases of doubt.

Publicising the clinic

A new clinic probably requires some publicity, especially since this area of medicine is unfamiliar to many doctors. A brief circular which explains the purpose of the clinic and the referral procedure can be sent to hospital staff and local family doctors. It is essential to include some indication of the sort of 'family' which it would be appropriate to refer; and probably helpful to give the telephone number of the clinic nurse or doctor who can be contacted for discussion. It may also be helpful to emphasize (if the clinic is set up this way) that the follow-up and continuing care of the patients and families will remain with their own clinicians, and that the role of the cancer family clinic is simply to advise. Presentation of familial cancer cases at hospital and regional postgraduate meetings is also an effective way to introduce the clinic and its personnel, and at the same time to educate your colleagues in its use.

Publicity in the community – for example by newspaper reports of the clinic, items on the health page of women's magazines – can be very effective. It allows family members who are concerned about their family history, but whose concerns have not been recognised by their doctors, access to information. Set against this is the possibility of inducing anxiety in people whose family history is in fact probably not very significant. Over-enthusiastic publicity may also raise unrealistic expectations of what the clinic can do. For this reason, it is essential to specify clearly the criteria for a family history of interest, erring on the side of caution, and to make it clear that individuals with such a family history only possibly – not certainly – may be at increased risk. One should try – though it may be difficult – to ensure that these details appear in the final version of any article. To avoid implications of advertising for personal gain, and to provide a 'filter' in case there should be a large (and largely inappropriate) response, it is also worth considering whether any media publicity should be in the name of an independent body – for example, a cancer charity or possibly the local health authority – to whom the public can respond in the first instance. Finally, to maintain the support of the clinical community, it may be wise to clarify any resource implications (for example, for breast screening) with the hospital authorities before an article appears.

Funding the clinic

Most of the familial cancer clinics in the UK have been established with research funds. Increasingly, however, inherited predisposition to cancer is being seen as a problem that should be addressed as part of a clinical service. It is likely that familial cancer clinics will either become integrated into the existing clinical genetics departments, or be developed as part of the service for specific cancers – for example, breast cancer. The effectiveness of familial cancer clinics in preventing deaths from cancer, or in reducing anxiety in individuals or families, is still unproven. Until now, the clinics have dealt mostly with rare inherited cancer syndromes. As they turn more to the common cancers, the resource implications will be considerable, and these have yet to be fully considered by the authorities. A clinic which is based on an active research programme and which is attempting to evaluate its effects in health service terms is likely to compete for funds more successfully than one which is not.

To make any commitment to the long-term follow-up of families, while new ones are continually accrued, is a recipe for an ever-expanding workload. To imply a long-term commitment when the clinic is based on short-term research funding is irresponsible.

THE CLINIC CONSULTATION

We each have our own style of clinic consultation, and this is adapted as the possibilities in familial cancer change. What follows is a discussion of some of the issues in running a clinic which I have found to be important, and my own current responses to them. Throughout, for convenience, I refer to 'the patient': this seems to me at least as acceptable as 'client' and less clumsy than 'consultand', although of course most of these individuals are not ill.

Preamble: why is the patient here?

I find it very helpful to establish at the outset how the patient has come to be sitting in the clinic. This can be the key to the conduct of the whole consultation. Some are there for the straightforward reason that they themselves are concerned about their family history and they want advice or reassurance. For many, that is not the case. They may want to help with research, or their doctor may have sent them along because the doctor thinks they should help with research, perhaps with only the barest explanation of what the clinic is about. Someone else – a doctor, or a relative – may have pressured them to come to the clinic 'to find out about their risks, and do something about it'. (Who has come with the patient? Do they have a lot to say?) Or they may have come not for themselves, but because of concern for their children. The clinic nurse may find out some of this before the clinic, but sometimes that is not possible. The worst outcome of a clinic consultation is for someone to be confronted with information that they did not want: to assume that everyone who sits in your clinic is there because they want to know **everything** you can tell them is likely, before long, to lead to disaster.

Reviewing the family history: more clues to what the patient thinks

The most organised clinics have the family history taken and reviewed before the patient sees the doctor, who then simply comments on it. This saves perhaps 20–30 min, and doubles the throughput of the clinic. While this is probably appropriate for a high-volume familial breast cancer clinic that aims to serve a population, it can bring disadvantages.

Even though the family history will already have been established to the extent needed for a clinic referral, I like to go through it all again from the start, drawing out the pedigree as I discuss it with the patient. This provides an invaluable opportunity to pick up signals about all sorts of things – the level of the patient's anxiety, what he or she is anxious about, the level of their understanding, what they are hoping the clinic will provide, the degree of detail and the form in which the information might best be given, relationships and pressures within the family (including the patient's spouse), who else in the family could or certainly should not be approached for information, as well as new or revised pieces of evidence which the patient has had time to remember or search out since the original contact. Over 9 years of a family cancer clinic, I believe that most of my errors of judgement were made when for some reason I gave advice without going through this preliminary step of acquaintance with the patient and family.

Explaining the implications of the history

There is much research to be done into the most effective way of communicating risks in a familial cancer clinic. The concepts are quite difficult – Mendelian inheritance, but the possibility that some 'families' do not have an inherited basis; incomplete penetrance; variable age at onset; the overall probabilistic view – and some people find them hard to deal with. The majority seem to appreciate a careful explanation of the steps in the assessment of their history, so that they can see for themselves how the risk estimates are arrived at, and the possible pitfalls along the way; possibly this also helps them understand the risks to other family members, in particular their children. For others, however, the detail is too much, and the uncertainty implicit in the reasoning probably unsettles rather than reassures.

The risks of cancer are, of course, related to age. They can be expressed as 'lifetime risk', or (which I find generally more helpful) risk by a certain age. It is worth remembering that the lifetime risk of breast cancer in the general population is about 1 in 12, a figure which is a shock to many women, in a way that the corresponding 1 in 70 risk by age 50 is not. The Mendelian/penetrance style of explanation tends to result in percentages; but 'odds of 4 to 1 against cancer by age 50' may be more easily understood, and be less frightening, than a '20% chance of cancer by age 50'. However, it is not clear that such numerical risks are useful at all. They certainly will mean different things to different people, and for many the statement that they are at 'no', 'little', 'moderate' or 'high' risk may be as good. The courses of action to be decided for breast cancer, for example generally resolve into 'do nothing', 'have screening', or 'have prophylactic surgery', which (in so far as these decisions are based on risk estimates at all, rather than on emotional response) would seem to correspond to risk categories of 'none', 'moderate' and 'high'.

One may ask whether it is always in the patient's best interests to confront them with a potentially worrying risk figure when it is clear either that they are apprehensive, or that the course of action (eg screening) is already decided. Depending what has been gleaned from the earlier discussion, I will sometimes avoid numerical risks, or bias my calculations by using figures from the end of the assumptions available to me. Another trap is the patient for whom the family history (often subtly exaggerated by the conversion of benign breast lumps into cancers, and so on) has become some kind of emotional bargaining counter for sympathy and support. The details of each diagnosis must of course be carefully verified to avoid inappropriate treatment of unaffected family members. But when the family history is found eventually to be insignificant, one should not expect that the patient will always be grateful or willingly reassured.

Course of action

It is useful to establish what possibilities the patient is already aware of, and what his or her preferences are. If the screening or treatment is to be carried out not by the family cancer clinic, but by the patient's own doctors, it is most important not to make a strong recommendation unless you know that the doctors concerned are likely to agree. If in doubt, contact them to discuss the matter. Similarly, it is helpful to know if other close relatives at similar risk have received advice elsewhere, and what advice this was: in a field where most recommendations are open to debate, and reassurance is at least a major objective, consistency of medical advice is important.

There is a school of thought that genetic counselling should be 'nondirective': that is, the patient is given the facts and makes his or her own decision. The uncertainties and complexities surrounding almost every aspect of the management of familial cancer may make this difficult or sometimes inappropriate. The patient or family may reasonably expect the help of the doctor to interpret and guide them through the choices available. This is something for each individual doctor to decide. Even if the patient is to be encouraged towards a particular decision, however, it is probably wise to explain the full range of choices that exist. Some – for example, the possibility of prophylactic mastectomy – may need to be carefully presented to avoid anxiety. However, this is probably the only time the patient will have the opportunity to hear a balanced account of the alternatives; and such is the media interest in this topic, it is better that the facts are presented fully in a balanced way by a knowledgeable doctor than later gleaned inaccurately from the press.

Communicating genetic advice

The amount of new information which will be presented in a 1 h familial cancer clinic appointment is likely to be overwhelming. It is important that the essential points are clearly grasped by the patient, and also by the doctors concerned with his or her care. Standard practice in most genetics clinics is to summarise the clinic discussion in a letter, often of 2–3 pages, which is sent to the patient, with copies (if the patient agrees) to the family doctor and relevant specialists. The patient is encouraged to telephone or write if anything is unclear. The letter will summarise the future action to be taken, and who is responsible: for example, that it was agreed the patient should discuss with her own doctor the arrangement for annual breast and ovarian cancer screening.

The letter can provide a record that the patient can give to her children when they are of a suitable age, thus recording and preserving the key genetic information that was found by the clinic, and placing the responsibility for seeking further advice in the hands of the family. It is important to bear in mind that the patient may also use the letter to approach other members of the family who may be at risk, or who have children at risk. While this can sometimes be useful, it can also be dangerous. This possibility should always be remembered when wording the letter, and it is probably a good idea to discuss the question of contacting relatives with the patient at the clinic, and to caution those that seem over-enthusiastic that others may not see the problem in the same way.

The question of contacting other branches of the family is a difficult one, which requires careful handling. Usually, it turns on how closely the patient is in touch, the patient's perception of whether contact would be welcome, and whether the information is likely to be of benefit. For some cancer syndromes where screening is effective, the arguments in favour will be strong; for others (notably at present breast and ovarian cancer) the benefits are less clear. In cases of doubt as to whether some harm may result from contacting a relative, a helpful (if time-consuming) strategy may be to identify the relatives' family doctors through NHS records, and discuss the question with them.

Privacy issues

The possibility that genetic information could be requested by third parties such as insurance companies or employers is currently a topic of great concern. For the moment, the consensus is that the right of the patient to confidentiality is total. This also applies to other family members. Great caution is needed when counselling different family members because some disclosure of the extent of the family history is obviously necessary, but details of individual medical histories, or annotated family pedigrees for example, should not be made available without the consent of the individuals concerned. As DNA testing becomes possible, further complexities will arise because of the implications of a test result in one individual for risks in other family members. These privacy issues are discussed in the recent Nuffield report on the ethics of genetic testing.

Follow-up

It has already been suggested that, except in special cases such as a familial breast cancer clinic where the aim is total care, the familial cancer clinic should not undertake any duty of follow-up, outside research studies. On the other hand, it should be made clear to the patients that the responsibility for follow-up is theirs. They are welcome to contact the clinic staff at any time – if they have new questions, if new cancers arise in the family which may change the risk implications, or if they want advice about new developments such as DNA testing or preventive regimes, eg tamoxifen. In the UK, there is a network of familial cancer clinics, and family members can be referred to the clinic closest to their home if they move away from the original clinic.

FUTURE PROSPECTS

As commoner, lower penetrance predisposing genes are identified for cancers, as for other common late onset diseases such as coronary heart disease and arthritis, much larger numbers of individuals can be identified potentially as at risk. How many people will want to be tested is not known. If there is evidence of benefit from screening or prevention, there seems no reason why genetic testing of this kind should be any less acceptable than blood pressure testing is now.

At this point, it seems likely that care of the familial aspects of these diseases will become just one facet of their general management. Perhaps each breast cancer unit will have its own familial cancer clinic staffed by genetic nurses and a breast cancer specialist who has an interest in the familial aspects of the disease. Alternatively, departments of preventive medicine may develop, to handle genetic testing, screening, prevention, and their evaluation on a population level. It will be interesting to see which of these approaches – or some other – evolves over the next decade.

REFERENCES

1   Biesecker BB, Boehnke M, Calzone K et al. Genetic counselling for families with inherited susceptibility to breast and ovarian cancer. J Am Med Assoc 1993; 269: 1970–1974.
2   Evans DGR, Fentiman IS, McPherson K, Asbury D, Ponder BAJ, Howell A. Familial breast cancer. BMJ 1994; 308: 183–187.

OTHER READING

Evans DGR, Ritiero G, Warrell D, Donnai D. Ovarian cancer family and prophylactic choices. J Med Genet 1992; 29: 416–418.
Evans DGR, Burnell LD, Hopwood P, Howell A. Perception of risk in women with a family history of breast cancer. Br J Cancer 1993; 67: 612–614.
Green J, Murton F, Statham H. Psychosocial issues raised by a familial ovarian cancer register. J Med Genet 1993; 30: 101–105.
Kash KM, Holland JC, Halpern MS, Miller DG. Psychological distress and surveillance behaviour of women with a family history of breast cancer. J Natl Cancer Inst 1992; 84: 24–30.
Lerman C, Daly M, Sands C et al. Mammography adherence and psychosocial distress among women at risk for breast cancer. J Natl Cancer Inst 1993; 85: 1074–1080.
Lynch HT, Watson P. Genetic counselling and hereditary breast/ovarian cancer. Lancet 1992; 339: 1181.
Nuffield Council on Bioethics (1993). Genetic screening: ethical issues.

Index Vol. 50 No. 3